PANCE PREP PEARLS

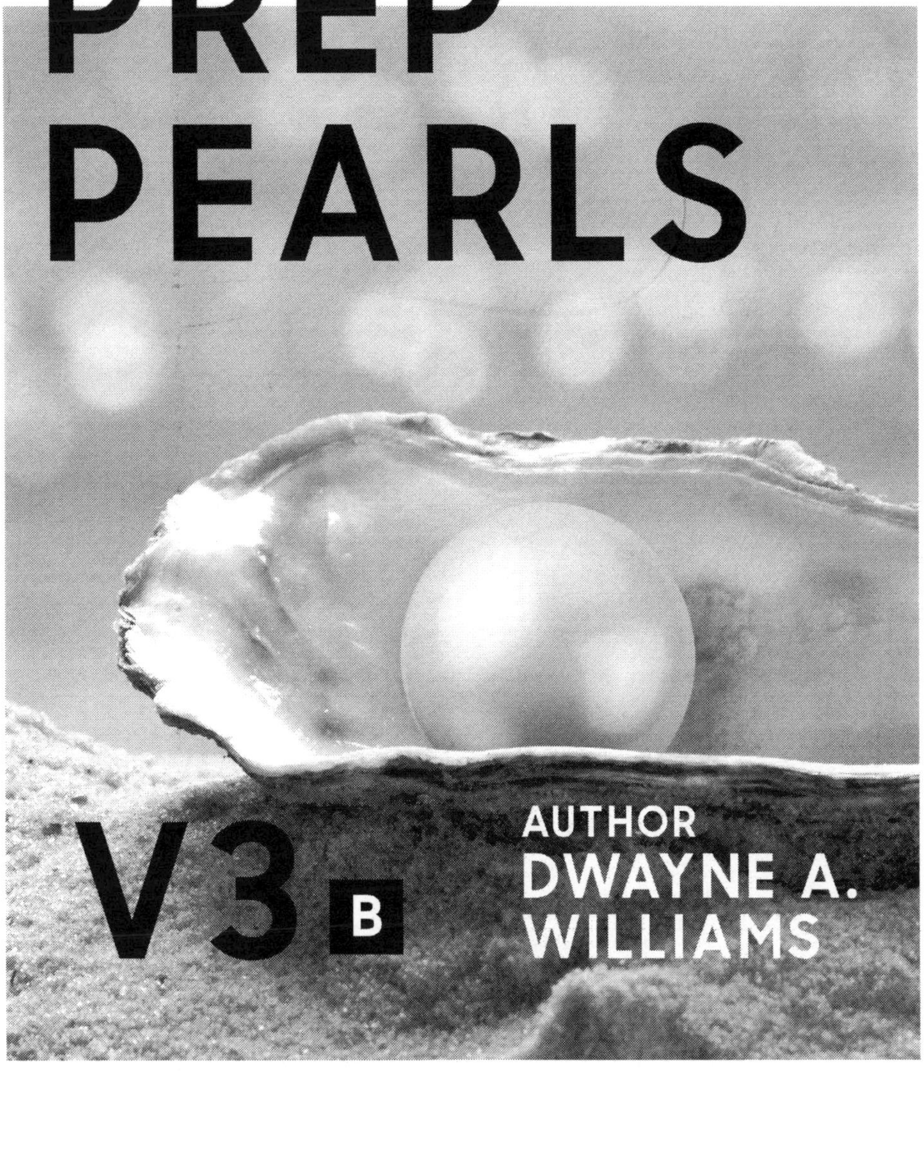

V3 B

AUTHOR
DWAYNE A. WILLIAMS

ISBN: 9781712913109
Imprint: Independently published
Kindle Direct Publishing Platform

Printed by Kindle direct publishing

DEDICATION

I would like to thank the Cornell and Long Island University Physician Assistant Programs for giving me the platform to teach. Thanks to my foundation teachers Marion Masterson, Medea Valdez, Gerard Marciano. A very special thanks to Stacey Hughes (words can't describe my gratitude to you), Sharon Verity and William Ameres for being my inspirational teachers as a student. To all those who contributed to making this profession great and to all my fellow educators who contribute to this field on so many levels.

Thanks to all of the owners of the photos. Your images helped to make this book a visual experience. Your contribution is invaluable. An extra special thanks to **Ian Baker**, the illustrator of most of the pictures in the book. You added a special touch to this project. Thanks Dr. Frank Gaillard and Jason Davis for your help during the process. Special thanks to **Kevin Young, Xiana Flowers & Kristen Risom** (the best illustrators I know!)

Special thanks to my parents Winifred & Robert Williams. Xiomara & Froylan Flowers (my second parents), Mercedes Avalon, Gilda Cain (the best nurse I know!) and my big brother Danilo Avalon.

To my gurus: Stacey Hughes, Tse-Hwa Yao, Ingrid Voigt, Dr. Antonio Dajer & Dr. Kenneth Rose.

Thanks to Isaak Yakubov (my Akim) for the Ultimate Mnemonic Comic Book and the amazing journey we have embarked on together. Thanks to Rachel Lehrer for allowing me to be a part of the FlipMed medical app project. I will make good on the promise I made to you.

Pamela Bodley, the world's best manager. You are the real boss lady!

Last but not least a very special thank you to my PPP warriors! I enjoy our interactions on social media and at conferences. This book would not have been the success it is without the support of each and every one you! YOU ARE A WARRIOR.....WARRIORS WIN!

PREFACE

STUDENTS

This book is designed for use in both didactic and clinical education. It is formatted to make you a rockstar on clinical rotations! It is a ***review book***, which means ***it is not meant to replace textbook-based education*** but as an additional study tool to enhance your knowledge base. Textbooks provide the foundation for understanding and learning medicine.

PRACTITIONERS

This book is purposed to increase your knowledge & retention of important clinical information and for use as a quick resource that is not time consuming.

THE STYLE OF PPP

Pance Prep Pearls is not written in the traditional style of a textbook but rather to feel like a collection of notes, drafts, charts, mnemonics and clinical pearls to make learning effective while entertaining. The use of bold and italics are to help you to organize the information and stress the importance of certain aspects of the disease states. The charts are designed for you to compare and contrast commonly grouped diseases and high-yield information. It is loaded with helpful algorithms to help you see the big picture on how to approach the disease.

I personally recommend that you use what I call the 5 P's of the ***Patient-Centered Learning Model*** as you study the different diseases:

1. **Pathophysiology:** imagine explaining the pathophysiology of a disease to your patient in 1 sentence (2 sentences maximum) in simple terms. Understanding the pathophysiology will often explain the clinical manifestations, physical examination findings, why certain tests are used and usually the treatment reverses the pathophysiology. This step is often skipped but is probably the most important (in terms of knowledge retention).
2. **Present** – based on the pathophysiology, how would this patient present? Know both the classic and the common findings and presentations (they aren't always the same).
3. **Pick it up**? – How would you diagnose the disease. Make sure to understand what is usually first line vs. gold standard (definitive diagnosis). Understand the indications and contraindications for each test.
4. **Palliate** – how do you treat (palliate) the disorder. Many people can list out the treatments but fail to remember first line treatments vs. alternative treatments. Make sure to understand the indications and contraindications of each treatment.
5. **Pharmacology** – understand the mechanism of action and understand why a medication is used for that disease. This helps to reinforce the pathophysiology as well as the presentation of the disease since the pharmacology often reverses the problem or treats the symptoms. A very important point is that if you see a medication that is used for different disorders, try to understand what connects the use of that drug to the different disorders.

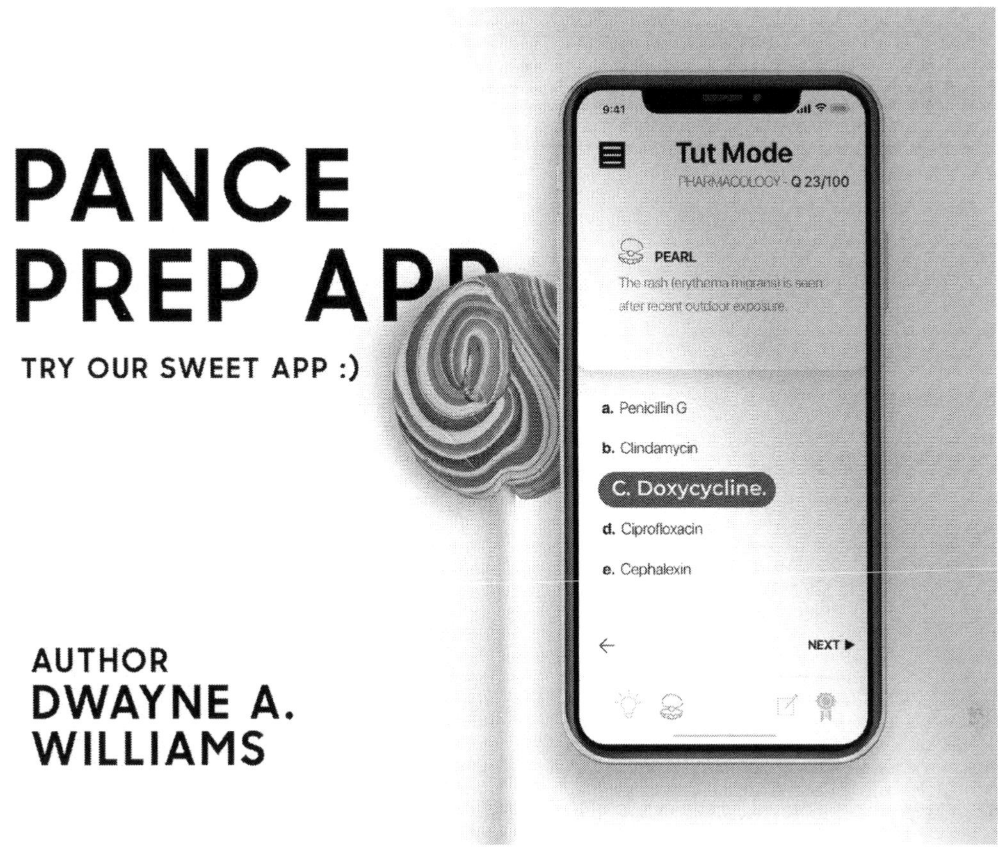

Over 8,600 clinically-based practice examination questions specifically formulated to enhance clinical skills and improve performance on examinations, such as the PANCE, PANRE, OSCES, USMLE, end of rotation examinations and comprehensive medical examinations.

This app will intuitively know your areas of weakness and give you a plan to improve your overall performance. Special clinical pearls, disease review, explanation of the answers, test taking strategies and much more.

3 modes,
Timed mode to simulate the exams
Tutor mode that allows you to review the disease states in addition to the questions and
improve mode to enhance your weak areas.

For every question in tutor mode, there is a feature for a hint to see if you are going in the right direction, answer explanation, a clinical pearl, and a bonus questions. Create your own examination based on organ systems or task areas. The ultimate study and exam preparation app!

TABLE OF CONTENTS

CHAPTER 7 – ENDOCRINE SYSTEM

ADRENAL DISORDERS

Zona Glomerulosa:	Aldosterone (Controls Na^+ balance)	Outer layer of cortex
Zona Fasciculata:	Cortisol	Middle Layer of cortex
Zona Reticularis:	Estrogens/Androgens	Inner Layer of Cortex

Think "GFR" for the layers of the cortex and "ACE" for the hormones they produce.

HYPOTHALAMIC - PITUITARY AXIS

The man (hypothalamus) turns on the thermostat (pituitary gland), which turns on the radiator (adrenal gland), which produces the heat (cortisol) to the desired temperature (homeostasis).

NEGATIVE FEEDBACK

When the heat (cortisol) becomes higher than the desired set temperature (homeostasis), this will cause the thermostat (pituitary gland) to shut off so that the radiator (adrenal gland) stops making heat (any new cortisol).

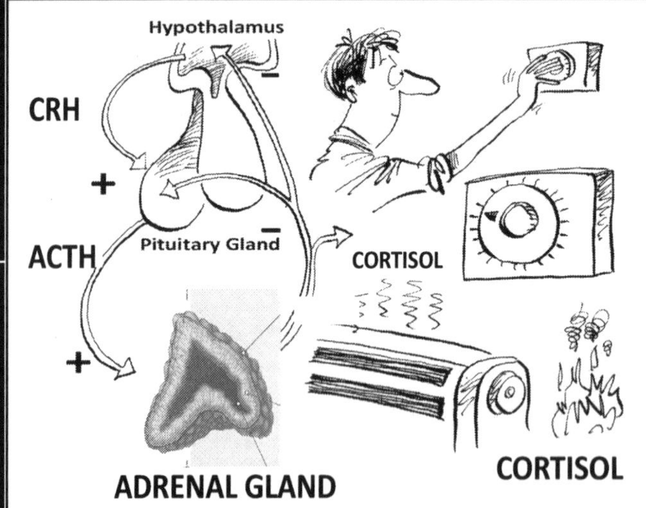

SECONDARY DISORDERS

Based on the feedback mechanisms, **secondary (pituitary gland)** & **tertiary (hypothalamic)** disorders have **LABS IN THE SAME DIRECTION**.

- **TSH-secreting PITUITARY adenoma**
  ↑TSH & ↑FreeT_4/T_3
- **Cushing's disease (PITUITARY adenoma)**
  ↑ACTH & ↑cortisol
- **Hypopituitarism:** low pituitary hormones & low target organ hormones

PRIMARY DISORDERS

Based on the feedback mechanisms, primary disorders have **LABS IN OPPOSITE DIRECTIONS** if the **problem is the target organ**:

Thyroid gland is the primary problem:

- **Graves', Toxic Goiter, Toxic adenoma**
  ↑FreeT_4/T_3 & ↓TSH
- **Hashimoto's, Thyroiditis**
  ↓FreeT_4/T_3 & ↑TSH

Ovaries are the primary problem:

- **Menopause:** ↓estrogen & ↑FSH/LH

Adrenal gland is the primary problem:

- **Addison's disease:** ↓cortisol & ↑ACTH
- **Adrenal adenoma:** ↑cortisol & ↓ACTH

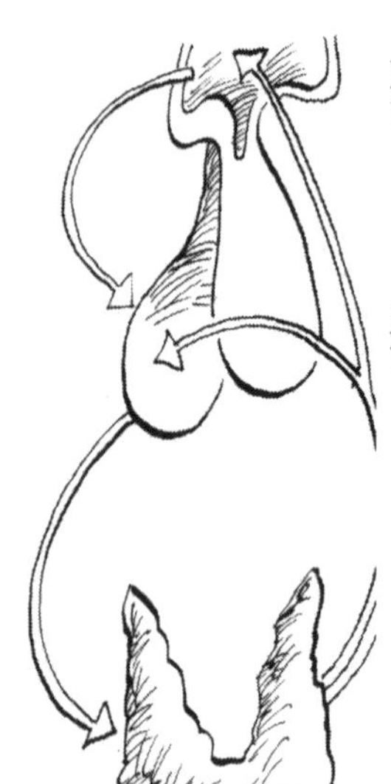

TERTIARY DISORDER
The **hypothalamus** is the problem

SECONDARY DISORDER
The **pituitary gland** is the problem

PRIMARY DISORDER
The **target organ** is the problem

Photo credit:
Shutterstock (used with permission).

CHRONIC ADRENOCORTICAL INSUFFICIENCY

- Disorder where the adrenal gland does not produce enough hormones.

SECONDARY

Pituitary failure of ACTH secretion (lack of cortisol only). Aldosterone intact due to renin angiotensin aldosterone system.

- Etiologies: **history of exogenous glucocorticoid use** (especially without tapering) **most common cause of secondary and overall insufficiency.** Hypopituitarism.

PRIMARY (ADDISON DISEASE)

Adrenal gland destruction (lack of cortisol AND aldosterone). Etiologies include:

- **Autoimmune most common cause in the US** (80%).
- **Infection** most common in developing countries (eg, Tuberculosis, HIV).
- Vascular: thrombosis or hemorrhage in the adrenal gland (Waterhouse-Friderichsen syndrome).
- Others: trauma, metastatic disease, medications (eg, **Ketoconazole,** Rifampin, Phenytoin, & Barbiturates).

CLINICAL MANIFESTATIONS

- Symptoms due to lack of cortisol – weakness, myalgias, fatigue. Nonspecific GI symptoms – weight or appetite loss, anorexia, nausea, vomiting, abdominal pain, & diarrhea. Headache, sweating, abnormal menstruation, mild hyponatremia, salt craving, hypotension. Hypoglycemia more common in secondary.

- **Primary (Addison's disease):** symptoms due to lack of sex hormones & aldosterone – **hyperpigmentation (increased ACTH** stimulates melanocyte-stimulating hormone secretion), **orthostatic hypotension.** Women may have loss of libido, amenorrhea, & loss of axillary pubic hair.

BASELINE LABS

- 8am ACTH, cortisol, & renin levels obtained. Increased renin, especially with primary.
- **Elevated ACTH in primary, decreased ACTH in secondary.**
- Labs: **Hypoglycemia. Primary (Addison) –** hyponatremia, **hyperkalemia,** & non-anion gap metabolic acidosis (due to decreased aldosterone).

SCREENING TEST

High-dose ACTH (Cosyntropin) stimulation test

- **Adrenal insufficiency if insufficient or absent rise in serum cortisol** (< 18 microg/dL) after ACTH administration.
- Normal response is rise in serum cortisol after ACTH administration.

MANAGEMENT

- **Glucocorticoid replacement: Hydrocortisone first-line.** Dexamethasone.
- Mineralocorticoid replacement (eg, **Fludrocortisone**) may be added **only in Primary (Addison's)**.

PATIENT EDUCATION

- Because cortisol is a "stress" hormone, people with chronic adrenal insufficiency must be treated with IV glucocorticoids & IV isotonic fluids before & after surgical procedures (mimicking the body's natural response).
- During illness/surgery/high fever, oral dosing needs to be adjusted to recreate the normal adrenal gland response to "stress" (eg, triple the normal oral dosing).
- Everyone should carry a medical alert tag as well as injectable form of cortisol for emergencies.

ADRENAL (ADDISONIAN) CRISIS (ACUTE ADRENOCORTICAL INSUFFICIENCY)

- **Acute adrenocortical insufficiency (Addisonian crisis)** is sudden worsening of symptoms in diagnosed or undiagnosed chronic adrenal insufficiency **precipitated by a "stressful" event** (eg, illness, surgery, trauma, volume loss, hypothermia, MI, fever, sepsis, hypoglycemia, steroid withdrawal etc.).
- The normal response to "stress" is a 3-fold increase in cortisol. These patients are unable to increase cortisol during times of stress to meet the demand.

ETIOLOGIES
- **Abrupt withdrawal of glucocorticoids (especially without tapering) most common cause.**
- Previously undiagnosed patients with Addison's disease subjected to "stress".
- Patients with known Addison disease that did not increase their dose during illness.
- Bilateral adrenal infarction (usually due to hemorrhage).

CLINICAL MANIFESTATIONS
- **Shock primary manifestation - hypotension, hypovolemia.** Nonspecific symptoms.

DIAGNOSIS
- Labs: **hyponatremia, hyperkalemia, hypoglycemia**. Cortisol and aldosterone (confirms diagnosis). ACTH, renin, CBC.
- Do not delay treatment while diagnostic testing is performed.

MANAGEMENT
- **Isotonic fluids (normal saline or D5NS) + IV hydrocortisone** (if known Addison) **or Dexamethasone** (if undiagnosed because it doesn't interfere with cortisol assays).
- Reversal of electrolyte disorders. Fludrocortisone.

ADRENAL INSUFFICIENCY LAB VALUES

	CRH	ACTH	Cortisol	CRH Stimulation Test (ACTH response)	Aldosterone	Renin
Hypothalamus (Tertiary)	Low	low	Low	Exaggerated, prolonged	Low	Normal/ low
Pituitary (Secondary)	High	**LOW**	**LOW**	Absent/↓ ACTH	Low	Normal/ low
Adrenal (Primary)	High	**HIGH**	**LOW**	↑ACTH	Low	High

- **Note that primary disorders, ACTH & cortisol go in opposite directions (same direction seen in 2ry/3ry).**

CUSHING'S SYNDROME LAB VALUES

	High Dose Suppression Test	ACTH
Cushing's Disease (Pituitary)	**Suppression of cortisol**	Increased
Ectopic ACTH-producing tumor	No suppression	Increased
Adrenal Tumor (cortisol producing)	No suppression	Decreased
Exogenous Steroids	No suppression	Decreased

Note that Cushing's disease is the only one that suppresses during high-dose suppression test.

CUSHING'S SYNDROME (HYPERCORTISOLISM)

Cushing's syndrome = **symptoms & signs** related to **cortisol excess.** 4 main causes:

Exogenous:
- **Long-term high-dose glucocorticoid therapy most common cause overall.**

Endogenous:
- **Cushing's disease:** **pituitary gland ACTH overproduction** (hyperplasia or adenoma) – **most common endogenous cause.**
- **Ectopic ACTH-producing tumor** (eg, **Small cell lung cancer**, Medullary thyroid cancer).
- **Adrenal tumor (adenoma)** - secretion of excess cortisol.

CLINICAL MANIFESTATIONS
- Proximal muscle weakness, **weight gain,** headache, oligomenorrhea, erectile dysfunction, polyuria, osteoporosis, & mental disturbances (from mild to psychosis).

PHYSICAL EXAMINATION
- Fat redistribution: central (truncal) **obesity, "moon facies"** (roundly shaped faces with puffiness & facial redness), **buffalo hump, supraclavicular fat pads, thin extremities.**
- Skin changes: thin skin (atrophy), **striae** (red or purple & 1 cm wide), easy bruising, decreased wound healing. Hyperpigmentation if increased ACTH.
- **Acanthosis nigricans** epidermal hyperplasia & thickening of the skin, especially around the neck & armpit with hyperinsulinemia.
- Androgen excess: hirsutism, oily skin, acne.
- **Hypertension.**

SCREENING TESTS: 3 options:
- 24-hour urinary free cortisol (*most specific*).
- Nighttime (11pm) salivary cortisol
- Low-dose (1 mg) overnight Dexamethasone suppression test.
  Elevated cortisol or no suppression with low dose Dexamethasone = Cushing's syndrome.

DIFFERENTIATING TESTS:

Baseline ACTH + High-dose Dexamethasone suppression test helps to distinguish Cushing's disease (pituitary) from other causes.
- **Cushing's disease: increased ACTH + suppression of cortisol on high dose**. *Cushing's disease is the only one of the 4 major causes that suppresses with high-dose dexamethasone.*
- Ectopic ACTH-producing tumor: increased ACTH + no suppression with high-dose Dexamethasone.
- Adrenal tumor & steroids: **decreased ACTH** + no suppression with high-dose Dexamethasone.

- Workup of suspected cause: after lab studies - Pituitary MRI (Cushing's disease) or sampling of petrosal sinus if MRI is negative; CT of the abdomen (Adrenal tumor); Chest imaging (ectopic ACTH-producing lung tumor).
- Labs: **hyperglycemia,** dyslipidemia, **leukocytosis. Hypokalemia** & metabolic alkalosis (are due to the aldosterone-like effects of cortisol).

MANAGEMENT
- **Corticosteroid use: gradual taper** (withdrawal) to prevent Addisonian crisis.
- **Cushing disease: Transsphenoidal resection.**
  Radiation therapy or Pasireotide can be used in inoperable pituitary tumors. Mifepristone
- Adrenal tumor: tumor excision.
- Ectopic tumor: resection if resectable. If unresectable, Ketoconazole or Metyrapone can be used.

PRIMARY HYPERALDOSTERONISM

Primary: renin-independent (autonomous).
- **Idiopathic** or idiopathic **bilateral adrenal hyperplasia most common** (60%).
- **Conn syndrome (adrenal aldosteronoma)** 40%. Located in the zona glomerulosa.
- Rare causes: unilateral adrenal hyperplasia, familial, or ectopic aldosterone secreting tumor.

Secondary: due to increased renin. Increased renin leads to increased aldosterone via the RAAS (renin angiotensin aldosterone system):
- Renal artery stenosis most common cause of secondary.
- Renal artery hypoperfusion (eg, CHF, hypovolemia, Nephrotic syndrome etc.).

CLINICAL MANIFESTATIONS
- Usually asymptomatic.
- **Triad of hypertension + hypokalemia + metabolic alkalosis.**
- Hypokalemia: proximal muscle weakness, **polyuria** (nephrogenic Diabetes insipidus), fatigue, constipation, decreased deep tendon reflexes, hypomagnesemia.
- Hypertension: may manifest as **headache** or flushing of the face (patients with primary are not usually edematous). Diastolic pressures tend to be more elevated than systolic pressures.
- **Primary hyperaldosteronism is a cause of secondary hypertension** – suspect in patients who develop hypertension at extremes of age (<30 years or > 60 years), not controlled on 3 blood pressure medications, or with the classic triad.

SCREENING TESTS
- **Plasma renin and aldosterone levels**: **aldosterone to renin ratio: ARR > 20:1** (high aldosterone + **low plasma renin levels) = Primary.** High plasma renin levels = secondary.
- Labs: **hypokalemia with metabolic alkalosis** (aldosterone promotes sodium retention at the expense of potassium and hydrogen excretion).
- ECG may show signs of hypokalemia (eg, T wave flattening followed by prominent U wave).

CONFIRMATORY TESTS
- Oral sodium loading test: high urine aldosterone = primary.
- Saline infusion test: no suppression of aldosterone levels = primary.
  Normal response is decrease in aldosterone levels.
- CT or MRI: to look for adrenal or extra-adrenal mass.
- Sample of venous blood draining from the adrenal – high aldosterone in primary (most accurate test to distinguish between adenoma vs. hyperplasia).

MANAGEMENT OF BILATERAL HYPERPLASIA
- Medical:
  Spironolactone or Eplerenone (they block aldosterone), **ACE inhibitors,** calcium channel blockers.
- Correct electrolyte abnormalities.

MANAGEMENT OF CONN SYNDROME
- **Surgical excision** + **Spironolactone** (blocks aldosterone).

PHEOCHROMOCYTOMA

- **Catecholamine-secreting adrenal tumor** (chromaffin cells).
- Rare (causes 0.1-0.5% of hypertension) but most common adrenal tumor in adults.
- May be associated with MEN syndrome II, Neurofibromatosis type 1, & von Hippel-Lindau disease.

- **90% benign.** Rule of 10s: 10% malignant, 10% bilateral, 10% seen in children, 10% extra-adrenal (paraganglioma).

PATHOPHYSIOLOGY
- **Secretes norepinephrine, epinephrine,** & dopamine **autonomously & intermittently** - triggers include surgery, exercise, pregnancy, medications (eg, tricyclic antidepressants, opiates, Metoclopramide, glucagon, & histamine).

CLINICAL MANIFESTATIONS
- **Hypertension is the most consistent finding** - may be temporary or sustained.
- **"PHE":**
  Palpitations
  Headache (most common symptom)
  Excessive sweating.

- Chest or abdominal pain, weakness, fatigue, weight loss (despite increased appetite), & pallor.

DIAGNOSIS
- Biochemical testing: plasma fractionated metanephrines confirmed by 24-hour urinary fractionated catecholamines including metabolites **(increased metanephrines & vanillylmandelic acid).**

- Imaging: MRI or CT of abdomen & pelvis to visualize adrenal tumor after biochemical testing.

- MIBG scanning – nuclear isotope that can detect tumors outside of the adrenal gland if CT or MRI is negative.

PREOPERATIVE MANAGEMENT
- **Nonselective alpha-blockade best initial therapy - PHEnoxybenzamine or PHEntolamine** 1-2 weeks **followed by beta blockers** or calcium channel blockers to control blood pressure prior to surgery. Think "PHE" for symptoms & management.

- **DO NOT initiate therapy with beta-blockade** to prevent unopposed alpha constriction during catecholamine release triggered by surgery or spontaneously, which could lead to life threatening hypertensive crisis.

- In patients with hypertensive crisis due to Pheochromocytoma, Phentolamine, Nitroprusside, or Nicardipine can be used to acutely lower the blood pressure.

MANAGEMENT
- **Complete adrenalectomy** after at least 1-2 weeks of medical therapy.

THYROID FUNCTION TESTS

TEST	DESCRIPTION	CLINICAL UTILITY
TSH	Thyroid stimulating hormone	• **BEST THYROID FUNCTION SCREENING TEST.** • Initial test for suspected thyroid disease. • Used to follow patients on thyroid hormone tx **- Low TSH ⇨ decrease dose of levothyroxine** **- High TSH ⇨ increase dose of levothyroxine** • Used with T_4 to manage patients with Grave's.
Free T_4 (FT_4)	**Free thyroxine** levels (metabolically active hormone)	• Ordered when TSH is abnormal to determine thyroid hyperfunction or hypofunction
THYROID ANTIBODIES	• **Anti-thyroid peroxidase Ab** • **Anti-Thyroglobulin Ab**	• Used to diagnose **Hashimoto's** thyroiditis **OR** other **autoimmune** thyroiditis
	• **Thyroid stimulating Ab (TSH receptor Ab)**	• **Specific for Graves' disease**
Free T_3	Serum triiodothyronine	• Useful to diagnose hyperthyroidism when TSH is low & T_4 is still normal.
FTI	Free Thyroxine Index	• Used in thyroid disease when the patient has protein abnormalities.

	TSH	FREE T4
PRIMARY Thyroid is the problem	• **INCREASED**	• **DECREASED**
	• In primary disorders, the labs are in **OPPOSITE** directions	
SECONDARY Pituitary gland is the problem	• **DECREASED**	• **DECREASED**
	• In secondary & tertiary disorders, the labs are in the **SAME** direction	
SUBCLINICAL	• **INCREASED** (hypothyroid)	• **NORMAL** (subclinical)
	• Management is to repeat TSH. • Thyroid hormone replacement may be needed if **TSH >10 mIU/L** to reduce cardiovascular risk.	

TERTIARY DISORDER
The **Hypothalamus** is the problem

SECONDARY DISORDER
The **Pituitary Gland** is the problem

PRIMARY DISORDER
The **target organ** is the problem

TSH is the initial test of choice for suspected hypothyroid or hyperthyroid conditions

RADIOACTIVE IODINE TEST (RAIU)	POSSIBLE DIAGNOSIS
DIFFUSE uptake	Graves' disease or TSH-secreting pituitary adenoma
Decreased uptake	Thyroiditis (eg, Hashimoto's, postpartum, DeQuervain)
Hot Nodule	Toxic Adenoma
Multiple Nodules	Toxic Multinodular goiter
Cold Nodules	Rule out malignancy

CLINICAL MANIFESTATIONS OF THYROID DISORDERS

	HYPOTHYROIDISM	HYPERTHYROIDISM
ETIOLOGIES	• **Iodine deficiency (dietary),** Cretinism • **Hashimoto's Thyroiditis** • Thyroiditis: Postpartum, deQuervain, Silent (lymphocytic) **later stage** • Pituitary Hypothyroidism • Hypothalamic Hypothyroidism • Riedel's Thyroiditis • Medications: **Lithium, Amiodarone, Apha interferon**	• **Grave's Disease** • Iatrogenic thyrotoxicosis • Thyroiditis: Postpartum, deQuervain, Silent (lymphocytic) **earlier stage** • Toxic Multinodular Goiter • Toxic adenoma • **TSH-secreting pituitary adenoma** • Medications: **Amiodarone** • Excess intake of T3, T4
CLINICAL MANIFESTATIONS		
CALORIGENIC	• **Decreased metabolic rate: in general, all metabolic processes are decreased, except for menstrual flow, which is increased.** • **Cold intolerance** (↓heat production) • Weight gain (despite ↓appetite)	• **Increased metabolic rate: In general, all metabolic processes are increased, except for menstrual flow, which is decreased.** • **Heat intolerance** (↑heat production) • Weight loss (despite ↑appetite)
SKIN	• Dry, thickened rough skin • **loss of outer 1/3 of eyebrow** • Goiter • **Nonpitting edema (myxedema)**	• **Skin warm, moist, soft, fine hair,** alopecia, easy bruising • Goiter
CNS	• **Hypoactivity:** Fatigue, sluggishness, memory loss, depression, ↓*DTR* • Hoarseness of voice	• **Hyperactivity:** anxiety, **fine tremors, nervousness,** fatigue, weakness, increased sympathetic
GI	• Constipation, anorexia	• Diarrhea, hyperdefecation
CVS	• **Bradycardia, ↓ cardiac output** • Pericardial effusion	• **Tachycardia, palpitations** • **High-output heart failure**

IATROGENIC HYPOTHYROIDISM

• Often due to treatment for hyperthyroidism with radioactive iodine or surgery (total or subtotal thyroidectomy) without subsequent thyroid hormone replacement.

• **Amiodarone:** contains iodine and may induce hypothyroidism (by the Wolff-Chaikoff effect) or hyperthyroidism (by the Jod-Basedow effect) depending on the underlying state of the patient.

• **Alpha-Interferon:** by stimulating the immune system in patients with baseline thyroid autoimmune predisposition (eg, patients with anti-TPO or anti-TG antibodies).

• **Lithium:** mechanism that causes hypothyroidism is poorly understood (may affect colloid).

CRETINISM

- **Untreated congenital Hypothyroidism.**

ETIOLOGIES
- **Lack of maternal iodine intake in developing countries.**
- **Dysgenesis of the thyroid gland** or defect in enzymes in developed countries.
- May be acquired if maternal TSH-receptor blocking antibodies passed into fetal circulation via the placenta.

CLINICAL MANIFESTATIONS
- **Mental developmental delays**, short stature.
- **Symptoms of hypothyroidism**: decreased metabolic rate, cold intolerance, dry thickened rough skin, constipation, weight gain despite decreased oral intake, menorrhagia, myxedema (eyelid and facial edema), weakness, & lethargy.
- **Goiter symptoms** in older children - *hoarseness* and *dyspnea* (tracheal compression).

PHYSICAL EXAMINATION
- **Coarse facial features, macroglossia, umbilical hernia, hypotonia (decreased DTRs)**, prolonged jaundice, feeding problems, & congenital malformations.

DIAGNOSIS
- **Primary hypothyroid profile: increased TSH + decreased free T4 or T3.**

MANAGEMENT
- **Levothyroxine** (synthetic T4).

SUBCLINICAL HYPOTHYROIDISM

- Hypothyroidism determined by laboratory tests **(isolated increased TSH)** in patients with little or no symptoms.
- Subclinical hypothyroidism may be associated with increased risk of cardiovascular disease, especially when the serum TSH concentration is > 10mU/L.

DIAGNOSIS
- **Isolated increased TSH** (hypothyroid) **+ normal free T4** and/or free T3 (subclinical).

MANAGEMENT
- Observation with follow up TSH.
- **Levothyroxine may be given if TSH 10mU/L or higher to prevent cardiovascular complications.**

HASHIMOTO THYROIDITIS

- **Most common cause of hypothyroidism in the US**. Increased incidence in **women 30-50y.**

PATHOPHYSIOLOGY
- **Autoimmune thyroid cell destruction** by anti-thyroid peroxidase & anti-thyroglobulin antibodies (and TSH receptor-*blocking* antibodies to a lesser extent).

CLINICAL MANIFESTATIONS
- **Symptoms of hypothyroidism** - decreased metabolic rate, fatigue, cold intolerance, dry thickened rough skin, constipation, weight gain despite decreased oral intake, menorrhagia, myxedema (eyelid and facial edema), weakness, & lethargy.
- Goiter symptoms: hoarseness and dyspnea (tracheal compression).
- Women may have galactorrhea (due to increased prolactin).

PHYSICAL EXAMINATION
- The thyroid gland may be atrophic, normal, or enlarged (goiter).
- **Bradycardia,** decreased DTR, **loss of outer 1/3 of eyebrows.**
- **Myxedema** – nonpitting edema (eg, periorbital, peripheral).

DIAGNOSIS
- **Primary hypothyroid pattern – increased TSH + decreased free T4** or T3. May be normal or subclinical in early disease.
- ⊕ **Antithyroid peroxidase and/or anti-thyroglobulin antibodies.**
- Radioactive uptake scan: diffuse decreased iodine uptake.
- Biopsy: rarely done - **lymphocytic infiltration** with germinal centers & **Hürthle cells** (enlarged epithelial cells with abundant eosinophilic granular cytoplasm).

MANAGEMENT: **Levothyroxine therapy.**

LEVOTHYROXINE

INDICATIONS
- **First-line management of Hashimoto thyroiditis** & subclinical hypothyroidism with TSH 10mIU/L or greater. Thyroid hormone replacement after thyroidectomy.

MECHANISM OF ACTION: synthetic thyroxine (T4). Half-life of 7 days.

MONITORING
- **Monitor TSH levels at 6-week intervals when initiating or changing the dose**.
- Increase the dose if TSH is high and decrease the dose if TSH is low.
- Low doses with small incremental increases should be used to initiate therapy in the elderly and patients with cardiovascular disease.
- During pregnancy, the dose needs to be increased.

INTERACTIONS
- Best taken in the morning on an empty stomach for optimal absorption.
- Multivitamins, aluminum, iron or calcium supplements, proton pump inhibitors should be taken 4 hours apart from Levothyroxine (they can decrease its effectiveness).
- May need to decrease the dose with anticoagulants, insulin, and oral hypoglycemics. Cholestyramine may increase T4 requirements.

ADVERSE EFFECTS: **overshoot can have adverse cardiovascular effects and cause Osteoporosis.**

EUTHYROID SICK SYNDROME

- **Abnormal thyroid function tests in patients with normal thyroid function.**
- **Most commonly seen with severe non thyroidal illnesses** (eg, sepsis, cardiac, malignancies, etc.).

PATHOPHYSIOLOGY
- Severe illness decreases peripheral conversion of T4 to T3.

DIAGNOSIS
- **Low T3 syndrome: decreased Free T3 & increased reverse T3 most common** (T3 is low due to illness-related decreased peripheral conversion of T4 into T3).
- Free T4 often normal or decreased in more severe disease.
- TSH may be normal, low, or high. TSH usually low with severe disease & increased in the recovery phase.

MANAGEMENT
- Endocrine consult. Because the cause is a nonthyroidal illness, *management is focused on the treating the underlying illness.*
- Thyroid hormone replacement is usually not indicated.

RIEDEL THYROIDITIS

- Rare chronic autoimmune thyroiditis characterized by **dense fibrosis that invades the thyroid & adjacent neck structures.**
- Part of the IgG4-related systemic disease.

CLINICAL MANIFESTATIONS
- Presents similar to thyroid malignancy - **"rock" hard, nontender, rapidly growing, fixed goiter** (moves poorly with swallowing).
- **Compression symptoms:** neck tightness or pressure, hoarseness, dysphagia, choking, coughing, increased respiratory rate from **airway compression**.
- Absence of cervical lymphadenopathy

DIAGNOSIS
- **IgG4 serum levels**, Euthyroid or hypothyroid (30%).
- Open thyroid biopsy: **dense fibrosis.** FNA insufficient test if suspected. Biopsy usually performed to rule out malignancy.

MANAGEMENT
- **Surgical** treatment to help reduce compression.

- **EXAM TIP**
- A "rock hard" thyroid is either indicative of Anaplastic thyroid cancer or Riedel thyroiditis
- A biopsy is needed to distinguish between the two.

MYXEDEMA COMA

- Rare, **extreme form of hypothyroidism** with a high mortality rate (>40%).
- **Most commonly seen in elderly women with long standing hypothyroidism during the winter.**

PATHOPHYSIOLOGY
- Usually an acute precipitating factor (infection, CVA, CHF, sedative/narcotic use) in a patient with longstanding hypothyroidism, discontinuation or noncompliance with Levothyroxine therapy, or failure to start Levothyroxine after treatment for hyperthyroidism.

CLINICAL MANIFESTATIONS
- **Severe signs of hypothyroidism** - **bradycardia,** obtundation (coma), **hypothermia,** hypoventilation, **hypotension,** hypoglycemia, hyponatremia.

DIAGNOSIS
- **Hypothyroid profile most common** - **increased TSH + decreased free T4** (free T4 and T3 levels may so low that it may be undetectable). Serum cortisol.

MANAGEMENT
- **IV Thyroid hormone replacement (Levothyroxine) + supportive** - ICU admission, **passive warming** (rapid warming contraindicated), IV normal saline. **IV Glucocorticoids** often given.

SUBACUTE (GRANULOMATOUS, DEQUERVAIN) THYROIDITIS

PATHOPHYSIOLOGY
- Unknown but **often follows antecedent viral respiratory tract infection or post-viral inflammation** (but it is not an autoimmune disease).
- **Hyperthyroidism is typically the initial presentation**, followed by euthyroidism, then hypothyroidism, followed by resolution & restoration of normal thyroid function.

CLINICAL MANIFESTATIONS
- **Painful thyroid gland** aggravated with head movements & swallowing. Usually starts lower neck & radiates to jaw & ear.
- Patients usually present in hyperthyroid phase due to acute neck pain.
- URI symptoms: fever, myalgias, malaise, fatigue.

PHYSICAL EXAMINATION
- **Diffusely tender goiter.**

DIAGNOSIS
- **High ESR + negative thyroid antibodies.**
- **Hyperthyroid profile early in the disease** (**decreased TSH + increased free T4**). May present in a euthyroid or later in a hypothyroid state.
- Adjunctive: Radioactive uptake scan - diffuse, decreased iodine uptake (similar to Hashimoto and Postpartum thyroiditis).
- Biopsy: **granulomatous** inflammation with **multinucleated giant cells** (rarely performed).

MANAGEMENT
- **Supportive**: reassurance it is self-limiting (95% return to euthyroid state).
- **NSAIDs or Aspirin for pain & inflammation.**
- Prednisone is an alternative if no response to NSAIDs or in severe pain.

GRAVES' DISEASE

- **Most common cause of hyperthyroidism in the US.**
- Highest incidence in women 20-40y.

PATHOPHYSIOLOGY
- **Autoimmune disease – TSH-receptor autoantibodies target & stimulate the TSH receptor** on the thyroid gland, leading to increased thyroid hormone production, thyroid gland enlargement, & hyperthyroidism.
- Ophthalmopathy: TSH-receptors autoantibodies activate retroocular fibroblasts and adipocytes, leading to orbitopathy (specific to Graves').

CLINICAL MANIFESTATIONS
- Symptoms of hyperthyroidism eg, palpitations, heat intolerance, tremors, weight loss, **atrial fibrillation** etc.
- **Specific to Graves':**
  - **Ophthalmopathy: proptosis, exophthalmos, lid lag,** diplopia, vision changes.
  - **Pretibial myxedema**: swollen red or brown patches on legs with non-pitting edema.

PHYSICAL EXAMINATION
- Diffusely enlarged nontender goiter, **thyroid bruit.**

DIAGNOSIS:
- **Primary hyperthyroid profile: decreased TSH + increased free T4** or T3.
- ⊕ **Thyroid-stimulating immunoglobulins (TSH-receptor antibodies)** hallmark.
- Radioactive uptake scan: diffuse, increased iodine uptake.

MANAGEMENT

Radioactive iodine:
- **Most common therapy used.** Ablates the thyroid within 6-18 weeks.
- May exacerbate ophthalmopathy initially. Contraindicated in pregnant & lactating women.

Thioamides:

Methimazole or Propylthiouracil.
- Mechanism of action: prevents thyroid hormone synthesis. Will often achieve a euthyroid state within 3-8 weeks. May be used in older patients or patients with cardiovascular disease. May also be used prior to more definitive treatment (eg, thyroidectomy or radioactive iodine). PTU also prevents peripheral conversion of T4 into T3.
- Adverse effects: agranulocytosis, aplastic anemia, and fulminant hepatitis. **Methimazole generally preferred** (less adverse effects but teratogenic in the first trimester).
- **Propylthiouracil preferred in the first trimester & for Thyroid storm.**

Beta-blockers (eg, **Propranolol**)
- Can be used to **rapidly ameliorate symptoms**, such as tremor, hypertension, atrial fibrillation, & tachycardia.

Ophthalmopathy
- **Glucocorticoids best initial therapy.** Radioactive iodine may exacerbate ophthalmopathy initially so Glucocorticoids usually employed prior to Radioactive iodine in severe ophthalmopathy.
- Decompressive therapy & orbital radiotherapy are other options.

TSH-SECRETING PITUITARY ADENOMA

- Benign pituitary adenoma that secretes TSH in an autonomous fashion.
- Rare cause of hyperthyroidism (<1% of all cases).

CLINICAL MANIFESTATIONS

- **Diffuse goiter** (95%).
- **Signs of hyperthyroidism** – anxiety, heat intolerance, weight loss despite increased appetite, fatigue, weakness, increased sympathetic output (tachycardia, palpitations, atrial fibrillation, fine tremor), diarrhea, increased metabolic rate, high-output heart failure, & oligomenorrhea.
- Compression of local structures: **bitemporal hemianopsia** (loss of outer visual fields of both eyes) due to **compression of the optic chiasm. Headache,** mental disturbances.

DIAGNOSIS

- **Secondary hyperthyroid profile: increased TSH AND increased free T4** (both in the **same direction**).
- Radioactive uptake scan: **diffuse increased uptake** (same as Graves').
- **Pituitary MRI** to detect the adenoma.
- Increased alpha subunit distinguishes it from TSH resistance syndrome.

MANAGEMENT

- **Transsphenoidal surgery** - definitive management.
- Somatostatin analogs may be used prior to surgery to restore euthyroidism.

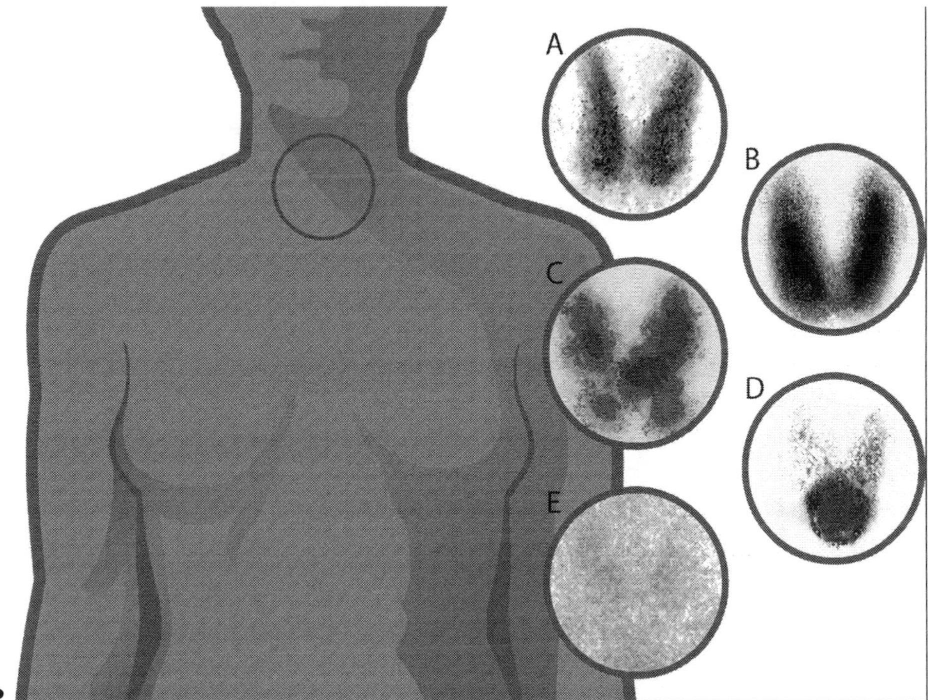

RADIOACTIVE UPTAKE SCAN

A. Normal thyroid gland
B. Graves' disease or TSH-secreting adenoma (diffuse increased uptake)
C. Toxic multinodular goiter (multiple areas of increased and decreased uptake)
D. Toxic adenoma (focal area of increased uptake – hot nodule)
E. Thyroiditis (diffuse decreased uptake)

TOXIC ADENOMAS

- **Single or multiple hyperfunctioning autonomous nodule(s).**
- Nontoxic usually asymptomatic. Toxic = symptoms of thyrotoxicosis.

CLINICAL MANIFESTATIONS

- **Signs of hyperthyroidism** - anxiety, heat intolerance, weight loss despite increased appetite, fatigue, weakness, increased sympathetic output (tachycardia, palpitations, atrial fibrillation, fine tremor), diarrhea, increased metabolic rate, high-output heart failure, & oligomenorrhea.
- Obstructive symptoms due to enlarged goiter - dyspnea, dysphagia, stridor, **hoarseness** if the goiter presses on the recurrent laryngeal nerve.

PHYSICAL EXAMINATION

- Palpable thyroid nodule.

DIAGNOSIS

- **Primary hyperthyroid profile decreased TSH + increased free T4** or T3. May be subclinical or normal.
- Radioactive iodine scan: **single or multiple areas of increased iodine uptake ("hot nodules"),** with decreased uptake in the surrounding normal tissue. Ultrasound.

MANAGEMENT

- **Radioactive iodine ablation** or surgery usually preferred over long-term anti-thyroid medications (Methimazole, Propylthiouracil).
- Surgery for compressive symptoms.

SUPPURATIVE THYROIDITIS

- Bacterial infection of the thyroid gland by Gram-positive bacteria **(*Staphylococcus aureus* most common)** or Gram-negative organisms. Pneumocystis, Mycobacterial, etc.
- Rare. Usually occurs in children.

CLINICAL MANIFESTATIONS

- **Thyroid pain & tenderness:** sudden onset of neck pain & tenderness to the thyroid gland. The pain is often worse with hyperextension and improves slightly with neck flexion. May radiate to the mandible, ears, or posteriorly. May have **overlying erythema to the skin.**
- **Fever, chills, pharyngitis,** dysphagia, dysphonia, hoarseness.

DIAGNOSIS

- Labs: **leukocytosis** & increased ESR. Thyroid function testing usually normal.
- **Fine needle aspiration** with Gram stain and culture.
- Thyroid ultrasound.

MANAGEMENT

- Antibiotics.
- Surgical drainage if fluctuant.

- **EXAM TIP**
- The only 2 causes of a **painful** thyroid are Subacute (Granulomatous, DeQuervain) and Suppurative thyroiditis

THYROTOXIC CRISIS (THYROID STORM)

- Rare, **potentially fatal** complication of untreated (or partially treated) **thyrotoxicosis** usually **after a precipitating event** (eg, surgery, trauma, infection, pregnancy).

- Only 1-2% of patients with hyperthyroidism present with thyroid storm (75% mortality)

CLINICAL MANIFESTATIONS
- **Hyperthyroid symptoms** & hypermetabolic state
  - **Cardiovascular dysfunction** eg, **palpitations, tachycardia, atrial fibrillation, CHF**.

  - **High fever** (104 – 106F), nausea, vomiting, **tremors.**

  - **CNS dysfunction** eg, agitation, delirium, psychosis, stupor, or coma, which later may progress to coma & hypotension.

- May have symptoms of hyperthyroidism – eg, warm and moist skin, hand tremor, ophthalmopathy.

DIAGNOSIS
- **Primary hyperthyroid profile** – **increased free T4 or T3 + decreased TSH** (may be so low it may be undetectable) most common pattern. Hyperglycemia may be seen.

MANAGEMENT
- **IV fluids + Propranolol + antithyroid medication** (eg, **Propylthiouracil**) **+ IV Glucocorticoids.**
  - Beta blockers (eg, Propranolol) reduces tachycardia and decreases adrenergic symptoms.

  - Anti-thyroid medications block the synthesis of new T3 and T4. **Propylthiouracil is preferred over Methimazole** because PTU also reduces peripheral conversion of T4 to T3.

  - Glucocorticoids reduce peripheral conversion of T4 to T3.

- This is **followed by oral or IV sodium iodide** (1 hour after PTU), iodinated radiocontrast agent.
  - Iodine solution blocks the release of thyroid hormone.
  - Iodinated radiocontrast agent Glucocorticoids reduce peripheral conversion of T4 to T3.

- Antipyretics given (**avoid Aspirin** because it can displace thyroid hormones off of carrier proteins).

- Cooling blankets.

HYPERTHYROID DISORDERS

TYPE	CAUSE	CLINICAL MANIFESTATIONS	DIAGNOSIS (not all tests need to be done)	MANAGEMENT
GRAVE'S DISEASE	***Autoimmune*** MC women 20-40y Circulating ***TSH receptor antibodies*** cause ↑thyroid hormone synthesis, release & thyroid gland growth ***worse with stress (ex. pregnancy, illness)*** ***Graves MC cause of hyperthyroidism**** (90%)	Clinical Hyperthyroidism • Diffuse, enlarged thyroid. • ***THYROID BRUITS**** • ***OPHTHALMOPATHY*: lid lag, exophthalmos/proptosis (exclusive to Grave)**** Hyaluronic acid deposition. ***Tx c steroids.*** Smoking & iodine may make ophthalmopathy worse. • ***PRETIBIAL MYXEDEMA**** Nonpitting, edematous, pink to brown plaques/nodules on shin (exclusive to Grave)	• ⊕ ***Thyroid- Stimulating Immunoglobulins (Ab)* most spp.*** ± Thyroid peroxidase & anti-TG Ab • **Hyperthyroid TFTs: ↑FT_4/FT_3 & ↓TSH** (± be subclinical) • **RAIU: ↑ *DIFFUSE uptake**** Normal Grave's Diffuse uptake seen in TSH-secreting pituitary adenoma also.	• ***Radioactive Iodine: MC therapy used.**** Destroys thyroid gland. Will need hormone replacement • ***Methimazole or PropylThioUracil*** • ***Beta blockers (ex. Propranolol) for symptomatic relief:**** tremors, anxiety, tachycardia, diaphoresis, palpitations, etc • ***Thyroidectomy:*** if compressive sx, no response to meds, If RAI is contraindicated (ex pregnancy)
TOXIC MULTINODULAR GOITER (TMG) (Plummer's Disease) ***TOXIC ADENOMA (TA)***	Autonomous functioning nodules ***MC in elderly*** One autonomous functioning nodule	**BOTH TMG & TA** Clinical Hyperthyroidism • Diffuse, enlarged thyroid • ***No skin/eye changes!*** • Palpable nodule(s) **Compressive sx:** • ***Dyspnea, dysphagia, stridor, hoarseness*** (laryngeal compression).	• **Hyperthyroid TFTs:** ↑ FT_4/T_3; ↓TSH (± be subclinical) • **RAIU: (PATCHY areas of both ↑ & ↓uptake) in TMG** TMG • **RAIU:** **↑LOCAL *uptake (hot nodule) in TA*** TA	**BOTH TMG & TA** • ***Radioactive Iodine: MC therapy*** • Surgery (subtotal thyroidectomy) if compressive symptoms present • ***Methimazole or PTU:*** - **MOA:** ***inhibit hormone synthesis. Methimazole preferred (less S/E)*** - ***S/E of both: agranulocytosis**** (so monitor WBC) & ***hepatitis.**** • ***PTU preferred in pregnancy.*** (especially 1st trimester) • ***Beta blockers for symptoms of thyrotoxicosis***
TSH SECERETING PITUITARY ADENOMA	Autonomous TSH secretion by pituitary adenoma	Clinical Hyperthyroidism • Diffuse, enlarged thyroid • ***Bitemporal Hemianopsia**** • Mental disturbances	• ***TFT's: ↑ FT_4/T_3; + ↑ TSH* (inappropriate TSH elevation in the setting of elevated FT_4/T_3 (same direction)**** • **RAIU: DIFFUSE uptake** • Pituitary MRI: adenoma	• **Transsphenoidal Surgery** to remove the pituitary adenoma

HYPOTHYROID DISORDERS

TYPE	CAUSE	CLINICAL MANIFESTATIONS	DIAGNOSIS	DURATION
HASHIMOTO'S thyroiditis (CHRONIC LYMPHOCYTIC) **MC cause of hypothyroidism in the US* – 6x MC in women**	***Autoimmune*** (Anti-thyroid Antibodies) (Ab)	Clinical Hypothyroidism • Painless, enlarged thyroid • May present in euthyroid state (rarely in hyperthyroid state)	• ***⊕Thyroid Ab present: thyroglobulin Ab, antimicrosomial & Thyroid Peroxidase Ab*** • ***TFTs (usually HypOthyroid)*** • ↓Radioactive I- uptake (usually not needed) • Bx: lymphocytes, germinal follicles, Hurthle	• Hypothyroidism usually permanent. • ***Levothyroxine therapy**** *Thyroid hormone replacement*
SILENT (LYMPHOCYTIC) THYROIDITIS	***Autoimmune*** (Anti-thyroid Ab)	Painless, enlarged thyroid. Thyrotoxicosis ⇨ hypothyroid (depends on when they present)	• ***⊕Thyroid Ab present:*** thyroglobulin Ab, antimicrosomial & Thyroid Peroxidase Ab • TFTs: Hyper/Hypothyroid (depends on when they present) • ↓Radioactive Iodine uptake on RAIU scan	• Return to euthyroid state within 12-18 months without treatment. **Aspirin** • ***No anti-thyroid meds**** • 20% possible permanent hypothyroidism
POSTPARTUM THYROIDITIS	***Autoimmune*** (Anti-thyroid Ab)	Painless, enlarged thyroid. Thyrotoxicosis ⇨ hypothyroid (depends on when they present)	• ***⊕Thyroid Ab present:*** thyroglobulin Ab, antimicrosomial & Thyroid Peroxidase Ab • TFTs (Hyper/Hypothyroid) (depends on when they present) • ↓Radioactive Iodine uptake on RAIU scan	• Return to euthyroid state in 12-18 months without treatment. **Aspirin,** NSAIDs • ***No anti-thyroid meds**** • 20% possible permanent hypothyroidism
de QUERVAIN'S THYROIDITIS (GRANULOMATOUS) PAINFUL SUBACUTE	***MC POST VIRAL*** * or viral inflammatory reaction. Associated with HLA-B35	***PAINFUL, tender neck/thyroid**** ***Clinical Hyperthyroidism*** (due to neck pain in acute phase) Thyrotoxicosis ⇨ hypothyroid (depend on when they present)	• ***↑ESR (hallmark)**** • ***NO thyroid Ab**** • ***TFTs (usually HypERthyroid)*** (depends on when they present) • ↓Radioactive Iodine uptake on RAIU scan	• Return to euthyroid state in 12-18 months without treatment. **Aspirin (for pain, inflammation, ↑'es T4)** • ***No anti-thyroid meds**** • 5% possible permanent hypothyroidism
MEDICATION-INDUCED	***AMIODARONE*** (contains iodine), ***LITHIUM*** **Alpha interferon**	Painless, enlarged thyroid. Thyrotoxicosis ⇨ hypothyroid (depend on when they present)		Often returns to euthyroid states when med is stopped, Corticosteroids
ACUTE THYROIDITIS (Suppurative)	***S. aureus MC*** (any organism may cause it)	May have ***PAINFUL, fluctuant*** thyroid. Usually very ill, ***febrile.***	Increased WBC count with left shift. Usually ***euthyroid***	Antibiotics Drainage if abscess present
RIEDEL'S THYROIDITIS	***Fibrous*** thyroid	***Firm hard 'woody' nodule (similar to anaplastic cancer)****	May develop hypothyroidism	Surgery may be needed

LEVOTHYROXINE: ***synthetic T_4.*** Monitor TSH levels @ 6 week intervals when initiating/changing dose. ***Slow, small increases in >50y & patients with cardiovascular disease.*** **Monitor elderly, patients with angina, MI, or CHF for adverse reactions** due to increased metabolic rate or withhold until cardiovascular status is stabilized. May need to lower doses of anticoagulants, insulin, and oral antihyperglycemics. Oral cholestyramine may increase T_4 requirements.

The MC cause of hypothyroidism in the US is Hashimoto's thyroiditis.* ***The MC cause of hypothyroidism worldwide is iodine deficiency.****

PAPILLARY THYROID CARCINOMA

- **Most common thyroid cancer** (>80%).
- **More common in women** but the prognosis is worse in men.
- Least aggressive type of thyroid cancer & excellent prognosis (high cure rate).
- Metastasis usually occurs local (cervical lymph nodes most common). Distant METS uncommon (when present, it usually involves the lungs or bone).

CLINICAL MANIFESTATIONS
- Usually presents as a painless thyroid nodule.

RISK FACTORS
- **Most common after radiation exposure** of the head & neck.
- Family history of thyroid cancer.

WORKUP
- Fine needle aspiration. Thyroid function tests usually normal.

MANAGEMENT
- **Thyroidectomy** (total or near total) usually followed by **postoperative Levothyroxine** to replace normal hormone production and to suppress tumor regrowth.
- Post-surgery radioiodine in some patients (high-risk and some intermediate risk disease).
- Post-treatment: may monitor Thyroglobulin levels, TSH, and ultrasound of the neck.

FOLLICULAR THYROID CARCINOMA

- Second most common type of thyroid cancer ~10%.
- More aggressive than Papillary but also slow growing.
- Most common 40-60y.

RISK FACTORS
- Increased incidence with iodine deficiency.
- Less often associated with radiation exposure (compared to papillary).
- Metastases: **distant METS more common than local METS** (hematogenous spread) – lung most common, liver, brain, bone. Think **Follicular** goes **FAR.**

DIAGNOSIS
- FNA with biopsy alone often cannot distinguish between follicular adenoma from carcinoma so definitive diagnosis is often made with postsurgical histologic testing.

MANAGEMENT
- **Thyroidectomy** (total or near total) usually followed by **postoperative Levothyroxine** to replace normal hormone production and to suppress tumor regrowth.
- Post-surgery radioiodine in some patients (high-risk and some intermediate risk disease).
- Post-treatment: may monitor Thyroglobulin levels, TSH, and ultrasound of the neck.

MEDULLARY THYROID CARCINOMA

- ~5% of all thyroid carcinoma
- **Derived from Calcitonin-synthesizing parafollicular C cells**
- 90% sporadic. **10% associated with MEN IIa or IIb** (associated with RET mutation).
- More aggressive. Local cervical node METS early in the disease with distant METS later in the disease.

LABS
- **Increased Calcitonin.**

MANAGEMENT
- **Total thyroidectomy** – may include dissection of lymph nodes and surrounding fatty tissue on the ipsilateral side. MTC does not take up iodine.
- May order urinary metanephrine levels to rule out Pheochromocytoma (Men II).
- Prognosis: worse than Papillary or Follicular.
- **Calcitonin levels are used to monitor for recurrence or residual disease**.

ANAPLASTIC THYROID CARCINOMA

- Rare. Most commonly seen in the elderly > 65y.
- **Most aggressive** of all thyroid cancers.
- **Poor prognosis**.

CLINICAL MANIFESTATIONS
- **Rapid growth, compressive symptoms** – dyspnea (may invade the trachea), dysphagia.

PHYSICAL EXAMINATION
- **"Rock" hard thyroid mass.** May be fixed.

MANAGEMENT
- **Most are not amenable to surgical resection.**
- External beam radiation or Chemotherapy.
- **Palliative tracheostomy** may be needed to maintain the airway.

THYROID NODULE

- **>90% of nodules are benign.** Most thyroid nodules in women are benign (follicular adenoma or cysts). Only 10% are malignant or suspicious.
- Risk factors: **extremes of age (very young or >60y), history of head & neck irradiation.**

BENIGN
- **Follicular adenoma (colloid) most common type of thyroid nodule** (50-60%).
- Adenomas, cysts, localized thyroiditis.

CLINICAL MANIFESTATIONS
- **Most are asymptomatic.**
- Compressive symptoms: difficulty swallowing or breathing, neck, jaw, or ear pain, hoarseness (recurrent laryngeal nerve impingement).
- Functional nodules: rare – presents with thyrotoxicosis.

PHYSICAL EXAMINATION
- Benign: **varied** - smooth, firm, irregular, sharply outlined, discrete, painless.
- Malignant: **rapid growth, fixed in place, no movement with swallowing** (Riedel's thyroiditis may also present like this).

WORKUP
- **Thyroid function testing:** often the **initial test done as part of the nodule workup**. If TSH is subnormal (subclinical or overt hyperthyroidism), order thyroid scintigraphy (radioactive iodine uptake scan).
  - **If TSH is normal or high, FNA with biopsy is indicated.**

- **Thyroid ultrasound:** usually performed after TFTs in patients with nodules (high-resolution ultrasound is the most sensitive test in the detection of the presence of a thyroid lesion). **Often used to determine if FNA with biopsy is needed**, help obtain a specimen during FNA with biopsy, used to see if nodule is cystic or solid, to monitor a suspicious nodule, or to see if a nodule is growing or shrinking.
  - US findings suspicious of cancer include irregular margins, hypoechoic, central vascularity, documented nodule growth.

- **Fine needle aspiration: best test to evaluate the etiology of a nodule** (may be guided by ultrasound).
  - **FNA performed in nodules >1.5 cm with normal TSH** or in highly suspicious nodules (eg, via ultrasound or examination).

- Radioactive iodine uptake scan: usually performed if the FNA is indeterminate or if low or subnormal TSH.
  - **Cold nodules (no or low iodine uptake) should be biopsied to rule out malignancy.**
  - Functioning (normal) or hot nodules have lower malignant potential.

MANAGEMENT
- **Surgical excision if thyroid cancer is suspected** or if an indeterminate FNA, especially with a cold scan.

- Observation + follow-up Ultrasound if surgery is not performed (usually every 6-12 months).

DIABETES MELLITUS

Type I DIABETES MELLITUS

- **Insulin deficiency due to pancreatic beta cell destruction.**
- These patients require exogenous insulin.
- **Onset usually < 30 years of age (3/4 is diagnosed in childhood)**. Peaks at 4-6 years of age then 10-14 years.
- Not associated with obesity.

ETIOLOGIES
- Type 1A (**Autoimmune**): **most common.** Often triggered by environmental factors (eg, infection). Increased with HLA DR3-DQ2 & DR4 genes.
- Type 1B = non-autoimmune beta cell destruction.

CLINICAL MANIFESTATIONS
- **Hyperglycemia without acidosis: most common initial presentation - polyuria, polydipsia, polyphagia.**
- Weight loss. Lethargy.
- **Diabetic ketoacidosis** second most common initial presentation **(more common in type 1)**, hyperglycemic hyperosmolar syndrome (more common in type 2).
- Silent (asymptomatic) incidental discovery.

Type II DIABETES MELLITUS

- Combination of **insulin insensitivity (resistance) & relative impairment of insulin secretion** (increased insulin levels early in the disease but may diminish with disease progression).

RISK FACTORS
- Likely due to **genetic & environmental factors** especially, especially **obesity greatest risk factor & decreased physical activity.** 90% of type II diabetics are overweight.
- Most common >40y.
- History of impaired glucose tolerance, **family history**, first degree relative, Hispanic, African-American, Pacific Islander, hypertension, dyslipidemia, delivery of baby >9 lbs, syndrome X, & insulin resistance: "CHAOS"- Chronic HTN, Atherosclerosis, Obesity (central), & Stroke.

CLINICAL MANIFESTATIONS
- Most are asymptomatic (may be an incidental finding).
- **Classic symptoms: polyuria, polydipsia, polyphagia.**
- **Poor wound healing, increased infections.** Hyperglycemic hyperosmolar syndrome.

GLUCOSE TEST	IMPAIRED TOLERANCE	DIABETES MELLITUS(mg/dL)	COMMENTS
FASTING PLASMA GLUCOSE	110 - 125	**≥ 126**	- Fasting at least 8 hours on **2 occasions.** - **GOLD STANDARD.**
2-HOUR GLUCOSE TOLERANCE TEST	≥140-199	**≥ 200**	- **Oral glucose tolerance test. (GTT).** - **3h GTT** gold standard in gestational diabetes
HEMOGLOBIN A1C	5.7 – 6.4 %	**≥ 6.5%**	Indicates average blood sugar **10-12 weeks prior** to measurement
RANDOM PLASMA		≥200	in a patient with classic diabetic symptoms or complications.

SCREENING: ADA: all adults ≥45 every 3 years OR any adult with BMI ≥25kg/m^2 & 1 additional risk factor.
USPSTF: (2015) any 40-70 year old that is overweight or obese (every 3 years).

INITIAL MANAGEMENT OF TYPE II DIABETES MELLITUS

- **Diet, exercise and lifestyle changes initial management of type II DM.**
  - Carbohydrates 50-60%; Protein 15-20%, 10% unsaturated fats.
- **Oral antihyperglycemic medications** initiated if unable to control glucose with lifestyle changes (eg, **Metformin initial therapy in most).**
- Metformin, Sulfonylureas, Meglitinides, TZDs, DPP-4 inhibitors, GLP-1 agonists, SGLT-2 inhibitors.
- Insulin may be needed if uncontrolled with other medications.

BIGUANIDES

METFORMIN

Mechanism of action:

- Major effect **is decreased hepatic glucose production** (by inhibiting gluconeogenesis). Increases insulin-mediated glucose utilization in peripheral tissues.
- Because it has **no effect on pancreatic beta cells, it is not usually associated with hypoglycemia.**
- Not associated with weight gain.

Indications:

- **Usually the first-line oral medication** in type II DM. Can decrease HgbA1C by 1.5% & glucose concentrations by approximately 20%.
- Additional benefits include **weight loss, decreased triglycerides, decreased cardiovascular risk**, & possible decreased cancer risk.

Adverse reactions:

- **GI complaints most common** - metallic taste, diarrhea, abdominal discomfort, anorexia, nausea.
- **Vitamin B12 deficiency** - decreased B12 absorption.
- **Lactic acidosis** tends to occur in patients predisposed to hypoxemia, hypoperfusion, heart failure, and severe renal or hepatic impairment.

Contraindications:

- **Severe renal or hepatic impairment**, heart failure, & excessive alcohol intake.
- **Metformin held before giving iodinated contrast** & may be resumed 48 hours with monitoring of creatinine.

SULFONYLUREAS

- **2nd-generation: Glipizide, Glyburide, & Glimepiride**
- 1st-generation: Tolbutamide, Chlorpropamide (not used as often due to higher adverse effect profile).

Mechanism of action:

- **Stimulates pancreatic beta cell insulin release (insulin secretagogue)** via mimicking the action of glucose, leasing to closure of the K-ATP channel of SUR1 receptor.
- **2nd-generation preferred because associated with less adverse effects** & shorter duration of action.

Indications:

- In addition to Metformin or as initial therapy in patients with contraindications to Metformin.
- Similar glycemic efficacy compared to Metformin.
- Short-acting Glimepiride or Glipizide safer in patients with chronic renal disease.

Adverse effects:

- **Hypoglycemia most common adverse effect** (especially with the long-acting 1st-generation) because insulin release is non glucose dependent.
- GI upset (reduced incidence if taken with food)
- Dermatitis (including photosensitivity, pruritus, erythema, rash, urticaria).
- Sulfonamide allergies, cardiac dysrhythmias, **weight gain.**
- CP450 system inducer (can lead to drug interactions).
- **Chlorpropamide has 2 unique adverse effects: hyponatremia** (increased ADH) & **Disulfiram reaction - flushing reaction after alcohol ingestion** (by inhibiting the metabolism of acetaldehyde).

MEGLITINIDES

Repaglinide, Nateglinide

Mechanism of action:

- **Stimulates pancreatic beta cell insulin release (insulin secretagogue** that is more glucose dependent, leading to **postprandial insulin release**).

Indications:

- May be used as monotherapy in patients with contraindications to Metformin or in combination with Metformin.
- Similar benefits of Sulfonylureas without the sulfa component (safe with sulfa allergies).

Adverse effects:

- **Hypoglycemia lower incidence compared to sulfonylureas**. Often administered with meals to decrease postprandial hyperglycemia.
- **Weight gain.**
- Nateglinide should not be used in chronic renal or liver disease because it is metabolized by the liver with active metabolites renally excreted.
- **Repaglinide is safer in patients with chronic renal disease** (principally metabolized by the liver).

THIAZOLIDINEDIONES

Pioglitazone, Rosiglitazone

Mechanism of action:

- **Increases insulin sensitivity** at the **peripheral receptor sites** (eg, **adipose, muscle, & liver**), leading to increased glucose utilization & decreased glucose production.
- No effect on pancreatic beta cells.
- Hemoglobin A1C falls at most 2% with monotherapy.

Adverse effects:

- **Peripheral edema & fluid retention, congestive heart failure**, & increased fractures (females).
- Hepatotoxicity LFTs should be monitored while on therapy.
- **Rosiglitazone is associated with higher incidence of cardiovascular events & atherogenic lipid profiles** (Pioglitazone usually preferred if TZD therapy is needed).
- Bladder cancer with Pioglitazone.

Contraindications:

- Heart failure (symptomatic, Class III or IV), history of bladder cancer, active liver disease, high-risk for fractures, pregnancy, Type I DM.

ALPHA-GLUCOSIDASE INHIBITORS

Acarbose, Miglitol

Mechanism of action:

- **Delays intestinal glucose absorption** (inhibits pancreatic alpha amylase and intestinal alpha-glucosidase hydrolase).
- Does not affect insulin secretion (not associated with hypoglycemia).
- Less potent than Metformin & Sulfonylureas.
- Can be used in patients with renal insufficiency.

Adverse effects:

- **GI: flatulence, diarrhea**, abdominal pain, **hepatitis**.
- Cautious use in patients with gastroparesis, inflammatory bowel disease, patients on bile acid resins.

GLUCAGON-LIKE PEPTIDE 1 RECEPTOR AGONIST

Liraglutide, Exenatide, Dulaglutide

Mechanism of action:

- **Mimics incretin**, leading to **increased glucose-dependent insulin secretion**, decreased glucagon secretion, & **delayed gastric emptying**. Administered via injection.

Indications:

- **Associated with weight loss & reduction of major cardiovascular events** (especially Liraglutide).
- Not associated with hypoglycemia when used as monotherapy.

Adverse effects:

- **GI** (nausea, vomiting, diarrhea). **Pancreatitis.**
- Small risk of hypoglycemia (usually in the setting of other hypoglycemic agents).

Contraindications:

- **History of Gastroparesis or Pancreatitis.**
- **Medullary thyroid carcinoma** or MEN 2 syndrome.

DPP4 INHIBITORS

Sitagliptin, Linagliptin, Saxagliptin

Mechanism of action:

- Dipeptidyl peptidase-4 (DPP-4) inhibition causes decreased degradation of Glucagon-like peptide-1 (GLP-1), increasing GLP-1 levels.
- This leads to increased insulin release, decreased glucagon, decreased hepatic glucose production, & increased uptake of glucose in the peripheral tissues.
- Not associated with hypoglycemia if not used with insulin secretagogues.

Indications:

- Monotherapy in patients who are intolerant of or have contraindications to other oral medications.
- Can be adjunctive therapy to those medications.

Adverse effects:

- Headache, **acute pancreatitis**, hepatitis, skin changes, joint pain, & renal dysfunction.

SGLT-2 INHIBITORS

"flozin" – Empagliflozin, Canagliflozin, Dapagliflozin

Mechanism of action:

- **Sodium-glucose transport (SGLT-2) inhibition** lowers renal glucose threshold, leading to **increased urinary glucose excretion.**
- SGLT2 is expressed in the proximal tubule & mediates reabsorption of approximately 90% of the filtered glucose load. They are relatively weak glucose-lowering agents.
- Not associated with hypoglycemia in the absence of therapies that otherwise cause hypoglycemia.

Indications:

- Most often used in combination with Metformin, Pioglitazone, Sitagliptin, or Insulin.
- Cardiovascular risk reduction: **improves cardiovascular outcomes and decreases the risk of heart failure (especially Empagliflozin).**
- Added benefit of **blood pressure & weight reduction.**

Adverse effects:

- **Transient nausea & vomiting**, thirst, abdominal pain. Acute kidney injury, bone fractures.
- **Urinary tract infections & yeast infections** (due to increased urinary glucose).
- May cause hypotension in patients on hypertensive medications (due to an osmotic diuresis).
- At the initiation of therapy, avoid hypoglycemia by monitoring HgbA1C.

Contraindications & cautions:

- Not used in Type I DM, type II with estimated GFR <60 mL.
- Canagliflozin & Ertugliflozin may be associated with increased risk of amputation.
- Cautious use with other medications that can cause dehydration (eg, NSAIDs, ACE inhibitors, ARBs, diuretics) and patients with low bone mineral density.

ANTI-HYPERGLYCEMIC AGENTS

	MECHANISM OF ACTION	SIDE EFFECTS/CAUTION
BIGUANIDES Metformin	• **Mainly ↓'es hepatic glucose production,** ↑'es peripheral glucose utilization • ↓GI intestinal glucose absorption, ↑insulin sensitivity **(no effect on pancreatic beta cells ⇨ no hypoglycemia, no weight gain** • **Usually 1st line PO medication** used to control Type II DM. **↓'es triglycerides.**	• **Lactic acidosis, Not given in patients c hepatic or renal impairment** Cr >1.5 • GI complaints common. **Macrocytic anemia** (↓B12), metallic taste. • **Metformin should be d/c'ed 24h before given iodinated contrast & resumed 48 hours afterwards with monitoring of creatinine.**
SULFONYLUREAS 1st gen: Tolbutamide, Chlorpropamide 2nd gen: Glipizide, Glyburide, Glimepiride	• **Stimulates pancreatic beta cell insulin release (insulin secretagogue – non glucose dependent)** • 2nd generation: less S/E (so preferred), shorter half-lives	• **Hypoglycemia most common.** • **GI upset** (reduced if taken c food), Dermatitis • **Disulfiram reaction**, sulfa allergy • Cardiac dysrhythmias, **weight gain** • CP450 inducer (drug-drug interactions)
MEGLITINIDES Repaglinide, Nateglinide	• **Stimulates pancreatic beta cell insulin release* (insulin secretagogue)**	• **Hypoglycemia** (less than sulfonylureas) • Weight gain
α - GLUCOSIDASE INHIBITORS: Acarbose Miglitol	• **Delays intestinal glucose absorption** (inhibits pancreatic alpha amylase and intestinal α - glucosidase hydrolase). • Does not affect insulin secretion.	• **Hepatitis** (↑LFT's), flatulence, diarrhea, abdominal pain. • Cautious use in patients c gastroparesis, inflammatory bowel disease, on bile acid resins.
THIAZOLIDINEDIONES Pioglitazone Rosiglitazone	• **↑ insulin sensitivity at the peripheral receptor site adipose & muscle.** • **No effect on pancreatic beta cells.**	• **Fluid retention & edema** (CHF), hepatotoxicity, bladder CA, fractures. • **Cardiovascular toxicity with Rosiglitazone.**
GLUCAGON-LIKE PEPTIDE 1 (GLP-1) AGONISTS: Exenatide, Liraglutide	• Mimics **incretin ⇨ ↑insulin secretion, delays gastric emptying, ↓ glucagon secretion.** No weight gain.	• Hypoglycemia (less than sulfonylureas b/c glucose dependent), pancreatitis. • **CI if history of gastroparesis**
DPP-4 INHIBITOR: Sitagliptin, Linagliptin	• Dipeptidylpeptase inhibition ⇨inhibition of degradation of GLP-1 ⇨ ↑ GLP-1	• Pancreatitis, renal failure, GI symptoms
SGLT-2 INHIBITOR: Canagliflozin Dapagliflozin	• SGLT-2 inhibition lowers renal glucose threshold ⇨ **↑urinary glucose excretion** SGLT = Sodium-Glucose Transport	• Thirst, nausea, abdominal pain, UTIs

TYPE OF INSULIN	ONSET	PEAK	DURATION	INSULIN COVERAGE
RAPID- ACTING **Lispro** (Humalog) **Aspart** (Novolog) Glulisine	5-15min	45-75m	2-4 hours	**Given at the same time of meal.** Often used with intermediate or long acting insulin.
SHORT- ACTING **Regular**	30m	2-4h	5-8h	**Given 30-60 minutes prior to meal.** Often used with intermediate or long acting insulin
INTERMEDIATE **NPH** **Lente**	2h	4-12h	8-18h	**Covers insulin for about half day (or overnight).** Often combined with rapid or short-acting insulin. NPH often given at bedtime
LONG ACTING **Detemir**	2h	3-9h	6-24h (dose dependent)	**Covers insulin for 1 full day (basal insulin)** Detemir 6-24 hours
Glargine	2h	No peak	20 - >24 h	• **Glargine causes fewer hypoglycemic episodes than NPH.** • **Long acting should not be mixed with other types of insulin** in the same syringe
PRE-MIXED: Humulin 70/30 (NPH/reg), Novolin 70/30, Novolog 70/30 (NPH, aspsart), Humulin 50/50				These are generally given twice daily before mealtime. 70/30 (NPH/Regular)

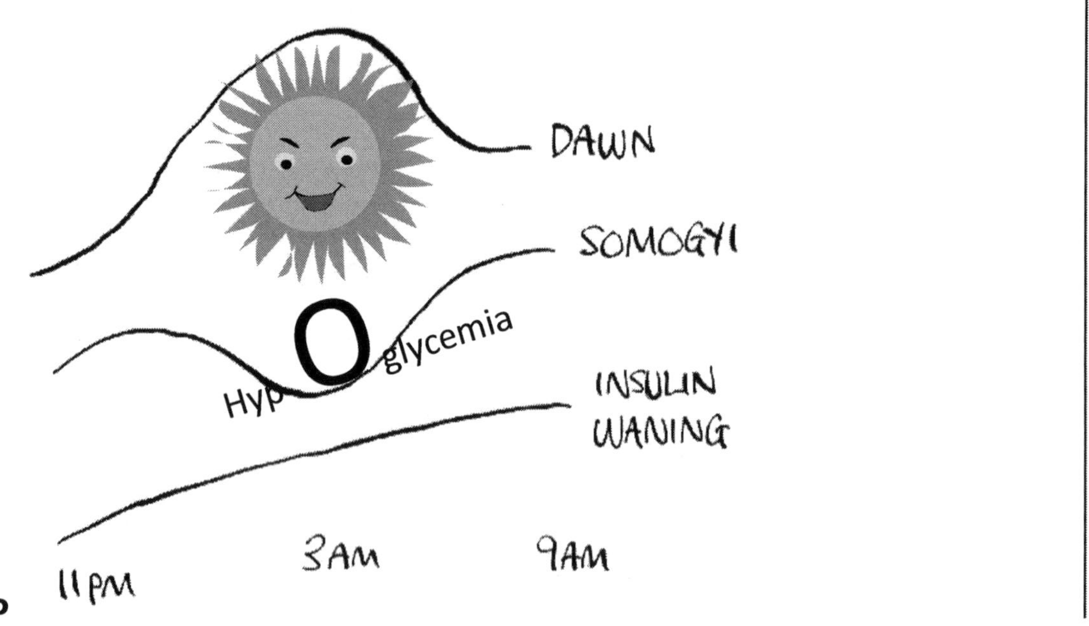

TIP

- In answering these questions, the 11pm dose is usually normal and the 8 am preprandial dose will be high.
- The key is what is the 3 am dose? If it rises with the sun at 3 am, it's the Dawn phenomenon
- If the 3am dose is l**O**w (Hyp**O**glycemia, then it is the S**O**m**O**gyi

SOMOGYI PHENOMENON

- **Nocturnal hypoglycemia followed by rebound hyperglycemia.**

Pathophysiology:

- Hyperglycemia occurs due to surge in growth hormone after early AM hypoglycemia.

Management:

Prevent hypoglycemia with any one:

- Decreasing nighttime NPH dose
- Move the evening NPH earlier
- Give a bedtime snack

DAWN PHENOMENON

- Normal glucose **until rise in serum glucose levels between 2am - 8 am**.

Pathophysiology:

- Results from decreased insulin sensitivity & **nightly surge of counterregulatory hormones** (during nighttime fasting).

Management:

Reduce early morning hyperglycemia with any one:

- **Bedtime injection of NPH** (to blunt morning hyperglycemia)
- Increase the NPH dose
- **Avoiding carbohydrate snack late at night**
- Insulin pump usage early in the morning.

INSULIN WANING

- Progressive rise in glucose from bed to morning (seen when NPH dose evening dose is administered before dinner).
- Due to ineffective dosing of NPH insulin.

Management:

- Move NPH insulin dose to bedtime or increase the evening dose.

HYPOGLYCEMIA

- **Blood glucose level 70 mg/dL or less**.
- A complication of the management of Diabetes mellitus. Usually due to too much insulin use, too little food, or excess exercise.

CLINICAL MANIFESTATIONS

- **Autonomic:** sweating, tremors, palpitations, nervousness, tachycardia, pallor, cool clammy skin.
- **CNS:** headache, lightness, confusion, slurred speech, dizziness, irritability, difficulty concentrating, blurred vision, nausea, syncope.

Management of mild to moderate:

- 15-20g fast-acting carbohydrate, fruit juice, hard candies.
- Recheck in 10-15 minutes.

Severe, unconscious, <40 mg/dL:

- **IV bolus of D50 or IV glucagon.** Glucagon SQ or IM if no IV access.
- If unknown cause, order C-peptide, plasma insulin levels & anti-insulin antibodies as part of the workup. **Elevated C-peptide seen in endogenous insulin production** (C-peptide is normal with exogenous insulin administration).

DIABETIC KETOACIDOSIS

- Consequence of **insulin deficiency & counterregulatory hormone excess.**
- Most commonly seen with Type I DM (due to insulin deficiency).

ETIOLOGIES

DKA is a response to stressful triggers:

- **Infection - most common cause** (eg, UTI or pneumonia) 30-40%.
- Discontinuation or inadequate insulin therapy, undiagnosed diabetics, MI, CVA, pancreatitis, etc.

CLINICAL MANIFESTATIONS

- Polyuria, polydipsia, nocturia, weakness, fatigue, altered mental status changes, nausea, vomiting, chest pain, **abdominal pain.**

PHYSICAL EXAMINATION

- Tachycardia, tachypnea, hypotension, decreased skin turgor, **fruity (acetone) breath**, & **Kussmaul respirations** (deep, continuous respirations).

DIAGNOSIS

- **Plasma glucose > 250** (usually not greater than 600), decreased arterial pH (<7.30) and bicarbonate (<22) due to high anion gap metabolic acidosis, increased serum osmolarity, **positive ketones in the urine** and serum.

MANAGEMENT

- **SIPS – Saline, Insulin (regular), Potassium repletion, S**earch for underlying cause.
- IV fluids: **critical initial step.**
  - **Isotonic 0.9% (Normal saline)** until hypotension & orthostasis resolves.
  - Then switch to ½ normal saline (0.45%).
  - When glucose levels become 250 mg/dL or less, use the D5 version of the current solution (to prevent hypoglycemia from Insulin therapy).

- Regular insulin: lowers serum glucose & switches body from catabolic to anabolic state (reduces ketones & fatty acid production as well as decreases gluconeogenesis).

- Potassium repletion: despite serum K+ levels, patients are always in a total body potassium deficit. **Correction of DKA will invariably cause hypokalemia.**
  - **Unless serum K+ is > 5.3 mEq/L, K+ repletion is recommended.**
  - If serum K+ is between 3.3 – 5.3 meq/L, IV KCl (20-30 mEq/L) is added to each liter of IV replacement fluid.
  - If serum K+ is < 3.3 mEq/L, IV potassium chloride (20-40 mEq/L) should be given.
  - If serum K+ > 5.3, delay replacement until K falls below 5.3. **Check serum K+ levels hourly.**

- Treatment goals: closing the anion gap in DKA determines complete management. **Bicarbonate levels more important than glucose levels in determining the severity of DKA.**

- Bicarbonate administration is only used in severe cases because it associated with complications (overcorrection, increased cerebral edema).

HYPEROSMOLAR HYPERGLYCEMIC STATE

- Consequence of **Insulin deficiency & counterregulatory hormone excess.**
- **HHS is more common with type II DM**, seen in older patients, associated with more severe dehydration and a higher mortality compared to DKA.

ETIOLOGIES
- DKA is a response to stressful triggers – **infection is the most common cause** (eg, **UTI or pneumonia**), undiagnosed diabetics, MI, CVA, pancreatitis, etc.

PATHOPHYSIOLOGY
- Illness leading to reduced fluid intake (infection most common) leads to **profound dehydration**, increased osmolarity, hyperglycemia, & total body potassium deficit.
- **HHS is not usually associated with severe ketosis or acidosis** because they make enough insulin to prevent ketogenesis.

CLINICAL MANIFESTATIONS
- **Hyperglycemia** increased thirst, polyuria, nocturia, weakness, fatigue, confusion, nausea, vomiting & **mental status changes.**

PHYSICAL EXAMINATION
- Tachycardia, tachypnea, hypotension, decreased skin turgor (dehydration), dry mouth & increased capillary refill time.

DIAGNOSIS
- **Increased osmolarity (>320), increased serum glucose** (**>600** mg/dL), absence of significant acidosis (arterial pH > 7.30 & serum bicarbonate > 15).

MANAGEMENT
- **SIPS – Saline most important component of treatment, Insulin (regular), Potassium repletion,** Search for the underlying cause.

	HHS	Mild DKA	Moderate DKA	Severe DKA
Plasma Glucose (mg/dL)	**>600**	**>250**	>250	>250
Arterial pH	**>7.30**	**<7.30**	7.0-7.24	<7.0
Serum Bicarbonate (mEq/L)	>15	**15-18**	10 to <15	<10
Ketones (Urine/Serum)	Small	**Positive**	Positive	Positive
Serum Osmolarity	**>320**	Variable	Variable	Variable

COMPLICATION OF DIABETES MELLITUS

CARDIOVASCULAR COMPLICATIONS

- Atherosclerosis - **Diabetes mellitus is considered a coronary artery disease equivalent.**
- Peripheral arterial disease
- Stroke - risk 2-4 x greater than the general population
- Congestive heart failure
- Cardiomyopathy
- **Hypertension** blood pressure goals in Diabetes mellitus < 140/90 mmHg. **ACE inhibitors or Angiotensin receptor blockers** if blood pressure 140/90 mmHg or greater or urine is positive for **microalbuminuria.**

Cardiovascular risk reduction:

- Aspirin used regularly in patients > 30 years.
- Statin medication indicated with LDL goal < 100 mg/dL.
- Reduce other cardiac risks.
- Hemoglobin A1C < 7.0%

DIABETIC NEUROPATHY

Many forms of diabetic neuropathy including:

SYMMETRIC POLYNEUROPATHY:

- **Most common type of diabetic neuropathy.**
- Progressive distal **sensory loss in a "stocking-glove" pattern (involving the distal lower extremities at first,** progressing to the hands) - loss of vibratory, proprioception, light touch, & temperature.
- Decreased ankle reflexes, gait abnormalities, and motor dysfunction can occur.
- May lead to **foot ulcer formation.**

AUTONOMIC:

- **Orthostatic (postural) hypotension**
- **Gastroparesis** (occurs after many years)
- Enteropathy (constipation or diarrhea).

CRANIAL MONONEUROPATHY

- Most commonly affecting extraocular muscles – **cranial nerve III** (oculomotor): **diplopia & ptosis with sparing of the pupils** (unlike other CN III palsies), VI (abducens), & IV (trochlear).
- CN VII (facial nerve) palsies.

PERIPHERAL MONONEUROPATHY

- **Median neuropathy most common (Carpal tunnel syndrome)**, ulnar neuropathy.

MANAGEMENT

- Optimal glucose control.
- **Pregabalin & Duloxetine** (SNRI) are FDA-approved. **Amitriptyline** (TCA) or **Gabapentin.**
- Second-line: Venlafaxine (SNRI) and topical agents (eg, Capsaicin cream & Lidocaine patches), alpha-lipoic acid, & transcutaneous electrical nerve stimulation.

SCREENING

- After initial screening, all diabetics should be **screened annually** by examining sensory function in the feet and assessing ankle reflexes.

DIABETIC GASTROPARESIS

- **Decreased GI motility & delayed gastric emptying** due to decreased ability of the gut to sense the stretch of the bowel walls in the absence of a mechanical obstruction.

PATHOPHYSIOLOGY

- Impaired neural control of gastric function (diabetic neuropathy).
- Decreased ability of the intestines to sense the stretch of the bowel walls (normally, stretch is the main stimulant for gastric motility).

CLINICAL MANIFESTATIONS

- **Nausea, vomiting, bloating, early satiety, upper abdominal discomfort**, & constipation in the setting of **longstanding Diabetes mellitus (years).**

PHYSICAL EXAMINATION

- May have epigastric distention or tenderness with a **succussion splash** but no rigidity or guarding.

DIAGNOSIS

- **Upper endoscopy** usually performed initially to rule out other causes of symptoms.
- **Nuclear gastric emptying scintigraphy:** **delayed gastric emptying** in the absence of structural obstruction.

MANAGEMENT

- **Improved glycemic control** & **dietary modification initial management** - small, frequent meals with soluble fiber and low in fat.
- **Prokinetics** **Metoclopramide or Erythromycin** or Domperidone. - they increase GI motility.
- Avoid medications that delay gastric emptying (eg, GLP1 agonist Exenatide & DPP4 inhibitors).

DIABETIC NEPHROPATHY

- **Diabetes mellitus is the most common cause of end stage renal disease.**

PATHOPHYSIOLOGY

- Progressive kidney deterioration leading to **microalbuminuria** (first sign of Diabetic nephropathy).

DIAGNOSIS

- Urine dipstick: positive dipstick for proteinuria = 24 hour urine protein loss between 30 and 300 mg.
- 24-hour urine for albuminuria.
- May have anemia & acidosis.
- Histology: **Kimmelstiel-Wilson lesion** - nodular glomerulosclerosis (**pink hyaline material** around the glomerular capillaries from protein leakage) – **pathognomonic of Diabetic nephropathy.**

MANAGEMENT

- **ACE inhibitors or ARBs** (reduces protein leakage & slows progression via efferent arteriole dilation).
- Low sodium diet. Strict glucose control.

SCREENING

- **Yearly screening for microalbuminuria**, BUN, & creatinine.

SYNDROME OF INAPPROPRIATE ADH (SIADH)

- Non-physiologic excess ADH from the pituitary gland or ectopic source leading to **free water retention & hyponatremia** due to the **kidney's inability to dilute the urine** to excrete the excess water.

ETIOLOGIES

- **CNS: most common – subarachnoid hemorrhage**, stroke, head trauma, meningitis, CNS tumors, post-op, hydrocephalus.
- **Pulmonary: Small cell lung cancer** (ectopic ADH), infection (eg, **Legionella pneumonia**). HIV.
- Medications: **anticonvulsants, Carbamazepine, Hydrochlorothiazide,** NSAIDs, Chlorpropamide, **antidepressants** (TCAs, SSRIs), high-dose **IV Cyclophosphamide, ecstasy** (MDMA), narcotics.
- Other: HIV. Endocrine: hypothyroidism & Conn syndrome.

CLINICAL MANIFESTATIONS

- Neurologic **symptoms of hyponatremia & cerebral edema** – confusion, lethargy, disorientation. Seizures or coma if severe.

DIAGNOSIS

- Dilutional labs:
  - **Normovolemic hypotonic hyponatremia** (usually **no signs of edema**).
  - **Decreased serum osmolarity,** hypouricemia, & decreased BUN.

- **Increased urine osmolarity (concentrated urine),** urine sodium > 20 mEq/L.
- Increased ADH levels.
- Diagnosis made in the absence of renal, adrenal, pituitary, thyroid disease, or diuretic use.

MANAGEMENT

- Treat the underlying cause. Rapid correction > 0.5 mEq/L/hour may lead to central pontine myelinolysis or osmotic demyelination.

- **Mild: water restriction** (eg, < 800ml – 1 liter daily).

- Moderate to severe: ADH receptor antagonists – Conivaptan, Tolvaptan.

- Severe hyponatremia (eg, obtunded, coma, or seizures): **IV hypertonic saline + Furosemide.**

- **Chronic: Demeclocycline** inhibits ADH.

DIABETES INSIPIDUS

- Inability of the kidney to concentrate urine, leading to **production of large amounts of dilute urine.**
- Central = No production of ADH; Nephrogenic = renal insensitivity to ADH.

2 TYPES

- Central: **no production of ADH (most common type).** Idiopathic most common, destruction of the posterior pituitary, head trauma, CNS tumor, infection, sarcoid granuloma.

- Nephrogenic: **partial or complete renal insensitivity to ADH.** Medications – **Lithium,** Amphotericin B, Demeclocycline. **Hypokalemia** or hypercalcemia (disrupts kidney concentrating ability), acute tubular necrosis, hyperparathyroidism.

CLINICAL MANIFESTATIONS

- **Polyuria (up to 20 liters daily) + polydipsia** (excessive thirst to maintain water balance).

- High-volume nocturia.

- **Neurologic symptoms of hypernatremia** (confusion, lethargy, disorientation, seizures or coma) can occur when water intake is less than urinary water loss.

PHYSICAL EXAMINATION

- Dehydration, hypotension, & rapid vascular collapse in severe cases.

DIAGNOSIS

- Labs:
  - **Increased serum osmolarity.**
  - **Decreased urine osmolality & specific gravity, increased urine volume.**
  - Hypernatremia if severe.

- **Fluid deprivation test: establishes the diagnosis of DI.**
  - Normal response = progressive urine concentration.
  - **DI = continued production of large amounts of dilute urine (low urine osmolality).**

- Desmopressin (ADH) stimulation test: distinguishes central from nephrogenic DI.
  - **Central = reduction in urine output + increase in urine osmolality** (response to ADH).
  - **Nephrogenic = continued production of large amounts of dilute urine** (no response to ADH).

MANAGEMENT OF CENTRAL DI:

- **Desmopressin (DDAVP) first-line** - intranasal injection or oral.
- Carbamazepine second line. Chlorpropamide.

MANAGEMENT OF NEPHROGENIC DI:

- Correct the underlying cause. Sodium & protein restriction.
- **Hydrochlorothiazide, Indomethacin, or Amiloride** if symptoms persist.
- Amiloride for Lithium-induced.

CALCIUM DISORDERS

- 99% of calcium is in bone. 1% in extracellular fluid. 50% of ECF Ca^{2+} is ionized (active) form.
- Normal calcium levels = 8.5-10 mg/dL. **Vitamin D required for intestinal Ca^{2+} absorption.**
- Ca^{2+} is important for bone, blood clotting, normal cellular function & neuromuscular transmission.
- Calcium is maintained within a normal range via 3 major hormones:

  Hypocalcemia stimulates **➊ ↑parathyroid hormone & ➋↑calcitriol (Vitamin D)** secretion: **↑'es blood** Ca^{2+} via ↑GI/kidney Ca^{2+} absorption & ↑bone Ca^{2+} resorption (via ↑osteoclast activity). Parathyroid hormone also inhibits phosphate reabsorption so phosphate is usually in the opposite direction of the PTH levels in primary parathyroid disorders.

  Hypercalcemia stimulates **➌ ↑Calcitonin secretion:** **↓'es blood** Ca^{2+} (↓Ca^{2+} GI/kidney absorption & ↑bone mineralization.

HYPERCALCEMIA

ETIOLOGIES

- **90% of cases** due to **Primary hyperparathyroidism or malignancy.**
- **Primary hyperparathyroidism most common cause overall** (parathyroid adenoma, multiple endocrine neoplasia, **Lithium therapy**).
- **Malignancy** due to PTH-related protein production.
- **Thiazide diuretics,** Hyperthyroidism, vitamin D or A intoxication, & granulomas (Sarcoidosis).

CLINICAL MANIFESTATIONS

- Most patients are asymptomatic.
- **Stones –** Nephrolithiasis (calcium oxalate & phosphate), **bones –** bone pain & fractures, **abdominal groans – ileus, constipation. Decreased DTR** & weakness (hypercalcemia decreases muscle contractions), **psychic moans** (eg, depression, anxiety, cognitive dysfunction), and increased vascular tone (hypertension).

DIAGNOSIS

- The first step is to repeat the measurement to verify in asymptomatic patients (and correct calcium for albumin).
- Ionized serum calcium more accurate than total serum calcium.
- **Intact PTH: once hypercalcemia is confirmed** to rule out 1ry hyperparathyroidism.
- **PTH-related protein often ordered if intact PTH is normal or low** (to rule out malignancy).
- 1,25 Vitamin D levels & 24h urinary calcium (calcium excretion usually elevated or high-normal in hyperparathyroidism & malignancy).
- ECG: may show **shortened QT interval**, prolonged PR interval, & QRS widening.

MANAGEMENT OF MILD (< 12 mg/dL):

- No immediate treatment needed. Treat underlying cause & increase water intake (promotes calcium excretion).

MANAGEMENT OF MODERATE (12-14 mg/dL):

- **IV fluids initial management of choice** if associated with significant symptoms (promotes excretion).
- IV loop diuretics (eg, **Furosemide**) can be added to promote calcium excretion.
- Calcitonin may be helpful adjunct in malignancy (faster onset of action compared to Bisphosphonates.
- **Bisphosphonates** (eg, Zoledronic acid or Pamidronate) may be given with Calcitonin in malignancy.
- Denosumab may be adjunct in malignancy-related hypercalcemia.
- Glucocorticoids in granulomatous disease.

HYPOCALCEMIA

ETIOLOGIES

- **Hypoparathyroidism most common cause overall** - autoimmune **destruction or removal of the parathyroid gland during neck surgery**.

- **Chronic renal disease** or liver disease (if PTH is increased – secondary hyperparathyroidism – increased PTH response to hypocalcemia).

- Vitamin D deficiency (Osteomalacia & Rickets).

- **Hypomagnesemia**, hyperphosphatemia, hypoalbuminemia.

- Medications: **diuretics**, calcium chelators (eg, high-citrate during blood transfusion), Bisphosphonates, Denosumab.

CLINICAL MANIFESTATIONS

- Most are asymptomatic.
- **Increased muscular contractions:** because hypocalcemia decreases excitation threshold, increased muscle & nerve excitability occurs – **muscle cramps, bronchospasm, finger or circumoral paresthesias, tetany - Chvostek sign** (facial spasm with tapping of the facial nerve), **Trousseau's sign** (inflation of BP cuff above systolic causes carpal spasm). **Increased DTR** & seizures.

- Cardiovascular: CHF, arrhythmias.
- Skin: dry skin, Psoriasis.
- GI: diarrhea, abdominal pain, or cramps.
- Skeletal: abnormal dentition, osteomalacia, osteodystrophy.

DIAGNOSIS

- Decreased free ionized calcium more accurate than total serum calcium. Order intact PTH, magnesium, phosphate, BUN, creatinine, & vitamin D metabolites.

- Albumin levels may be needed to correct calcium for hypoalbuminemia:
  Corrected Ca = [0.8 x (normal albumin 4.4 – patients albumin)] + serum Ca.

- ECG: **prolonged QT interval classic.**

MANAGEMENT

- Mild: **oral Calcium + Vitamin D.** K+ & Mg+ repletion may be needed.

- **Severe or symptomatic: IV calcium gluconate** or IV calcium carbonate.

PRIMARY HYPERPARATHYROIDISM

- Excess parathyroid hormone (PTH).

ETIOLOGIES
- **Parathyroid adenoma most common cause** (80-85%), parathyroid hyperplasia or enlargement.
- **Lithium**
- MEN I and IIa. Malignancy is rare.

MEN 1	Hyperparathyroidism	Pituitary Tumors	Pancreatic Tumors
Men 2A	Hyperparathyroidism	Pheochromocytoma	Medullary Thyroid Carcinoma

CLINICAL MANIFESTATIONS
- **Most are asymptomatic**.
- **Signs of hypercalcemia:** "stones, bones, abdominal groans, psychic moans." – nephrolithiasis, painful bones, fractures, ileus, constipation, nausea, vomiting, weakness, **decreased deep tendon reflexes.**

DIAGNOSIS
- **Triad: hypercalcemia + increased intact PTH + decreased phosphate.**
- **Increased 24-hour urine calcium excretion**, increased vitamin D.
- Ancillary: may have osteopenia on bone scan. Imaging studies to detect parathyroid adenoma (ultrasound or nuclear scanning).

MANAGEMENT
- **Parathyroidectomy definitive management.**
- Vitamin D & Calcium supplementation post parathyroidectomy to prevent hypocalcemia.
- Cinacalcet inhibits the release of PTH in patients that are not surgical candidates.
- May be observed in mild cases.
- Management of severe hypercalcemia: IV fluids. May need Furosemide added if severe.

HYPOPARATHYROIDISM

ETIOLOGIES
- **The 2 most common causes are post neck surgery (eg, thyroidectomy, parathyroidectomy) or autoimmune** destruction of the parathyroid gland.
- Radiation therapy
- **Hypomagnesemia**, congenital Pseudohypoparathyroidism, DiGeorge syndrome (parathyroid hypoplasia).

CLINICAL MANIFESTATIONS
- **Signs of hypocalcemia: increased muscle contraction** - carpopedal spasm, perioral numbness, tetany, Trousseau sign (carpopedal spasms when the blood pressure cuff is inflated), Chvostek sign (tapping of the cheek causes facial spasm), mental irritability, increased deep tendon reflexes.

DIAGNOSIS
- **Triad of hypocalcemia + decreased intact PTH + increased phosphate.**
- ECG: prolonged QT interval (increased risk of arrhythmias).

MANAGEMENT
- **Calcium supplementation + activated Vitamin D** (eg, **Calcitriol**).
- Acute symptomatic hypocalcemia: **IV Calcium gluconate.**

	HYPOcalcemia	HYPERcalcemia
ETIOLOGIES	• **HYPOCALCEMIA with ↓PTH:** ***Hypoparathyroidism MC overall cause*** of ↓Ca^{+2}* - **Hypoparathyroidism:** parathyroid gland destruction ***(autoimmune, post surgical)**** • **HYPOCALCEMIA with ↑PTH:** -***Chronic renal dz MC cause if ↑PTH,* Liver dz.*** -***Vitamin D deficiency*** (Osteomalacia & Rickets). ↑*PTH* in response to hypocalcemia - ***Hypomagnesemia,*** ↑phosphate. *Hypoalbuminemia* -High citrate states: ex. blood transfusion -Acute pancreatitis, rhabdomyolysis. Meds: PPIs	• ***90% of cases of hypercalcemia are due to:*** ***PRIMARY HYPERPARATHYROIDISM OR MALIGNANCY!**** • **PTH-mediated:** - ***Primary hyperparathyroidism:* MC cause overall*** ***Triad: ❶ ↑Ca +❷ ↑intact PTH + ❸ ↓phosphate**** - *MEN I & IIa*, 3ʳʸ hyperparathyroidism • **PTH-independent:** - ***Malignancy (secretes ↑PTH-related protein), ↓intact PTH*** - Vitamin D excess (granulomatous dz, vitamin intoxication) - Vitamin A excess, milk alkali syndrome, ***thiazides*, lithium****
CLINICAL MANIFESTATIONS	Hypocalcemia ↓'es excitation threshold for heart, nerves & muscle ⇨ ***less stimulus needed for activation/contraction.*** • ***Neuromuscular:*** muscle cramping, bronchospasm, syncope, seizures, ***finger/circumoral paresthesias*** • **Tetany:** ***Chvostek's sign:*** facial spasm with tapping of the facial nerve. ***Trousseau's sign:*** inflation of BP cuff above systolic BP causes carpal spasms. ↑***DTR*** • **Cardio:** CHF, arrhythmias. Skin: dry skin, psoriasis • **GI:** ***diarrhea, abdominal pain/cramps.*** • ***Skeletal:*** abn. dentition, osteomalacia, osteodystrophy	Hypercalcemia ↑'es excitation threshold for heart, nerves & muscle ⇨ ***stronger stimulus needed for activation/contraction.*** • ***Most patients are asymptomatic.*** ±Arrhythmias • **Stones:** ***kidney stones*** (hypercalciuria ⇨ calcium oxalate & phosphate stones), ***Nephrogenic DI: polyuria***, nocturia. • **Bones:** ***painful bones, fractures*** (due to ↑bone remodeling). • **Abdominal groans:** ***ileus, constipation,**** (decreased contraction of the muscles of the GI tract), nausea, vomiting. • **Psychic moans:** weakness, fatigue, AMS, ↓***DTR***, depression or psychosis may develop. Blurred vision.
LAB FINDINGS	• ↓***ionized Ca^{2+}*** & total serum Ca^{2+} (<8.5mg/dL) • ±↑Phosphate, ↓Magnesium. Check PTH, BUN/Cr	• ↑***ionized Ca^{2+}*** (most accurate), ↑Total serum Ca^{2+} (>10mg/dL) • PTH-related protein, 1,25 vitamin D levels, 24h urinary calcium
ECG FINDINGS	• ***PROLONGED QT INTERVAL****	• ***SHORTENED QT INTERVAL,**** *prolonged PR interval, QRS widening.*
MANAGEMENT	**Severe/symptomatic:** • ***Calcium gluconate IV**** or IV calcium carbonate - Ca^{2+} carbonate must be given via central line **Mild:** • ***PO Calcium + Vitamin D (Ergocalciferol, Calcitriol)*** Calcitriol if renal disease b/c no renal conversion needed • *K^{+} & Mg^{+2} repletion may be needed in some cases.* • Corrected Ca^{2+} in patients with low serum albumin: *[0.8 x (nml albumin(4.4) - pts albumin)] + serum Ca^{2+}*	**Severe/symptomatic:** • ***IV saline* ⇨ Furosemide*** (Lasix) ***1st line.*** Loop diuretics enhance renal Ca^{2+} excretion. ***Avoid Hydrochlorothiazide* (causes ↑Ca)*** • ***Calcitonin, Bisphosphonates in severe cases (IV Pamidronate)*** • Steroids: Vitamin D excess, malignancy (ex. myeloma), granulomas. **Mild:** • No treatment needed for mild hypocalcemia. Tx underlying cause.

ANTERIOR PITUITARY TUMORS

PROLACTINOMA

- Benign tumor (adenoma) of the lactotroph cell.
- **Most common type of pituitary adenoma.**

PROLACTIN FUNCTIONS

- Prolactin responsible for lactation, suppression of pregnancy during lactation, & suppression of gonadotropin-releasing hormone, leading to decreased FSH & LH.

- **Dopamine inhibits prolactin release.**

MANIFESTATIONS IN WOMEN

- **Due to hypogonadism** (oligomenorrhea, **amenorrhea**, infertility).
- **Galactorrhea (rare)**.
- Local compression - headache & visual changes.

MANIFESTATIONS IN MEN

- **Hypogonadism** - erectile dysfunction, **decreased libido**, **infertility**, & rarely gynecomastia.
- Local compression can cause **headache** or visual changes.

PHYSICAL EXAMINATION

- Pituitary tumors can compress the optic chiasm, leading to **bitemporal hemianopsia.**

DIAGNOSIS

- Endocrine studies: **increased prolactin, decreased FSH, and LH.**

- **TSH**, growth hormone, & ACTH levels ordered because Prolactinomas can cause hypersecretion or hyposecretion of other hormones.

- **MRI study of choice to look for sellar lesions & pituitary tumors** (small adenomas may not be visible).

MANAGEMENT

- **Dopamine agonists (eg, Cabergoline or Bromocriptine) first-line treatment** for both symptomatic macro and microadenomas (Cabergoline is better tolerated).

- Watchful waiting may be employed if asymptomatic.

- Transsphenoidal surgery usually reserved for Prolactinomas refractory to medical management or large adenomas (>3 cm) in women who wish to become pregnant.

- Radiation therapy rarely used.

SOMATOTROPH ADENOMA

- **Growth hormone-secreting pituitary adenoma** that leads to **acromegaly** in adults or **gigantism** in children (if it occurs before epiphyseal closure).

PATHOPHYSIOLOGY
- Growth hormone (GH) is a counterregulatory hormone that increases glucose.
- Increased growth hormone stimulates increased hepatic production of insulin-like growth factor.

CLINICAL MANIFESTATIONS
- **Diabetes mellitus or glucose intolerance.**
- **Enlargement of soft tissues, cartilage and bone** - hands, feet, skull, tongue, forehead, & jaw aka macrognathia (**increased ring, shoe, & hat size**), carpal tunnel syndrome, obstructive sleep apnea, increased spaced between teeth, coarse facial features.
- **Headache common**, visual symptoms (eg, **bitemporal hemianopsia)**, deepened voice, thickened moist skin (doughy). Skin tags, weight gain, arthralgias.
- **Hypertension**, kidney stones, and **colonic polyps.**

DIAGNOSIS
- Screening: **insulin-like growth factor initial test of choice.**
- Confirmatory: **oral glucose suppression test - increased growth hormone levels seen in acromegaly** (normal response is GH suppression).
- **MRI imaging test of choice** to evaluate for sellar or pituitary lesions (after laboratory confirmation).

MANAGEMENT
- **Transsphenoidal surgery management of choice** for removal of active or compressive tumors.

Medical:
- Indications: either an adjunct to surgery or when surgery is not possible.
- **Octreotide or Lanreotide first-line medical management** (somatostatin inhibits GH release).
- Cabergoline or Bromocriptine – dopamine agonists (dopamine inhibits GH release).
- Pegvisomant - GH receptor antagonist that inhibits insulin like growth factor release.

Radiation therapy:
- Reserved for cases not responsive to surgical or medical management.

CORTICOTROPH ADENOMA

- **ACTH-secreting pituitary adenoma** that leads to **hypercortisolism (Cushing's syndrome).**
- Also known as **Cushing's disease.**

CLINICAL MANIFESTATIONS
- Proximal muscle weakness, **weight gain,** headache, oligomenorrhea, erectile dysfunction, polyuria, osteoporosis, & mental disturbances (from mild to psychosis).

DIFFERENTIATING TESTS
- The presence of an **increased baseline ACTH + suppression of cortisol on high-dose Dexamethasone suppression distinguishes Cushing's disease** from other causes of Cushing's syndrome (Hypercortisolism).
- **MRI of the pituitary imaging test of choice.**
- Sampling of the petrosal sinus if MRI is negative (MRI may miss small tumors).

MANAGEMENT: **Transsphenoidal resection is the treatment of choice**

ANTERIOR HYPOPITUITARISM

- Pituitary destruction or deficient hypothalamic pituitary stimulation. Congenital or acquired - tumor, infiltrative disease, bleeding into pituitary (eg, Sheehan's syndrome), pituitary infarction, radiation therapy.

CLINICAL MANIFESTATIONS
- Can be any combination of growth hormone deficiency (dwarfism, metabolic derangements in adults), hypothyroidism, & gonadotropin deficiency.

DIAGNOSIS
- **Both target hormones and pituitary hormones are decreased - same direction = secondary (pituitary) problem or tertiary (hypothalamus) problem.**
  - TSH and Free T4 are both decreased if secondary hypothyroidism
  - ACTH and cortisol are both decreased if secondary hypocortisolism

MANAGEMENT
- Hormone replacement therapy.

GROWTH HORMONE DEFICIENCY

- Deficiency in pituitary production of growth hormone (GH).

ETIOLOGIES
- Congenital or acquired (eg, tumor, infiltrative disease, bleeding into pituitary - Sheehan's syndrome), pituitary infarction, or radiation therapy.

CHILDREN OR INFANCY:
- **Short stature,** growth delays, **dwarfism, fasting hypoglycemia**.

ADULTS
- Mild-moderate central obesity, increased blood pressure, **dyslipidemia**, decreased bone mass in men, decreased cardiac output, muscle wasting, increased inflammatory markers and impaired concentration.

DIAGNOSIS
- Arginine and sleep stimulation test – no change in GH release if hypopituitarism.
- Measurements of basal GH levels do **not** distinguish between normal and subnormal GH secretion.

HYPERPROLACTINEMIA

ETIOLOGIES
- Pathologic: **Prolactinoma most common cause, hypothyroidism (increased TRH stimulates prolactin)**, acromegaly, cirrhosis, & renal failure.
- Pharmacologic: **dopamine antagonists - 1st and 2nd-generation antipsychotics**, such as **Risperidone, Haloperidol**, Metoclopramide, Promethazine, & Prochlorperazine because dopamine is an inhibitor of prolactin. SSRIs, TCAs, Cimetidine, Verapamil, & estrogen.
- Physiologic: pregnancy, stress, & exercise.

PATHOPHYSIOLOGY: prolactin inhibits gonadotropin-releasing hormone, leading to hypogonadism.

MANIFESTATIONS IN WOMEN
- **Hypogonadism** - oligomenorrhea, **amenorrhea**, infertility, vaginal dryness. **Galactorrhea** (rare).

MANIFESTATIONS IN MEN
- **Hypogonadism** - erectile dysfunction, decreased libido, **infertility,** & rarely gynecomastia.

WORKUP: **serum prolactin, TSH,** beta-hCG, BUN, creatinine, & LFTs.

MANAGEMENT
- Depends on cause.
- Medication-induced: discontinue offending drugs.
- **Dopamine agonists** (eg, **Cabergoline & Bromocriptine**) inhibit prolactin.
- Surgical or radiation therapy may be needed in some cases of refractory Prolactinomas.

HYPOGONADISM

- Decrease in either or both of the primary function of the testes (testosterone and sperm production).

ETIOLOGIES
- Primary: hypergonadotropic – decrease function of Leydig cells (decreased testosterone synthesis), seminiferous tubule dysfunction, alcoholic liver disease.
- Secondary: hypogonadotropic - disorder of the pituitary gland or the hypothalamus (eg, pituitary adenoma, craniopharyngioma). Affects both spermatogenesis and Leydig function.

CLINICAL MANIFESTATIONS
- Adolescents: failure to undergo or complete puberty (decreased secondary male characteristics).
- Adults: decreased libido, energy, body hair, & muscle mass; osteoporosis, gynecomastia, infertility.

DIAGNOSIS
- **Morning serum total testosterone:** decreased. If subnormal, testosterone levels should be repeated along with FSH and LH to distinguish primary from secondary:
  - Primary: decreased testosterone + normal FSH (if limited to Leydig cells) or high FSH (seminiferous tubule dysfunction).
  - Secondary: decreased testosterone + decreased FSH and LH (same direction) or normal FSH.
- Sex hormone-binding globulin. Semen analysis if hypogonadism is part of a fertility workup.

MANAGEMENT
- Testosterone replacement therapy if testosterone deficiency seen on 3 separate occasions (eg, gel).
- Infertility: in vitro fertilization with sperm extracted from the testes if Primary. Gonadotropin therapy or pulsatile gonadotropin releasing hormone therapy (if pituitary function is normal).

METABOLIC SYNDROME (SYNDROME X, INSULIN RESISTANCE SYNDROME)

- Syndrome of multiple metabolic abnormalities that increase the risk for complications such as diabetes mellitus & cardiovascular disease.

- Also known as syndrome X or Insulin resistance syndrome.

PATHOPHYSIOLOGY

- **Insulin resistance is the key component.**

- Free fatty acids are released, which causes an increase in triglyceride & glucose production as well as reduction in insulin sensitivity, leading to insulin resistance & hyperinsulinemia.

- The high levels of insulin cause sodium reabsorption, leading to hypertension.

DIAGNOSIS

ATP III criteria: at least 3 of the following 5:

1. ↓HDL: <40 mg/dL in men & < 50 mg/dL in women.
2. ↑Blood pressure: ≥135 systolic or ≥85 mmHg diastolic (or drug treatment for Hypertension).
3. ↑Fasting triglyceride levels: ≥150 mg/dL (or drug treatment for high triglycerides).
4. ↑Fasting blood sugar: ≥ 100 mg/dL (or drug treatment for high glucose).
5. ↑Abdominal obesity: waist circumference >40 inches in men & >35 inches in women.

MANAGEMENT

- Lifestyle: weight reduction, exercise and increased physical activity, diet (rich in fruits, vegetables, lean poultry, fish, whole grains). Weight loss.

WEIGHT LOSS MEDICATIONS:

- **Phentermine** (3 months short-term use only). Sympathomimetic with unknown mechanism of action.

- **Phentermine/Topiramate** (no restriction on treatment duration).
  Adverse effects: insomnia, constipation, palpitations, headache, paresthesias.

- **Lorcaserin:** selective serotonin agonist (5-HT2C receptor) that induces satiety.

- **Orlistat:** inhibits fat absorption.

- Bariatric surgery may be used in some patients.

MULTIPLE ENDOCRINE NEOPLASIA I

- Rare inherited disorder of 1 or more overactive endocrine gland tumors – **3 Ps (Parathyroid, Pancreas, & Pituitary).**
- Also known as Wermer's syndrome. Associated with Menin gene defect.
- Most tumors are benign (especially before 30 years).

CLINICAL MANIFESTATIONS

3 Ps:

- **Parathyroid: Hyperparathyroidism most common** (parathyroid adenoma)
- **Pancreatic tumors** (2nd most common) – **Gastrinomas (ZES)**, Insulinomas, Glucagonomas, VIPomas, Somatostatinomas.
- **Prolactinomas.**
- Other tumors include carcinoid tumors, nonfunctioning polypeptide malignant tumors, lipomas.

DIAGNOSIS

- Genetic testing and studies for suspected tumors.

MANAGEMENT

- Tumor specific.

Screening in patients with MEN I:

- **PTH + calcium, gastrin, & prolactin.**

MULTIPLE ENDOCRINE NEOPLASIA II

- Rare inherited disorder of 1 or more overactive endocrine gland tumors due to RET proto-oncogene.

MEN 2A (90%)	**medullary thyroid carcinoma**	**Pheochromocytoma**	**Hyperparathyroidism**
MEN 2B (5%)	**medullary thyroid carcinoma**	**Pheochromocytoma**	**Neuromas, Marfanoid**
Familial MTC:	**medullary thyroid carcinoma**		

MEN IIb:

- **Medullary thyroid carcinoma, Pheochromocytoma, Neuromas, & Marfanoid habitus.**
- Men IIb associated with more aggressive form of medullary thyroid carcinoma (may present in infancy).
- Mucosal neuromas of the lips, tongue, eyelids, conjunctiva, nasal & laryngeal mucosa.
- Marfanoid habitus, including high arched palate, pectus excavatum, & scoliosis.

DIAGNOSIS

- Genetic testing for RET proto-oncogene.
- Imaging depends on tumor presentation.

SCREENING IN PATIENTS WITH MEN II:

- **Calcitonin, epinephrine, PTH, & calcium.**

CHAPTER 8 - RENAL SYSTEM

DIURETICS

MANNITOL

MECHANISM OF ACTION

- **Osmotic diuretic** – increases urine volume by **drawing fluid from intracellular compartment & increasing tubular osmolarity** (Mannitol is freely filtered but minimally reabsorbed).
- **The proximal tubule is the main site of action.**
- Given IV (poor oral absorption).

4 MAIN INDICATIONS

- **Treatment of increased intracranial pressure**
- **Treatment of refractory increased intraocular pressure**
- Promotes diuresis in the oliguric phase of acute kidney injury
- Increases excretion of toxic metabolites. Mannitol increases urine output within 5-10 minutes of administration.

ADVERSE EFFECTS

- **Pulmonary edema** (due to increased fluid shifts), hypotension, tachycardia, hypernatremia, & hypokalemia.
- Monitor input, urine output, blood pressure, pulse, & electrolytes during administration.

CONTRAINDICATIONS

- Anuria, dehydration, progressive heart failure, & significant electrolyte abnormalities.

ACETAZOLAMIDE

MECHANISM OF ACTION

- **Carbonic anhydrase inhibitor** in the **proximal tubule, leading to sodium & bicarbonate diuresis.**

INDICATIONS

- **Reduces intraocular pressure in Glaucoma**
- **Reduces intracranial pressure**
- Acidifies the blood in patients with metabolic alkalosis, **Alkalinizes the urine**
- Mild diuretic, Altitude sickness.

ADVERSE EFFECTS

- **Hyperchloremic metabolic acidosis** (due to increased loss of bicarbonate),
- Hypokalemia
- **Sulfa allergies**
- **Kidney stones** (calcium phosphate)
- Numbness, tinnitus & vomiting.

CONTRAINDICATIONS

- Severe kidney or hepatic dysfunction.

LOOP DIURETICS

Furosemide, Bumetanide, Torsemide.

MECHANISM OF ACTION

- **Strongest class of diuretics: inhibits water, Na+, K+, Cl-** transport as well as Ca+ and Mg+ absorption across the **thick ascending limb of the Loop of Henle,** leading to a dilute urine.
- Increased prostaglandin synthesis, improving renal blood flow.

INDICATIONS

- **Hypertension, edema** (eg, pulmonary or peripheral edema due to CHF, Nephrotic syndrome, & Cirrhosis), hypercalcemia, & hypermagnesemia.

ADVERSE EFFECTS

- **Decreased electrolytes (hypokalemia, hypocalcemia, hypomagnesemia,** hypochloremia, & hyponatremia), dyslipidemia, **ototoxicity** (especially with high-doses, rapid IV administration or renal insufficiency), **sulfa allergy,** acute interstitial nephritis, **hypochloremic metabolic alkalosis, hyperuricemia** (can precipitate Gout), **and hyperglycemia.**
- NSAIDs may decrease their efficacy.
- **Ethacrynic acid is a medication similar to Furosemide that can be used if sulfa allergy** (does not contain sulfonamide) **& safe in patients with Gout. Associated with higher risk of ototoxicity** compared to Furosemide.

THIAZIDE DIURETICS

Hydrochlorothiazide, Chlorthalidone, Chlorothiazide
Thiazide-like: Indapamide, Metolazone

MECHANISM OF ACTION

- Blocks NaCl & water reabsorption at the **early distal convoluted tubule (diluting segment).** This leads to diuresis and inability to produce a dilute urine.
- **Thiazides also decrease urinary calcium excretion.**

INDICATIONS

- **Hypertension** (eg, no comorbidities, African-Americans, osteoporosis & elderly), peripheral edema, & **Nephrogenic diabetes insipidus** (decreases ability to produce dilute urine).

ADVERSE EFFECTS

- Most common - hypokalemia, hypomagnesemia, hypochloremia. Increased **GLUC**ose **(increased Glucose, Lipids, Uric acid, Calcium).**
- **Hypercalcemia,** Thiazides are the diuretics most likely to cause **hyponatremia**.
- Sulfa allergies & metabolic alkalosis.

POTASSIUM-SPARING DIURETICS

Spironolactone, Eplerenone

MECHANISM OF ACTION

- **Aldosterone receptor antagonist** in the distal cortical collecting tubule (increasing sodium and water excretion while conserving potassium & hydrogen ions).

INDICATIONS

- Primary hyperaldosteronism, heart failure (decreases mortality), cirrhosis-related ascites, weak diuretic (used primarily in combination with loop or thiazide diuretic to minimize potassium loss), & antiandrogenic (female hirsutism).

ADVERSE EFFECTS

- **Hyperkalemia,** normal anion gap metabolic acidosis.
- **Anti-androgen effects: gynecomastia,** erectile dysfunction, & decreased libido.
- Eplerenone associated with lower incidence of anti-androgenic effects.

Amiloride, Triamterene

MECHANISM OF ACTION

- Directly decrease sodium channel activity in the cortical collecting duct but do not affect the aldosterone receptor.

INDICATIONS

- hypertension, CHF, lithium-induced polyuria.
- Not associated with anti-androgenic effects.

ADVERSE EFFECTS

- **Hyperkalemia,** non-anion gap metabolic acidosis.
- Triamterene associated with urine crystal formation.

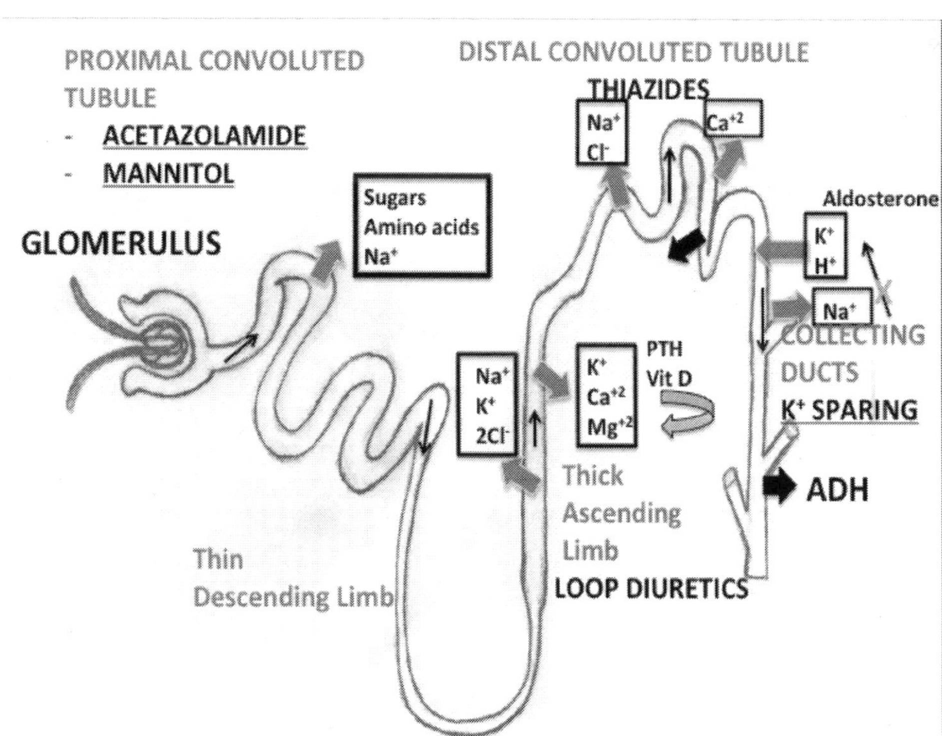

DIURETIC	MECHANISM OF ACTION	INDICATIONS	SIDE EFFECTS & CONTRAINDICATIONS
PROXIMAL TUBE DIURETIC			
MANNITOL	***Osmotic diuretic:*** ↑'es urine volume by ↑'ing tubular fluid osmolarity (since mannitol is filtered but not easily reabsorbed).	• ***Intracranial HTN*** (↓'es intracranial CSF pressure) • Oliguria (trauma, shock) • Glaucoma, Acute kidney injury	**S/E:** ***PULMONARY EDEMA**** (due to ↑fluid shift) **CI:** anuria
ACETAZOLAMIDE	*CARBONIC ANHYDRASE INHIBITOR* in the ***proximal tubule*** ⇨ ***$NaHCO_3$*** diuresis. ***Mild diuretic, acidifies the blood*** in patients with metabolic alkalosis	• ***Glaucoma*** (↓'es intraocular pressure), • ***Intracranial HTN*** (↓'es intracranial CSF pressure) • Urinary alkalinization • Metabolic alkalosis	• ***Hyperchloremic metabolic acidosis*** (due to loss of bicarbonate). • Hypokalemia, ***sulfa allergies*** • ***Kidney stones*** (calcium & phosphate)
LOOP DIURETICS			
FUROSEMIDE (Lasix) **BUMETANIDE** (Bumex) TORSEMIDE	Inhibits water, ***Na^+-K^+-Cl^-*** transport across thick ascending ***LOOP OF HENLE*** ⇨ dilute urine ***(strongest class of diuretics)**** ***↑PG synthesis*** ⇨ ***↑renal blood flow***	• ***HTN*** • ***Edema:*** pulmonary edema, CHF, nephrotic syndrome, cirrhosis. • ***Hypercalcemia***	• ***Hypokalemia/hypocalcemia/↓ Mg*** • ***Hyperglycemia & Hyperuricemia (caution in DM, gout).**** • ***Ototoxicity, Sulfa allergy*** • Acute Interstitial Nephritis (all sulfa drugs) • Hypochloremic metabolic alkalosis • NSAIDs decrease its efficacy
ETHACRYNIC ACID	***Similar action to furosemide*** *(but does not contain sulfonamide)*	• ***Diuresis in pts c sulfa allergy*** • ***Can be used in pts with gout***	• *More ototoxicity compared to Lasix*
THIAZIDE DIURETICS			
HYDROCHLOROTHIAZIDE Chlorthalidone Indapamide Metolazone Chlorothiazide	***Blocks NaCl & water reabsorption*** at the early ***distal diluting tubule.*** ⇨ ***diuresis & inability to produce dilute urine**** *Lowers urinary Ca^{+2} excretion.*	• ***HTN*** (if no comorbidities, elderly, African Americans). • Nephrolithiasis • ***Nephrogenic DI*** ***HCTZ ↓'es ability to dilute urine****	• ***HypOnatremia,* HYPERCALCEMIA,* hypokalemia,*** hyperlipidemia. • ***Hyperuricemia & hyperglycemia***, therefore ***caution in pts c DM, gout.*** • ***Sulfa allergies,*** Metabolic alkalosis. Sexual dysfunction
POTASSIUM SPARING			
SPIRONOLACTONE **EPLERENONE**	***Inhibits aldosterone-mediated Na/H_2O absorption in cortical collecting tubule*** while facilitating the reabsorption of K^+ (potassium-sparing). Weak diuretic	• ***CHF (reduces mortality)*** • Most useful in combo with loop to minimize K loss. • ***Hyperaldosteronism***	• ***Hyperkalemia,* metabolic acidosis*** (K^+ & H^+ not exchanged for Na^+). • ***Spironolactone causes gynecomastia* (anti-androgen effects)***
TRIAMTERENE **AMILORIDE**	***Blocks Na^+ within cortical collecting tubule***	• Lithium-induced nephrogenic DI	• ***Hyperkalemia,* metabolic acidosis**

NEPHROTIC SYNDROME

- Kidney disease characterized by **proteinuria, hypoalbuminemia, hyperlipidemia, & edema.**

PRIMARY ETIOLOGIES

- **Minimal change disease: most common cause in children.** May occur in the setting of viral syndrome, allergies, or Hodgkin disease. Loss of negative charge of basement membrane promotes proteinuria.

- Membranous nephropathy: **most common 1ry cause in Caucasian males > 40y.** May be seen with SLE, viral hepatitis, malaria, medications (eg, Penicillamine), hypocomplementemia.

- Focal segmental glomerulosclerosis: in the setting of HTN, Heroin, HIV. **African-Americans**.

SECONDARY ETIOLOGIES

- **Diabetes mellitus most common secondary cause in adults**, Systemic lupus erythematosus, Amyloidosis, Hepatitis, Sjögren syndrome, Sarcoidosis, medications, infections, & malignancy.

CLINICAL MANIFESTATIONS

- **Generalized edema (especially periorbital in children) usually worse in the morning.**
- May develop **frothy urine.** Ascites & anasarca if severe.
- Anemia, **DVT** (loss of protein C, S, & antithrombin III + liver production of more clotting proteins).

DIAGNOSIS

- **UA: initial test** - proteinuria causing "foamy urine", lipiduria.
  - Microscopy: **oval Maltese cross-shaped fat bodies (fatty casts)**.

- Protein measurements:
  - Urine **albumin: creatinine ratio. 24-hour urine protein > 3.5g/day gold standard**.

- Hypoalbuminemia, hyperlipidemia.

- Renal biopsy: definitive diagnosis/most accurate test (not usually needed).
  - Minimal change disease: no visible cellular changes seen on simple light microscopy but **podocyte damage seen on electron microscope** (loss, fusion of the foot processes). Not usually needed.

  - Membranous nephropathy: **thick basement membrane**.

MANAGEMENT

- **Glucocorticoids: first-line for Minimal change disease.** FSGS (steroid responsiveness important determinant of prognosis). Other immunomodulators (eg, Cyclophosphamide, Cyclosporine, Tacrolimus).

- Edema reduction: diuretics (eg, Thiazides or loop diuretics); 1 liter fluid & sodium restriction.

- **Proteinuria reduction: ACE inhibitors or Angiotensin receptor blockers** (efferent arteriolar dilation, reduces renal blood flow, GFR, and protein loss).

- Hyperlipidemia: diet modifications & statin therapy.

ACUTE GLOMERULONEPHRITIS (AGN)

- Immunologic inflammation of the glomeruli, leading to protein & RBC leakage into the urine.
- Characterized by **hypertension, hematuria (RBC casts), azotemia**, & **proteinuria (edema).**

ETIOLOGIES

- **IgA NEPHROPATHY (BERGER'S DISEASE): most common cause of acute Glomerulonephritis. Often affects young males within days** (24-48 hours) **after URI or GI infection** (due to IgA immune complexes). IgA is the first-line of defense in respiratory & GI secretions, so infections may cause IgA overproduction.
- **POST-INFECTIOUS: most common after group A *Streptococcus*** 10-14 days after **skin** (eg, **Impetigo**) or pharyngeal infection (may occur after any infection). Classically: **2-14y boy with facial edema** up to 3 weeks **after Strep with scanty, cola-colored/dark urine** (hematuria & *oliguria).* ↑anti-streptolysin (ASO) titers, Low serum complement (C3).
- **MEMBRANOPROLIFERATIVE/MESANGIOCAPILLARY:** due to SLE, viral hepatitis (eg, **HCV,** HBV), hypocomplementemia, cryoglobulinemia.
  Membranoproliferative usually present with a **mixed nephritic-nephrotic picture**.
- **RAPIDLY PROGRESSIVE GLOMERULONEPHRITIS (RPGN): associated with poor prognosis (rapid progression** to end stage renal disease – weeks/months). **Crescent formation on biopsy** (crescents formed due to fibrin & plasma protein deposition collapsing the crescent shape of Bowman's capsule)**.**

Any cause of AGN can present with RPGN. The following 2 ONLY PRESENT with RPGN:

- **GOODPASTURE'S DISEASE: ⊕ anti-GBM antibodies.** antibodies against type IV collagen of the glomerular basement membrane (GBM) in kidney & lung alveoli.
  - Presents with **Acute glomerulonephritis + hemoptysis.**
- **VASCULITIS:** characterized by lack of immune deposits & ⊕ ANCA antibodies.
  - Microscopic Polyangiitis (vasculitis of small renal vessels): ⊕ P-ANCA.
  - Granulomatosis with Polyangiitis (Wegener's): necrotizing vasculitis ⇨ ⊕ C-ANCA.

CLINICAL MANIFESTATIONS

- **Hematuria hallmark (cola or tea-colored urine)**
- **Edema** (peripheral & periorbital)
- Fever, abdominal or flank pain, malaise, oliguria (acute kidney injury).

Physical examination:

- **Hypertension common,** periorbital & facial edema, peripheral edema.

DIAGNOSIS

- UA: **hematuria, RBC casts,** dysmorphic RBCs (acanthocytes), **proteinuria** (usually < 3g but can be in the nephrotic range), high specific gravity (> 1.020 osm).
- **Increased BUN & creatinine.**
- Renal biopsy gold standard (not needed in most cases).
  - Ig A nephropathy: **IgA mesangial deposits** on immunostaining.
  - Poststreptococcal: hypercellularity, ↑monocytes/lymphocytes, **immune humps** of IgG, IgM, & C3.
  - Goodpasture syndrome: linear IgG deposits in the glomerular basement membrane.

MANAGEMENT

Usually self-limited with a good prognosis (except for rapidly progressive forms).

- **IgA nephropathy or proteinuria: ACE inhibitors,** ± Corticosteroids.
- Edema, hypervolemia or hypertension: Loop diuretics (edema); HTN (beta-blockers, CCBs).
- Post streptococcal AGN: Supportive, ± Abx. Lupus nephritis: Steroids or Cyclophosphamide.
- Rapidly progressive AGN or severe disease: Corticosteroids plus Cyclophosphamide.

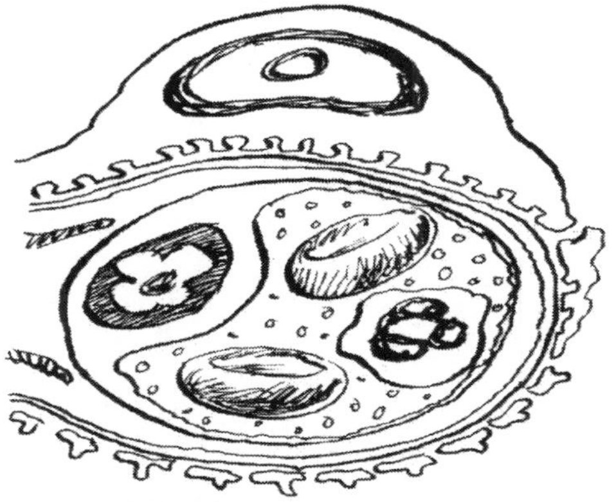	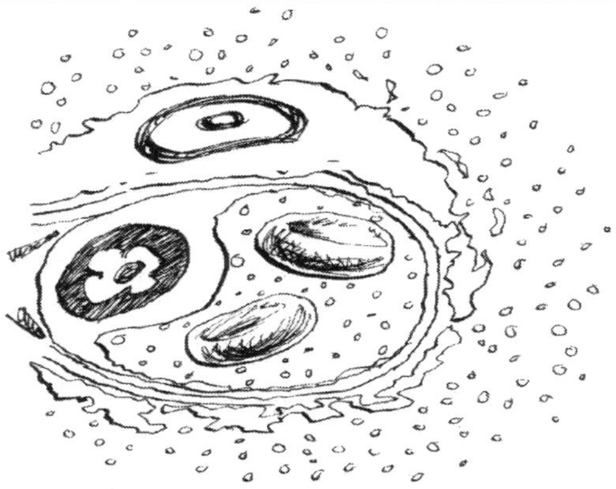	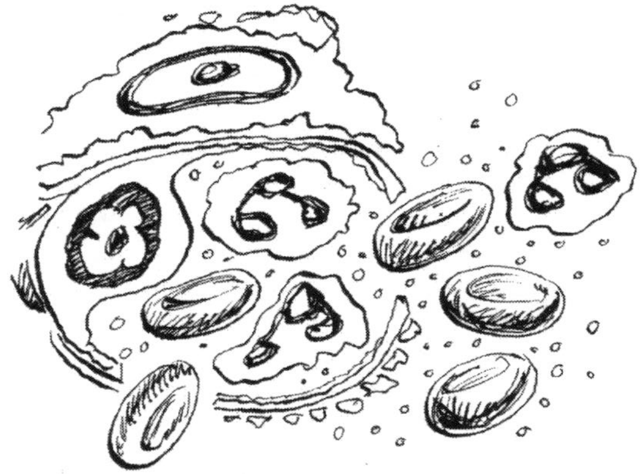
NORMAL GLOMERULUS impermeable to proteins, blood cells etc. Function of the glomerulus is to produce urine.	**NEPHROTIC SYNDROME:** Glomerular damage ⇨ ↑***urinary protein loss***	**GLOMERULONEPHRITIS (NEPHRITIC SYNDROME):** ***Immune-mediated glomerular inflammation*** ⇨ glomerular damage ⇨ ↑***urinary protein AND RBC loss***

	NEPHROTIC SYNDROME	NEPHRITIC SYNDROME (GLOMERULONEPHRITIS)
PATHOPHYSIOLOGY	Glomerular damage ⇨ ↑***urinary protein loss***	***Immune-mediated glomerular inflammation*** ⇨ glomerular damage ⇨ ↑***urinary protein & RBC loss***
HALLMARKS	***Proteinuria, hypoalbuminemia, edema, hyperlipidema, hallmark****	***Proteinuria, HTN, azotemia, oliguria, hematuria (RBC casts) hallmark****
CLINICAL MANIFESTATIONS	• ***EDEMA PREDOMINANT FEATURE*** (peripheral, periorbital) especially in children • ±↑BUN/Cr (varying degrees) • Dyspnea, ***transudative pleural effusion**** • ***DVTs,*** Frothy urine	• ***HEMATURIA, HTN**** • ***Azotemia:*** *↑BUN/creatinine* • ***Oliguria:**** *<400ml urine/day* • ***Fever, abdominal/flank pain**** • Edema (not as much as in NephrOtic)
URINALYSIS	• **PROTEINURIA >3.5g/DAY*** • Urine dipstick protein (3+ or 4+) • **FATTY CASTS,** ***oval fat bodies "maltese cross"****	• Proteinuria <3.5g/day • ***Hematuria**** • ***RBC CASTS****
BIOPSY	• ***Hypocellular*** • Minimal Change disease: normal on light microscopy, loss of podocytes on electron microscopy. Associated with loss of negative glomerular basement membrane (GBM) charge which further facilitates albumin loss (albumin has negative charge)	• ***Hypercellular**** (↑WBCs , mesangial cells) • Immune complex deposition • ***Crescent-shape*** of glomerulus on biopsy = ***rapidly progressing glomerulonephritis****

Mixed Nephrotic/Nephritic picture = hematuria (nephritic) + nephrotic range protein >3.5g/day.

ACUTE KIDNEY INJURY (AKI) ACUTE RENAL FAILURE

- ❶ ↑serum creatinine >50% or ❷ ↑blood urea nitrogen/BUN (azotemia).
- **RIFLE Criteria:** 3 progressive levels of AKI:
  Risk, Injury, Failure with 2 outcome determinants: Loss & End stage renal disease.
- Phases of AKI: oliguric (maintenance) phase (↓urine output <400mL/d, azotemia, hyperkalemia, metabolic acidosis) ⇨ diuretic phase (↑urine output, hypotension, hypokalemia) ⇨ ***recovery.***

3 TYPES: ❶ PRErenal ❷ POSTrenal (BOTH rapidly reversible) or ❸ INTRArenal (intrinsic).

PRERENAL

- Characterized by **decreased renal perfusion** with nephrons still structurally intact.
- May lead to intrinsic injury (Acute tubular necrosis) if not corrected.
- Most common type of acute kidney injury overall (40-80%) but ATN most common type in hospitalized patients.

ETIOLOGIES

Reduced renal perfusion hallmark

- **Hypovolemia** renal volume loss (eg, diuretic therapy), GI loss (diarrhea or vomiting), or blood loss.
- Afferent arteriole vasoconstriction (eg, **NSAIDs,** IV contrast).
- Efferent arteriole dilation (eg, **ACE inhibitors, Angiotensin receptor blockers).**
- **Hypotension**. Relative hypovolemia (eg, CHF with decreased pump function).

DIAGNOSIS

Evidence of water & electrolyte conservation:

- Increased BUN > increased creatinine (**BUN: creatinine ratio >20:1**).
- Fractional excretion of sodium **(FENA) < 1%** & urine sodium <20
- Concentrated urine: high urine specific gravity (> 1.020) & increased urine osmolarity (>500 mOsm/kg).

MANAGEMENT

- **Volume repletion** to restore volume & renal perfusion (rapidly responds to treatment).

POSTRENAL AZOTEMIA

- Also known as **Obstructive uropathy.**
- Pathophysiology: characterized by **obstruction of the passage of urine**.
- Rare cause of acute kidney injury because both kidneys need to be obstructed.

ETIOLOGIES

- Kidney stones (eg, ureteral), tumors, bladder outlet obstruction (Benign prostatic hypertrophy or Prostate cancer), & sloughed off renal papillae.

CLINICAL MANIFESTATIONS

- Usually asymptomatic, change in urine output, hypertension, and rarely pain.

DIAGNOSIS

- Increased creatinine usually associated with bilateral kidney involvement.
- **Ultrasound often the initial imaging test to look for signs of obstruction & hydronephrosis**.
- Depending on the cause or site of obstruction, catheterization, CT scan, MRI or pyelography may be useful.

MANAGEMENT

- **Removal of the obstruction** (readily reversible if corrected quickly).

INTRINSIC RENAL FAILURE

ACUTE INTERSTITIAL NEPHRITIS

- A type of intrinsic acute kidney injury characterized by an inflammatory or allergic response in the interstitium with sparing of the glomeruli & blood vessels.

ETIOLOGIES

- **Drug hypersensitivity most common** (70%) – especially **NSAIDs** & selective COX-2 inhibitors, **Penicillins, sulfa drugs** (Sulfonamides, Furosemide & Thiazides), Cephalosporins, Ciprofloxacin, Rifampin & Allopurinol.
- Infections (15%) - Strep, Legionella, CMV, EBV, HIV etc.
- Idiopathic 8%.
- Autoimmune 6% - SLE, Sarcoidosis, Cryoglobulinemia.

CLINICAL MANIFESTATIONS

- **Fever, eosinophilia**, **maculopapular rash,** & arthralgias.

DIAGNOSIS

- Urinalysis: **WBC casts** & eosinophiluria.
- Eosinophilia (via Hansel or Wright stain) & increased serum IgE.

MANAGEMENT

- Removing the offending agent allows for spontaneous recovery.
- Most recover kidney function within 1 year.

ACUTE TUBULAR NECROSIS (ATN)

- A type of intrinsic acute kidney injury characterized by acute destruction & necrosis of the renal tubules of the nephron.
- **Most common type of intrinsic acute kidney injury** (50%).

Ischemic:

- Prolonged prerenal azotemia associated with hypotension or hypovolemia.

Nephrotoxic:

- Exogenous: **contrast dye (immediate), Aminoglycosides,** & Vancomycin (average 5-10 days of use), Cyclosporine, NSAIDs.
- Endogenous: uric acid precipitation (tumor lysis syndrome), myoglobinuria (Rhabdomyolysis), lymphoma, leukemia, Bence-Jones proteins (Multiple myeloma).

DIAGNOSIS

- Urinalysis: renal tubular **epithelial cell casts & granular (muddy brown) casts** (sloughing off of tubular cells into the nephrons).
- Unlike prerenal, the sodium & water reabsorptive abilities are lost in ATN, leading to **low urine specific gravity** (**isosthenuria** = inability to concentrate urine), **low urine osmolarity** < 500 mOsm/kg, increased **FENA > 2%,** increased urine sodium > 40 mEq/L, & BUN: creatinine ratio < 15:1.

MANAGEMENT

- **Remove offending agent(s) & IV fluids first-line.**
- No proven therapy proven to benefit ATN. N-acetylcysteine may be added to Normal saline in contrast-induced cases.
- Furosemide may be used if patient is euvolemic and not urinating.
- Most patients return to baseline in 7-21 days.

ACUTE GLOMERULONEPHRITIS see page 460.

VASCULAR:

Microvascular: TTP, HELLP syndrome, DIC.

Macrovascular: aortic aneurysm, renal artery dissection, renal artery or vein thrombosis, malignant hypertension, atheroembolic disease (associated with **ischemic digits/blue toe syndrome** or **livedo reticularis** especially post catheterization, CABG, AAA repair).

URINALYSIS: most important noninvasive test regarding the possible etiologies.

URINARY PATTERN	
RBC CASTS, with hematuria, dysmorphic red cells	**Acute glomerulonephritis (AGN)** or **vasculitis.**
MUDDY BROWN (GRANULAR) OR EPITHELIAL CELL CASTS	**ATN (acute tubular necrosis)**
WHITE BLOOD CELL CASTS, pyuria (free WBC cells)	**AIN (acute interstitial nephritis)** or **Pyelonephritis**
WAXY CASTS: acellular with sharp edges	Narrow waxy casts: **CHRONIC** ATN/ Glomerulonephritis Broad waxy casts: **end stage renal disease** (tubal dilation).
FATTY CASTS: "maltese crosses", oval fat bodies	**Nephrotic syndrome** (due to hyperlipidemia).
HYALINE CASTS	**Nonspecific (may be seen in normal urine).** Tamm- Horsfall proteins secreted by tubular epithelial cells.
Normal or Near Normal UA: few cells with little or no casts	Acute Kidney injury: **prerenal or postrenal.** Hypercalcemia, multiple myeloma.
Hematuria & pyuria (excluding red cell casts)	**UTI,** acute interstitial nephritis (AIN), glomerular disease, vasculitis.
Hematuria alone	See hematuria section (page 366).
Pyuria alone	**MC due to infection**; sterile pyuria in tubulointerstitial disease.

	PRERENAL	**ATN**
Creatinine (Cr)	Increases slower than 0.3mg/dL/day	Increases at 0.3-0.5 mg/dL/day
UNa, FeNa	**↓Urine Na⁺ <20; FeNa⁺ <1%**	**↑Urine Na⁺ >40;** FeNa⁺ >2%
URINALYSIS (UA)	**Normal UA** **HIGH SPECIFIC GRAVITY (↑UOsm)**	**EPITHELIAL CELLS, GRANULAR CASTS.*** **LOW SPECIFIC GRAVITY**
Response to volume replacement	**Creatinine rapidly improves c IVF**	Creatinine won't improve much
Blood Urea Nitrogen (BUN)/Cr	**↑BUN: Cr >20:1**	10-15:1

$$\text{FENA \%} = \frac{\text{Urinary conc Na}}{\text{Plasma Na}} \times \frac{\text{Plasma creatinine}}{\text{Urine creatinine}} \times 100$$

CELLULAR CASTS: cells that make it into the tubules clump together & take the shape of the tubules as they travel through the nephron.

The type of cast is helpful to figure out the possible type of kidney injury:

ACUTE TUBULAR NECROSIS
- **Epithelial cell & Muddy brown casts**

ACUTE INTERSTITIAL NEPHRITIS
- **White blood cell casts**

ACUTE GLOMERULONEPHRITIS
- **Red blood cell casts**

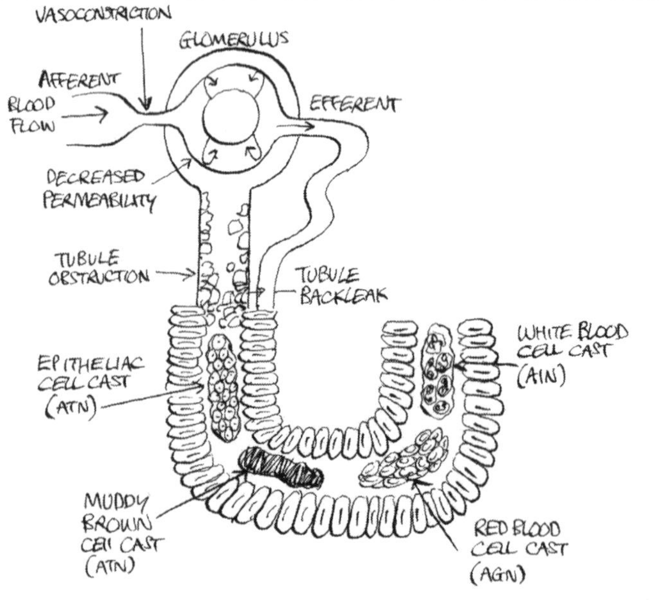

ADULT POLYCYSTIC KIDNEY DISEASE

- **Autosomal dominant disorder** due to mutations of either genes PKD1 (85-90%) or PKD2 (10-15%). Causes 10% of end stage renal disease.
- Multisystemic progressive disorder characterized by **formation & enlargement of kidney cysts & cysts in other organs** (eg, **liver most common, spleen, & pancreas**).

PATHOPHYSIOLOGY
- Vasopressin stimulates cystogenesis and eventually end stage renal disease (ESRD) over time.
- Patients usually present in the 30-40s.

CLINICAL MANIFESTATIONS
- Renal - **abdominal & flank pain**, nephrolithiasis, urinary tract infection, & **hematuria.**
- Extrarenal manifestations: **cerebral "berry" aneurysms** (can cause Subarachnoid hemorrhages), hepatic cysts, **Mitral valve prolapse**, & **colonic diverticula** (Diverticulosis).

PHYSICAL EXAMINATION
- **Palpable flank masses** or large palpable kidneys. **Hypertension.**

DIAGNOSIS
- Urinalysis: hematuria, decreased urine concentrating ability, & proteinuria.
- **Renal ultrasound most widely used diagnostic imaging test.**
- CT scan or MRI more sensitive than ultrasound.
- Genetic testing may be performed once diagnosed.

MANAGEMENT
- Simple cyst: observation, periodic reevaluation. ACE inhibitors, angiotensin receptor blockers (HTN).
- Multiple cysts: supportive, **increase fluid intake** - fluids decreases vasopressin (reducing vasopressin-induced cystogenesis) & HTN control.

	HYPOphosphatemia	**HYPERphosphatemia**
ETIOLOGIES	• **↑Urinary PO_4 excretion:** **1ry Hyperparathyroidism**, **Vitamin D deficiency** • **Internal PO_4 redistribution:** respiratory alkalosis, excessive IV Glucose, treatment for DKA, refeeding syndrome in ETOHics (insulin shifts phosphate intracellularly). • **Decreased intestinal absorption:** antacids, phosphate binders	• **Renal failure most common** - **↓Ca^{+2}, ↑Phosphate, ↑iPTH** • **1ry Hypoparathyroidism** - **↓Ca^{+2}, ↑Phosphate, ↓iPTH** • Vitamin D intoxication - ↑Ca^{+2}, ↑Phosphate, ↓iPTH • Iatrogenic, DKA • Rhabdomyolysis, Tumor lysis
CLINICAL	• **Diffuse muscle weakness, flaccid paralysis (due to ↓ATP)**	• **Soft tissue calcifications** • Most asymptomatic, heart block
MANAGEMENT	Treat the underlying cause. **Phosphate repletion:** if symptomatic or serum PO_4 <2.0mg/dL • potassium phosphate • sodium phosphate	• **Renal failure: phosphate binders: Calcium acetate** (PhosLo), **Calcium carbonate, Sevelamer** (Renagel) • Decrease dietary phosphate: dairy products, dark colas. • Hydration, Acetazolamide

CHRONIC KIDNEY DISEASE & END STAGE RENAL DISEASE

Chronic kidney disease: progressive functional decline **≥3 months-years evidence by:**

1. Proteinuria
2. Abnormal urine sediment
3. Abnormal serum/urine chemistries
4. Abnormal imaging studies
5. Inability to buffer pH
6. Inability to make urine
7. Inability to excrete nitrogenous waste
8. ↓ synthesis of Vitamin D/Erythropoietin

CHRONIC KIDNEY DISEASE STAGING

Stage 0: At risk patients: DM, HTN, chronic NSAID use, Africa-American/Hispanic/Asian), age >60, SLE, s/p kidney transplant, family history of kidney disease. **Normal GFR, normal urine.**

Stage 1: Kidney damage with normal GFR (or >90)
Kidney damage = proteinuria, Abnormal UA, serum, imaging
Stage 2: GFR 89-60
Stage 3: GFR 59-30 (3a 59-45) (3b 44-30)
Stage 4: GFR 29-15
Stage 5: GFR <15 End Stage Renal Disease (ESRD) = uremia requiring dialysis and/or transplant.
Normal Glomerular Filtration Rate (GFR) 120-130

Albuminuria
A1 = ACR <30mg/g
A2 = ACR 30-300mg/g
A3 = ACR ≥300mg/g

ETIOLOGIES

- **Diabetes mellitus most common cause of End-stage renal disease.**
- **Hypertension second most common.**
- Glomerulonephritis, Polycystic kidney disease, & rapidly-progressive glomerulonephritis.

CLINICAL MANIFESTATIONS

- Uremia: nausea, vomiting, fatigue, malaise, metallic taste, hiccups, altered mentation, irritability, muscle cramps and easy bruising, fluid overload, encephalopathy, pericarditis.

DIAGNOSIS

Proteinuria: **single best predictor of disease progression.**

- **Spot Urine Albumin/UCreatinine Ratio (ACR) preferred over 24h urine collection.** Spot test estimates grams of protein loss/day.
- Increased BUN and creatinine
- Urinalysis: abnormal sediment: may have RBC casts, WBC casts etc. **Broad waxy casts seen in ESRD** (taking the shape of dilated & damaged tubules). Urine dipstick
- Estimated GFR: CKD-Epi most accurate, MDRD. Cockcroft-Gault used for Creatinine clearance (eg, "renally" dosing medications excreted by the kidney).
- Renal ultrasound: **small kidneys classic** (large kidneys in diabetic nephropathy, PKD).

MANAGEMENT

- Hypertension: **blood pressure goal <140/90 mmHg.** ACE inhibitors or Angiotensin receptor blockers in early disease.
- Proteinuria: **ACE inhibitors or Angiotensin receptor blockers in early disease.**
- Diabetes control: **Hemoglobin A1C goal < 7.0%** if predialysis & not at risk for hypoglycemia.
- Hyperlipidemia: LDL <100 mg/dL, triglycerides <150 mg/dL, HDL >50 mg/dL.
- Renal osteodystrophy: low calcium + high phosphate. Managed by active vitamin D (Calcitriol) + phosphate binders (eg, Calcium Acetate, Calcium carbonate); Lanthanum or Sevelamer used if both calcium & phosphate levels are elevated.
- Hypocalcemia & Osteomalacia: replace vitamin D and calcium.
- Dialysis: end stage disease (stage 5), acidosis, electrolyte imbalances, ingestion, overload (volume) and uremia. Renal transplant for some end-stage renal disease.
  Dialysis indicated if GFR 10mL/min or less and/or serum creatinine ≥ 8mg/dL.
  (In diabetics, if GFR 15ml/min or less and/or serum creatinine of ≥ 6 mg/dL).

RENAL OSTEODYSTROPHY

- Bone disorders **(Osteitis fibrosa cystica** & **Osteomalacia)** associated with **Chronic kidney disease.**

PATHOPHYSIOLOGY

- Failing kidneys do not eliminate phosphate properly (**increased phosphate**) & simultaneously poorly synthesize vitamin D.
- This leads to hypocalcemia and compensatory increase in PTH (secondary hyperparathyroidism) and decreased bone mineralization by osteoclast activity (PTH pulls the calcium from the bones).

CLINICAL MANIFESTATIONS

- **Bone & proximal muscle pain (in the context of uremia).**
- Pathologic fractures & chondrocalcinosis.

DIAGNOSIS

- **Hypocalcemia + increased phosphate + increased intact PTH (secondary hyperparathyroidism).**

- Increased alkaline phosphatase. Vitamin D levels vary.

- Radiographs: **Osteitis Fibrosa Cystica - periosteal erosions, bony cysts** with thin trabeculum & cortex, **"salt & pepper" appearance of the skull** (punctate trabecular bone resorption in the skull).

- Biopsy: **cystic brown tumors –** describes the appearance of hemosiderin (not an actual tumor).

MANAGEMENT

- **Phosphate binders** decrease phosphate and add calcium (eg, **Calcium carbonate & Calcium acetate)**. **Sevelamer** used if both calcium & phosphate levels are elevated. Phosphate goal <5.5.

- Supplementation: **active forms of vitamin D** (eg, **Calcitriol**) & calcium.

- Cinacalcet (lowers PTH).

CLASSIC BONE DISEASES				
RESULT	CALCIUM	PHOSPHATE	PTH	ALKALINE PHOSPHATASE
HYPOPARATHYROIDISM	• Decreased	• Increased	• Decreased	• Increased
PRIMARY HYPERPARATHYROIDISM	• Increased	• Decreased	• Increased	• Increased
SECONDARY HYPERPARATHYROIDISM Associated with RENAL OSTEODYSTROPHY	• Decreased	• Increased	• Increased	• Increased
OSTEOMALACIA Due to Vitamin D deficiency	• Decreased or normal	• Decreased or normal	• Increased	• Increased
OSTEOPOROSIS	• Normal	• Normal	• Normal	• **Normal** • May increase with an acute fracture
PAGET DISEASE OF THE BONE	• Normal	• Normal	• Normal	• Markedly elevated

HORSESHOE KIDNEY

- Fusion of one pole of each kidney – most commonly fused at the lower poles.
- The fusion may be associated with entrapment of the inferior renal artery.

RISK FACTORS

- May be associated with other congenital urologic abnormalities (eg, **ureteropelvic junction obstruction most common,** vesicourethral reflux) or genital abnormalities (eg, bicornuate or septate uterus in girls as well as cryptorchidism & hypospadias in boys).
- May also be seen in Turner syndrome and Trisomy 13, 18, & 21.

COMPLICATIONS

- Urine stasis leads to **increased risk for Pyelonephritis & kidney stone formation.**
- Increased risk of renal malignancies – **Renal cell carcinoma most common** (45% of tumors), Transitional cell cancer, and Wilms tumor.

CLINICAL MANIFESTATIONS

- **Majority are asymptomatic** and seen as an incidental finding (eg, antenatal ultrasound).
- Hematuria or pain due to infection or obstruction. Renal calculi (20%).
- Hydronephrosis (due to vesicourethral reflux or ureteropelvic junction obstruction).

DIAGNOSIS

- Ultrasound to detect horseshoe kidneys & evaluate for hydronephrosis. Serum creatinine.
- **CT urography best initial test to evaluate anatomy and relative renal function.**
- Voiding cystourethrogram to detect vesicourethral reflux.
- Radionuclide renal scan can differentiate true obstruction from passively dilated systems.

MANAGEMENT

- Majority of cases require no treatment. UTI or Hydronephrosis treated with antibiotics.
- Patients with obstruction should be referred to a urologist.

HYDRONEPHROSIS

- Urinary tract obstruction leading to **dilatation of the collecting system in one or both kidneys.**
- Pathophysiology: characterized by **obstruction of the passage of urine**.

ETIOLOGIES

- Kidney stones (eg, ureteral), tumors, bladder outlet obstruction (Benign prostatic hypertrophy or Prostate cancer), & sloughed off renal papillae.

CLINICAL MANIFESTATIONS

- Usually asymptomatic, change in urine output, hypertension, hematuria, and rarely pain.

DIAGNOSIS

- UA: often benign but may show hematuria. Labs: may have increased serum creatinine.
- Ultrasound: **initial imaging of choice – dilatation of the collecting system in one or both kidneys**.
- CT scan: indicated with those with flank pain and suspected nephrolithiasis or in patients whom visualization of the ureters is needed.

MANAGEMENT

- **Removal of the obstruction** (readily reversible if corrected quickly). May lead to urinary tract infections and possible end-stage renal disease.

RENOVASCULAR HYPERTENSION (RENAL ARTERY STENOSIS)

- Hypertension secondary to **renal artery stenosis** of 1 or both kidneys.
- **Most common cause of secondary hypertension.**

PATHOPHYSIOLOGY

- Decreased renal blood flow leads to activation of the renin-angiotensin-aldosterone system.

ETIOLOGIES

- **Atherosclerosis most common in the elderly.**
- **Fibromuscular dysplasia most common cause in women < 50 years.**

CLINICAL MANIFESTATIONS

- Suspect in patients with headache & hypertension <20 years or > 50 years, severe HTN, HTN resistant to 3 or more drugs, **abdominal bruit** or if patient develops **acute kidney injury after the initiation of ACE Inhibitor therapy.**

DIAGNOSIS

- Diagnostic testing is only indicated if a corrective measure is to be performed if clinically relevant disease is discovered.
- Noninvasive options include **CT angiography**, MR angiography, & Duplex Doppler ultrasound. CT and MR angiography give better sensitivity, specificity, and anatomic detail than Doppler ultrasonography.
- **Renal catheter arteriography: definitive (gold standard).** Revascularization can be performed during the same procedure if stenosis is present. Not used in patients with renal failure.

SURGICAL MANAGEMENT

- **Revascularization definitive management** (eg, angioplasty or bypass).
- **Angioplasty with stent** performed if creatinine > 4.0, increased creatinine with ACE inhibitor treatment or >80% stenosis.
- Bypass may be performed if angioplasty is unsuccessful.

MEDICAL MANAGEMENT

- **ACE inhibitors or Angiotensin receptor blockers** (inhibits aldosterone II–mediated vasoconstriction). However, **ACE inhibitors & ARBs are contraindicated if bilateral stenosis or in patients with a solitary kidney** because they can lead to Acute kidney injury in these patients (markedly reduced renal blood flow & GFR).
- Add-on therapy to ACE or ARBs include Thiazide diuretics (eg, Indapamide, Chlorthalidone), long-acting calcium channel blocker, or mineralocorticoid receptor antagonist.

HYPERKALEMIA

ETIOLOGIES

- **Pseudohyperkalemia:** due to **hemolysis** – **venipuncture** especially if the patient clenches fist during venipuncture or the tourniquette is left on too long, lab error (lysis of the cells). Suspect in asymptomatic patients with elevated potassium, **thrombocytosis or leukocytosis** & no ECG changes (can leak out into lab specimen).
- Decreased renal K+ excretion – **acute or chronic renal failure** (especially end stage renal disease).
- Hypoaldosteronism – Primary adrenal insufficiency (Addison disease). Drugs that block aldosterone, such as **ACE inhibitors, Angiotensin receptor blockers, Spironolactone, Eplerenone** (K+ sparing diuretics).
- Medications: K+ supplementation, NSAIDs, Cyclosporine, Heparin, Trimethoprim, Other K+ sparing diuretics (Amiloride & Triamterene), Beta-blockers, & Digoxin.
- Tissue destruction: (releases K+ from cells) - rhabdomyolysis, burns, or tumor lysis syndrome.
- K^+ extracellular redistribution: **metabolic acidosis** (eg, DKA), insulin deficiency, catabolic states, Mannitol.

CLINICAL MANIFESTATIONS

Hyperkalemia affects muscle contraction and cardiac conduction, it does not cause seizures.

- Neuromuscular: **weakness** (progressive ascending), fatigue, paresthesias, **paralysis.**
- Cardiovascular: palpitations, **cardiac arrhythmias (potentially life-threatening)**.
- GI: abdominal distention, **ileus** (paralyzes intestinal muscles).

DIAGNOSIS

- Serum potassium >5.0 mEq/L. Check labs for potential causes - glucose (hyperglycemia), bicarbonate (acidosis), CBC (hemolysis), CK (rhabdomyolysis).
- ECG: **tall peaked T waves earliest manifestations**, QT interval shortening, **wide QRS,** prolonged PR interval, P wave flattening, **sine wave** followed by arrhythmias.

MANAGEMENT

- Mild or no ECG changes: recheck K+ levels to rule out hemolysis from venipuncture.

- Pseudohyperkalemia: repeat the sample.

MANAGEMENT IF SIGNIFICANTLY ELEVATED **or ECG changes**

- **IV Calcium gluconate** (or Calcium chloride) **to stabilize the myocardium** (does not lower levels but protects against arrhythmias). Address causes.

- **Potassium-lowering agents**
  - **Parenteral insulin with glucose**
  - High-dose **beta-2 agonists** are quick-acting.
  - Sodium polystyrene sulfonate (removes K+ from the body via bowel movement - works in hours).
  - IV saline with a loop diuretic.
  - Patiromer (oral potassium binder).

- Bicarbonate (not usually used). Dialysis.

HYPOKALEMIA

ETIOLOGIES

- Urinary or GI losses: **diarrhea, vomiting,** laxative abuse, **diuretic therapy** (including **loop diuretics**, thiazides, & carbonic anhydrase inhibitors). Increased mineralocorticoid activity (eg, Hyperaldosteronism).

- Increased intracellular K+ shift: **metabolic alkalosis** (hydrogen ions leave the cell in exchange for potassium entering the cells), medications (insulin therapy, beta 2 agonists, chloroquine, vitamin B12 treatment, & Amphotericin B). Hypothermia.

- **Hypomagnesemia** (low magnesium opens magnesium-dependent potassium channels, spilling potassium into the urine), Licorice.

- Type I (classic distal) and type II (proximal) renal tubular acidosis. Hyperthyroidism. Genetic defects (Liddle's, Bartter & Gitelman syndromes).

CLINICAL MANIFESTATIONS

- Hypokalemia affects muscle contraction and cardiac conduction, it does not cause seizures.

- **Neuromuscular – severe muscle weakness,** paralysis, **decreased deep tendon reflexes, ileus,** nausea & vomiting.

- Cardiovascular: palpitations & arrhythmias. **Polyuria** (causes nephrogenic diabetes insipidus). May cause rhabdomyolysis or myoglobinuria.

DIAGNOSIS

- Serum electrolytes (including Magnesium levels).

- ECG: **T wave flattening (earliest change) followed by prominent U wave** development. PVCs & ST depressions.

MANAGEMENT

- **Oral potassium chloride mainstay of treatment.**

- Severe: slow IV Potassium chloride (usually 10 – 20 mEq/L/hr given). Peripheral infusions > 40 mEq/L/hr may lead to burning, sclerosis, or phlebitis.

- **It may be difficult to replete potassium in patients with concurrent hypomagnesemia without magnesium repletion.**

HYPERMAGNESEMIA

- **Renal insufficiency** (hypermagnesemia is rare in the absence of renal insufficiency).
- **Iatrogenic excess IV magnesium administration** (eg, in the management of asthma, preeclampsia, eclampsia, torsades de pointes, & arrhythmias).
- **Lithium**. Adrenal sufficiency, milk alkali syndrome.
- Ingestion of magnesium-containing substances (eg, vitamins, antacids).

CLINICAL MANIFESTATIONS

- **Decreased deep tendon reflex first sign,** nausea, vomiting, skin flushing, **weakness,** lightheadedness, AMS, ileus (due to GI hypomotility), somnolence, & **respiratory depression**.
- Increased magnesium levels have **calcium channel blocker-like effects: conduction defects, bradycardia**, & **hypotension** that may be refractory to fluids & pressors.

DIAGNOSIS

- Serum electrolyte levels
- ECG: may be similar to hypomagnesemia: prolonged QT &/or PR interval, wide QRS complex.

MANAGEMENT

- Mild: in the presence of normal renal function, cessation of Mg+2-containing sources will normalize Magnesium levels.
- Severe: **IV Calcium gluconate stabilizes the cardiac membranes** in patients with ECG changes. **IV fluids + Furosemide** enhance renal Mg+2 excretion.
- Dialysis for severe or refractory cases.

HYPOMAGNESEMIA

ETIOLOGIES

- GI losses: **malabsorption** (eg, **chronic alcoholism,** Celiac disease, small bowel bypass, **prolonged diarrhea** or vomiting, & laxatives).
- Renal losses: **thiazide & loop diuretics**. Diabetes mellitus, renal tubular acidosis.
- Endocrine: Hypoparathyroidism, Hyperaldosteronism.
- Medications: **proton pump inhibitors** (eg, **Omeprazole**) > 5 years**,** Amphotericin B, Cisplatin, Cyclosporine, & Aminoglycosides.

CLINICAL MANIFESTATIONS

- **Neuromuscular hyperexcitability similar to hypocalcemia – tetany, increased deep tendon reflexes (one of the first clinical signs), Trousseau & Chvostek signs, tremor,** muscle cramps, weakness & seizures. Altered mental status, lethargy, vertigo.
- **Cardiovascular:** arrhythmias & palpitations. Psychiatric: dementia or psychosis.

DIAGNOSIS

- Serum electrolytes.
- ECG: prolonged QT interval, prolonged PR, QRS widening, atrial or ventricular fibrillation, ventricular tachycardia.

MANAGEMENT

- Mild: oral Magnesium oxide.
- Severe or Torsades: **IV Magnesium sulfate** or chloride. Mg sulfate preferred in Torsades.
- **Hypocalcemia or Hypokalemia may be induced by hypomagnesemia & may be refractory to correction until magnesium is repleted.**

HYPERNATREMIA

- **Increased serum sodium** (> 145 mEq/L) **due to increased free water loss,** hypotonic fluid loss, or hypertonic sodium gain (iatrogenic).

ETIOLOGIES
- Diarrhea, diuretics, sweating, burns, fever, insensible loss, **Diabetes insipidus.**

PATHOPHYSIOLOGY
- **Sustained hypernatremia seen when appropriate water intake not possible or impaired** (eg, infants, elderly, debilitated patients) or impaired thirst mechanism.

CLINICAL MANIFESTATIONS
- **Neurological symptoms** are primarily due to shrinkage of brain cells from dehydration – **thirst most common initial symptom,** confusion, lethargy, disorientation, fatigue, nausea, vomiting, muscle weakness.

- Seizures, coma, brain damage, & respiratory arrest if severe.

- Symptoms vary with degree and rapidity of hypernatremia.

PHYSICAL EXAMINATION
- Dehydration: **dry mouth or mucous membranes, decreased skin turgor,** tachycardia, hypotension.

DIAGNOSIS
- Serum studies: serum sodium, urine osmolarity, serum osmolarity, assess volume status. **Hypernatremia nearly always associated with hyperosmolality.**

- Urine studies: urine sodium is elevated if renal loss or decreased if extrarenal loss. Urine osmolality is increased (concentrated) if extrarenal or decreased (dilute urine) if diabetes insipidus.

MANAGEMENT
- **Hypotonic fluids** (eg, pure water oral, D5W, 0.45% NS, 0.2% saline). **Preferred route is oral** (or feeding tube if present).

- **Isotonic fluids if hypovolemic** (Normal saline or Lactated ringers) then switch to hypotonic fluids to correct the hyponatremia once volume is repleted.

- **Rapid correction** (> 0.5 mEq/L/hr) can result in *cerebral edema.*

HYPONATREMIA

- Serum sodium < 135 mEq/L due to **increased free water.**
- Type is determined by **serum osmolality & volume status.**
- Clinically significant hyponatremia is **hypotonic hyponatremia.**

HYPERTONIC HYPONATREMIA:
- Due to hyperglycemia or Mannitol infusion.

ISOTONIC HYPONATREMIA:
- lab error due to hyperproteinemia or hypertriglyceridemia.

Hypotonic hyponatremia: clinically significant hyponatremia. 3 types determined by volume status:
- **Hypovolemic:** renal volume loss – **diuretics,** ACE inhibitors. Extrarenal volume loss - GI loss (diarrhea or vomiting), burns, fever, pancreatitis.
- **Isovolemic: SIADH,** hypothyroidism, adrenal insufficiency, reset hypothalamic osmostat, water intoxication (primary polydipsia), MDMA (ecstasy), tea & toast syndrome, beer potomania.
- **Hypervolemic: edematous states** - Congestive heart failure, Nephrotic syndrome, Cirrhosis.

CLINICAL MANIFESTATIONS
- **Neurologic symptoms: primarily due to cerebral edema** - confusion, lethargy, disorientation, fatigue, nausea, vomiting, & muscle cramps. Seizures, coma or respiratory arrest if severe.
- Symptoms vary with degree & rapidity of hyponatremia.

DIAGNOSIS: 3 steps: this helps determine the cause and the effective treatment.
- Step 1 – **measure serum sodium.**
- Step 2 - **serum osmolality.**
- Step 3 – **assess volume status** (if hypotonic/decreased osmolality).

MANAGEMENT
- In general, with the exception of severe cases, **correction of serum sodium > 0.5 mEq/L/hour can lead to central pontine myelinolysis (demyelination),** leading to permanent neurologic damage.
- When treating hyponatremia, it is important to consider **volume status**, degree and severity of symptoms and duration & magnitude of the hyponatremia. There are 4 treatments you need to know:
- **Isovolemic** hypotonic hyponatremia: **water restriction.** Treat the underlying cause.
- **Hypovolemic** hypotonic hyponatremia: **volume replacement - Normal (0.9%) saline.** Treat the underlying cause.
- **Hypervolemic** hypotonic hyponatremia: **volume removal – diuretics, sodium + water restriction.** Treat the underlying cause.
- Severe hyponatremia (eg, obtunded, coma or seizures): **IV hypertonic saline + Furosemide** (regardless of the volume status, stabilization of the patient is paramount if severe).

HYPERVOLEMIA	HYPOVOLEMIA	ISOVOLEMIA
peripheral and presacral edema	**poor skin turgor**	absence of the
pulmonary edema	**dry mucous membranes**	signs of hyper-
jugular venous distension	**flat neck veins**	or hypovolemia
hypertension	**hypotension**	
decreased hematocrit	increased hematocrit	
decreased serum protein	increased serum protein	
decreased BUN: creatinine	**increased BUN: creatinine ratio >20:1**	

UNa <20 mEq/L

HYPONATREMIA

Critical hyponatremia:
Tx c hypertonic saline
+ Loop diuretic

***Note: all have ↑ADH**
•SIADH: inappropriate
•The rest: appropriate

Serum Osm **(STEP 1)**

- **Low**
  - **HYPOTONIC HYPONATREMIA**
  - **(TRUE)**
- **Normal**
  - **Lab Error**
  - (↑Protein, ↑Triglycerides)
- **High**
  - **Hyperglycemia**
  - Mannitol

ECF Volume **(STEP 2)**

Low (HYPOVOLEMIA)

RENAL LOSS (UNa > 20)
- *Diuretics*
  - ***Thiazides***
  - K-sparing
- ACE-I, ARBs
- IV RTA, Hypoaldosteronism

EXTRA RENAL LOSS (UNa <10), FeNa <1)
- Bleeding
- Burns
- GI (N/V, diarrhea)
- Pancreatitis

Mgmt: Normal Saline (correct the volume)

Normal (ISOVOLEMIA)
- **SIADH, post op**
- Hypothyroidism
- Adrenal Insufficiency
- Reset Osmostat
- Water Intoxication
  1° Polydipsia

Mgmt: Water Restriction

High (HYPERVOLEMIA)

Una <20
- **CHF, Cirrhosis**
- **Nephrosis**

UNA >20
- **Acute/Chronic Renal failure**
- **Mgmt: H_2O/salt restriction**

REVIEW OF HYPERNATREMIA

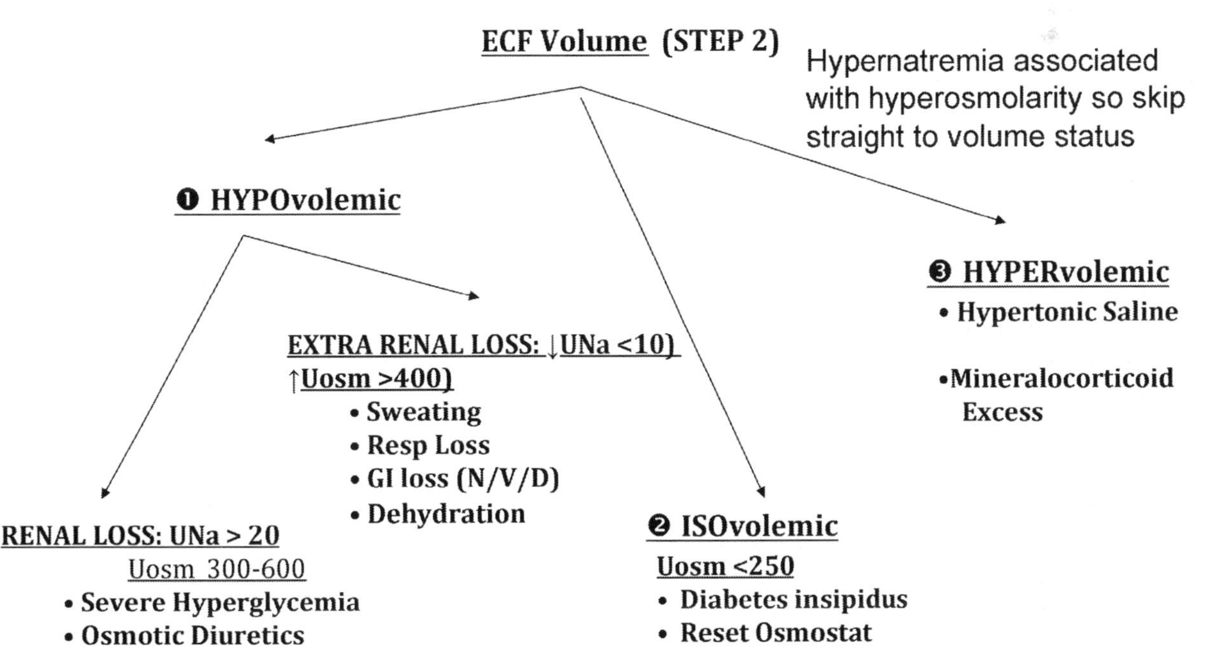

	HYPOnatremia	HYPERnatremia
ETIOLOGY	• Due to ❶ ***impaired kidney free water excretion (increased ADH secretion)*** where the kidney is unable to make dilute urine in the setting of ❷ ↑'ed ***water intake.*** • Remember Na disorders are a problem with water handling (not total body sodium)!!	• ***MC caused by net water loss*** (free water loss, hypotonic fluid loss) or *hypertonic sodium gain (iatrogenic).* • ***Sustained hypernatremia seen when appropriate water intake is not possible/***impaired (ex. infants, elderly, debilitated patients) or impaired thirst mechanism.
CLINICAL MANIFESTATIONS	• Symptoms vary with degree & rapidity of hyponatremia. • ***CNS dysfunction due to cerebral edema:**** hypotonicity shifts water intracellularly ⇨ cerebral edema. - Nonspecific neuro sx: fatigue, headache, nausea, vomiting, muscle cramps, lethargy, AMS, ↓DTR. - Neuro Complications: seizures, coma, permanent brain damage, death, respiratory arrest.	• Symptoms vary with degree and rapidity of hypernatremia. • ***CNS dysfunction:*** hypertonicity shifts water out of cells ⇨ ***shrinkage of brain cells.*** - Confusion, lethargy, coma, muscle weakness, lethargy, seizures
LAB FINDINGS	• ***Serum Na <135.*** May order urine Na & urine osmolality.	• ***Serum Na >145.*** May order urine Na & urine osmolality.
MANAGEMENT	• **Hypotonic Hyponatremia:** - ***ISOvolemic: H_2O restriction.**** (<1.5L/d). Tx cause. - ***HYPERvolemic: H_2O + Na restriction.**** - ***HYPOvolemic: normal saline*** (volume expansion decreases hypovolemic stimulus for ADH secretion). • **Hypertonic Hyponatremia:** ***normal saline until hemodynamically stable*** ⇨ switch to ***½ normal saline*** • **Severe (Iso or Hyper) volemic Hyponatremia:** - ***Hypertonic saline + Furosemide**** (rapidly ↑'es Na).	• ***HYPOTONIC FLUIDS:*** - ***Preferred route is oral*** (or feeding tube if present). - ***Only hypotonic fluids are appropriate:*** Ex. pure water orally, D5W, 0.45%NS, 0.2% saline. - except for cases of frank circulatory compromise, 0.9% normal saline is unsuitable for hypernatremia!
CORRECTION	• ***Correct ≤0.5mEq/L/h*** *to* ***PREVENT DEMYELINATION.****	• ***Correct ≤0.5mEq/L/h*** *to* ***PREVENT CEREBRAL EDEMA.****
	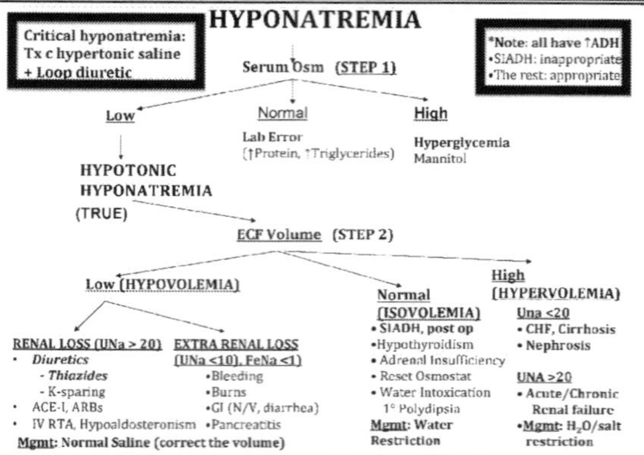 **HYPONATREMIA** Critical hyponatremia: Tx c hypertonic saline + Loop diuretic *Note: all have ↑ADH • SIADH: inappropriate • The rest: appropriate Serum Osm (STEP 1) Low → HYPOTONIC HYPONATREMIA (TRUE) Normal: Lab Error (↑Protein, ↑Triglycerides) High: Hyperglycemia, Mannitol ECF Volume (STEP 2) Low (HYPOVOLEMIA): RENAL LOSS (UNa > 20) • *Diuretics* - *Thiazides* - K-sparing • ACE-I, ARBs • IV RTA, Hypoaldosteronism EXTRA RENAL LOSS (UNa <10), FeNa <1) • Bleeding • Burns • GI (N/V, diarrhea) • Pancreatitis Mgmt: Normal Saline (correct the volume) Normal (ISOVOLEMIA): • SIADH, post op • Hypothyroidism • Adrenal Insufficiency • Reset Osmostat • Water Intoxication 1° Polydipsia; Mgmt: Water Restriction High (HYPERVOLEMIA): Una <20 • CHF, Cirrhosis • Nephrosis; UNA >20 • Acute/Chronic Renal failure • Mgmt: H_2O/salt restriction	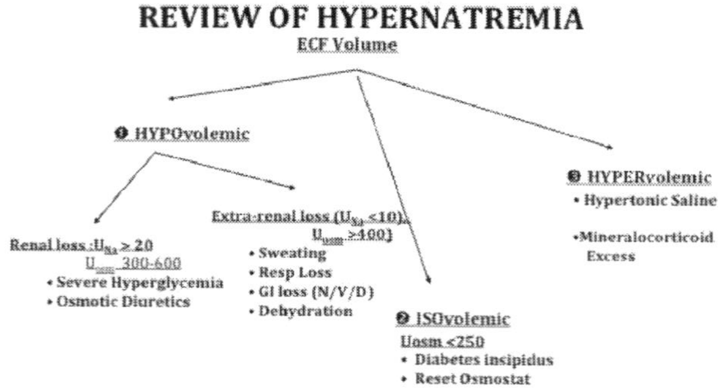 **REVIEW OF HYPERNATREMIA** ECF Volume ❶ HYPOvolemic Renal loss: U_{Na} > 20, U_{osm} 300-600 • Severe Hyperglycemia • Osmotic Diuretics Extra-renal loss (U_{Na} <10), U_{osm} >400) • Sweating • Resp Loss • GI loss (N/V/D) • Dehydration ❷ ISOvolemic: Uosm <250 • Diabetes insipidus • Reset Osmostat ❸ HYPERvolemic • Hypertonic Saline • Mineralocorticoid Excess

	HYPOmagnesemia	HYPERmagnesemia
ETIOLOGIES	• **GI losses**: ***Malabsorption: ETOHics,**** Celiac disease, small bowel bypass, diarrhea, vomiting, laxatives. • **Renal losses:** - ***Diuretics:*** thiazides, loop diuretics. - Diabetes mellitus, renal tubular acidosis. - **Meds**: ***proton pump inhibitors (omeprazole),*** Amphotericin B, Cisplatin, Cyclosporine, Aminoglycosides.	• RARE. 2 MC causes ❶ ***renal insufficiency*** or ❷ ***increased Mg intake*** (ex. overcorrection of hypomagnesemia). - ***Acute or chronic renal failure***: ↓Mg excretion. - **Iatrogenic**: excess IV Mg administration in the treatment of asthma, eclampsia, torsades de pointes. - Excess ingestion of Magnesium: vitamins, antacids, milk alkali syndrome. - Lithium toxicity, Adrenal sufficiency.
CLINICAL MANIFESTATIONS	• **Neurovascular**: AMS, lethargy, weakness, muscle cramps, vertigo, seizures, ***↑DTR, tetany.**** • **Hypocalcemia*:** Trousseau's & Chvostek's signs are due to impaired PTH secretion/release because magnesium is needed to make parathyroid hormone. • **Cardiovascular:** arrhythmias, palpitations (due to hypomagnesemia & associated hypokalemia).	• Nausea, vomiting, skin flushing, dizziness, muscle weakness, AMS, ***↓DTR (hyporeflexive).**** • Severe: hypotension, bradyarrhythmias, AV conduction blocks, respiratory depression, tachyarrhythmias.
LAB FINDINGS	• *Hypomagnesemia. ± hypokalemia & hypocalcemia*	• *Hypermagnesemia. ± hyperkalemia & hypercalcemia*
ECG FINDINGS	• ***Prolonged PR & QT interval***, wide QRS, A-fib, V-fib, Ventricular tachycardia (R on T), ***Torsades**** R ON T PHENOMENON TORSADES DE POINTES	• Similar to hypomagnesemia Prolonged PR & QT interval, wide QRS • May show ECG signs of hyperkalemia • Arrhythmias
MANAGEMENT	**MILD** • **Oral Magnesium**: ex. Magnesium oxide. **SEVERE** • ***IV Magnesium Sulfate.*** Also used in ***Torsades de pointes**** • Hypocalcemia & hypokalemia associated with hypomagnesemia are often refractory to treatment until magnesium is repleted.*	**MILD TO MODERATE:** • ***IV fluids + Furosemide*** (Lasix): enhances renal magnesium excretion. Also used if severe **SEVERE** • ***Calcium Gluconate:**** antagonizes the toxic effects of magnesium & stabilizes the cardiac membrane. • Dialysis in severe cases.

	HYPO kalemia	HYPER kalemia
ETIOLOGIES	• Increased urinary/GI losses: ***MC causes - diuretic therapy,* vomiting, diarrhea.*** RTA: classic distal (Type I), proximal (II) • Increased intracellular shifts: ***metabolic alkalosis,**** β-2 agonists, hypothermia, Chloroquine use, vitamin B12 tx, insulin. • Hypomagnesemia. • Decreased potassium intake: very rare unless superimposed with another cause.	• **↓Renal excretion:** ***acute or chronic renal failure*** (especially if on dialysis & coupled with increased K^+ intake (ex bananas). ***↓aldosterone: hypoaldosteronism, adrenal insufficiency.*** • ***Meds: K^+ supplements, K^+-sparing diuretics, ACEI/ARB's, digoxin, β-blockers, NSAIDs,*** Cyclosporine. • ***Cell lysis:*** rhabdomyolysis, burns, hypovolemia, thrombocytosis, tumor lysis syndrome, leukocytosis (intracellular release of K^+ from cell lysis). • K^+ redistribution: ***metabolic acidosis**** (DKA), catabolic states • ***Pseudohyperkalemia: venipuncture MC,*** lab error.
CLINICAL MANIFESTATIONS	• **Neuromuscular**: severe muscle weakness (including respiratory), rhabdomyolysis, ***nephrogenic DI: POLYURIA**** (affects renal concentrating ability), myoglobinuria, cramps, nausea/vomiting, ileus, ***↓DTR.*** • **Cardiovascular:** palpitations, arrhythmias.	Serum levels & symptoms not consistent. Rapidity in serum K^+ change influences symptoms more than levels. • **Neuromuscular:** weakness (progressive ascending), fatigue, paresthesias, flaccid paralysis. • **Cardiovascular:** palpitations, cardiac arrhythmias. • **GI:** abdominal distention, diarrhea.
LAB FINDINGS	• BMP: potassium < 3.5 mEq/L. Magnesium, glucose, bicarbonate ordered in the workup.	• ***Potassium >5.0*** mEq/L. Glucose, bicarbonate part of the workup. • ±CBC (hemolysis), ±CK (rhabdomyolysis).
ECG FINDINGS	• ***T wave flattening*** *(earliest change)* ⇨***prominent U wave**** ±Hypomagnesemia changes Prominent U wave	• ***Tall peaked T waves**** ⇨ ***QR interval shortening, wide QRS,*** prolonged PRI ⇨ ***P wave flattening*** ⇨sine wave ⇨ arrhythmias. Peaked T waves
MANAGEMENT	• ***Potassium replacement:*** KCl oral if possible IV KCl given for rapid treatment/severe sx. • *High dose KCl given in central line.* ***Hypokalemia associated with ↑risk of digoxin toxicity.**** • Potassium sparing diuretics: *Spironolactone, Amiloride* • ***If hypomagnesemia present, it may be hard to replenish potassium*** *(so tx hypomagnesemia)* • Use nondextrose IV solutions (because dextrose induced insulin release will shift K^+ into cells).	Repeat blood draw to verify not from hemolysis during blood draw (since venipuncture may cause cell lysis). • ***IV Calcium gluconate:* stabilizes the cardiac membrane*** used for ***severe symptoms, K^+ > 6.5, ⊕ significant ECG findings***. Given over 30-60min. Given simultaneously with other tx for hyperkalemia. • ***Insulin (with glucose): insulin shifts K^+ intracellularly*** glucose given to prevent hypoglycemia from insulin. • Sodium polystyrene sulfonate (***Kayexalate***): ***enhances GI potassium excretion. Lowers total body K^+*** • ***$Beta_2$ agonists***: 4-8 times dosing use for asthma. 12-20mg via nebulizer. • Bicarbonate: not usually given unless metabolic acidosis also present • Loop diuretics, Fludrocortisone (synthetic mineralocorticoid). • Dialysis if severe.

LUNGS: CO_2 regulation via respiratory rate (min-hours). Acidosis stimulates ↑respiration (to blow off excess CO_2). Alkalosis depresses respiration (to retain CO_2).

KIDNEYS:

- **generates new HCO_3^- by eliminating H^+** from body (adds one HCO_3^- for every H^+ secreted)
- **reabsorbs virtually all filtered HCO_3^-:** at the **proximal tubule**.
  ↑HCO_3^- reabsorption seen with ↑PCO_2, hypovolemia, hypokalemia.

Anion Gap Metabolic Acidosis	Non-Gap Metabolic Acidosis	Acute Respiratory Acidosis	Metabolic Alkalosis	Respiratory Alkalosis
"MUDPILERS" **M**ethanol **U**remia **D**KA/Alcoholic KA **P**ropylene glycol **I**soniazid, Infection **L**actic Acidosis **E**thylene Glycol **R**habdo/**R**enal Failure **S**alicylates	**"HARDUPS"** **H**yperalimentation **Acetazolamide** **R**enal Tubular Acidosis **Diarrhea** **U**retero-Pelvic Shunt **P**ost-Hypocapnia **S**pironolactone	anything that causes hypoventilation, i.e.: "CHAMPP" CNS depression (drugs/CVA) Hemo/Pneumothorax Airway Obstruction Myopathy Pneumonia Pulmonary Edema	**"CLEVER PD"** **C**ontraction **L**icorice* **E**ndo* (Ex Conn's, Cushing's) **V**omiting **E**xcess Alkali* **R**efeeding Alkalosis* **P**ost-hypercapnia **D**iuretics*	**"CHAMPS"** anything that causes hyperventilation, i.e.: **C**NS disease **H**ypoxia **A**nxiety **M**ech Ventilators **P**rogesterone **S**alicylates/Sepsis
Too much acid or little Bicarbonate	**Too much acid or little Bicarbonate**	**Anything that decreases respiration**	**Little acid or too much bicarbonate**	**Anything that causes hyperventilation**

HIGH ANION GAP METABOLIC ACIDOSIS

↑Anion Gap acidosis: the acid in blood dissociates into H^+ & an anion not routinely measured (the H^+ is buffered by HCO_3^- leaving the unmeasured anion to accumulate in serum, creating the AG)

$$H\mathbf{Ua} + NaHCO_3 \Rightarrow Na\mathbf{Ua} + H_2CO_3 \Rightarrow CO_2 + H_2O$$

NORMAL GAP METABOLIC ACIDOSIS (HYPERCHLOREMIC)

Normal Gap Acidosis: lost HCO_3^- is replaced by Cl^- (a measured anion) so there is no change in AG but there is an accumulation of Cl^- concentration. In other cases (diarrhea, type II RTA) there is loss of $NaHCO_3$ and the kidney tries to preserve volume by retaining NaCl (same overall sequelae).

$$HCl + NaHCO_3 \Rightarrow NaCl + H_2CO_3 \Rightarrow CO_2 + H_2O$$

METABOLIC ALKALOSIS

- **↑HCO_3^- (serum) with ↑pH** requires generating & maintenance factors.

ETIOLOGIES (GENERATING FACTORS)

1. **Loss of H^+ from GI tract/kidneys: vomiting/NG suction (loss of gastric HCl** that is perpetuated by EFCV depletion), chronic diarrhea (also perpetuated by EFCV depletion), loop diuretics.
2. **Exogenous alkali or contraction alkalosis:** diuresis ⇨ excretion of HCO_3^- poor fluid ⇨EFCV "contracts" around stable level of HCO_3^- ⇨ ↑HCO_3^- concentration.
3. **Post hypercapnia:** rapid correction of respiratory hypercapnia (eg, mechanical ventilation) ⇨ transient excess HCO_3^- until kidney can excrete it.

RESPIRATORY ACIDOSIS

Anything that decreases respiration.

1. **Acute Respiratory failure: CNS depression** (opioids, sedatives, trauma), cardiopulmonary arrest, pneumonia.
2. **Chronic respiratory failure:** COPD, obesity, neuromuscular disorders (ex. Myasthenia gravis, Guillain-Barré syndrome etc).

RESPIRATORY ALKALOSIS

1. **Hyperventilation:** CNS disorders, pain, anxiety, salicylates, progesterone, pregnancy, hepatic failure, stimulation of pulmonary receptors (pneumonia, asthma).

SIMPLIFIED 3-STEP APPROACH TO ACID BASE DISORDERS

Normal Values: Na: 135-145; Cl: 105, HCO_3^-: 24 (22-26); P_{CO2} = 40 (35-45); AG 10-12; pH = 7.35-7.45, PO_2: 80-100

Step 1: Identify the most *apparent* disorder ✓pH

pH normally 7.35 – 7.45. If in normal range, still check PCO_2 & HCO_3. If abnormal, a disorder may be present.

If pH > 7.45 ⇨ Alkalosis

If pH < 7.35 ⇨ Acidosis

Step 2: Look at P_{CO2} is it normal, low or high??

Normal P_{CO2} 35-45

- ***If P_{CO2} is in going in the opposite direction as the pH, then the 1ry disorder is respiratory.***
- Think **RO**ME (In primary **R**espiratory disorders, P_{CO2} & pH are in **O**pposite directions).
- Respiratory compensation: in primary metabolic disorders, if the P_{CO2} is going in the same direction as the pH, then there is partial respiratory compensation (full compensation if the pH is normal).

Step 3: ***Look at [HCO_3^-] it normal, low or high?***

Normal *[HCO_3^-]* 22-26

- ***If [HCO_3^-] is in going in the same direction as the pH, then the 1ry disorder is metabolic.***
- Think RO**ME** (In primary **M**etabolic disorders, HCO_3 & pH are in the same/**E**qual direction).
- Metabolic compensation: in primary respiratory disorders, if the [HCO_3^-] is going in the opposite direction as the pH, then there is a partial metabolic compensation (full compensation if the pH is normal).

Perform step 4 & 5 ONLY if the primary disorder is metabolic acidosis.

Step 4: If metabolic acidosis is present, calculate the anion gap.

Anion gap (AG) = Na - (Cl^- + $HCO3^-$) Normal anion gap 10 - 12

Step 5: If a high anion gap is present in step 4, perform step 5 - calculate the **Delta Ratio** to look for the presence of additional disorders.

(Measured AG – 12)/(24 – measured bicarbonate)

$$\frac{\text{Measured anion gap} - \text{Normal AG (use 12)}}{\text{Normal Bicarb (use 24)} - \text{measured HCO3}}$$

- If 1-2 ⇨ pure elevated anion gap metabolic acidosis only.
- <1 ⇨ normal anion gap metabolic acidosis is also present.
- >2 ⇨ metabolic alkalosis or compensated chronic respiratory acidosis is also present.

EXAMPLE 1: 21 year old with Type I DM presents with nausea vomiting, fruity breath.

pH: 7.29 paCO2: 22 HCO3: 13 Na: 134 Cl: 91 HCO3: 12

CASE 1: pH: 7.45	paCO2: 56	HCO3: 37		
CASE 2: pH: 7.29	paCO2: 58	HCO3: 22		
CASE 3: pH: 7.32	paCO2: 34	HCO3: 14	Na: 135 Cl: 109 HCO3: 14	
CASE 4: pH: 7.49	paCO2: 42	HCO3: 36		
CASE 5: pH: 7.36	paCO2: 58	HCO3: 29		
CASE 6: pH: 7.25	paCO2: 25	HCO3: 10	Na: 140 Cl: 77 HCO3: 10	
CASE 7: pH: 7.48	paCO2: 28	HCO3: 18		
CASE 8: pH: 7.28	paCO2: 26	HCO3: 11	Na: 129 Cl: 100 HCO3: 10	

EXAMPLE 1 explained: 21 year old with Type I DM presents with nausea vomiting, fruity breath.

Na: 134	Cl: 91	BUN: 29	pH: 7.29	pCO2: 22
K: 5.8	HCO3: 13	Cr: 1.6	HCO3: 12	glucose: 780

Step 1: Identify the most *apparent* disorder ✓pH

pH normally 7.35 – 7.45. **pH = 7.29** ↓⇨***Acidosis***

Step 2: Look at P_{CO2} is it normal, low or high??

Normal P_{CO2} 35–45. **pCO2: 22**↓ Normal [HCO_3^-] 22-26. **HCO3: 12**↓

- Think RO**ME** (In primary **M**etabolic disorders, HCO_3 & pH are in the same/**E**qual direction) = ***primary metabolic acidosis.***
- In primary metabolic disorders, if the P_{CO2} is going in the same direction as pH (which it is in this example), then there is partial respiratory compensation.

Perform step 4 & 5 ONLY if a metabolic acidosis is the primary disorder (which it is in this example)

Step 4: If metabolic acidosis is present, calculate the anion gap.

AG = Na - (Cl^- + $HCO3^-$) Normal anion gap 10 – 12. 134 – (91 + 13) = 30 = ↑***AG acidosis***

Step 5: If high anion gap is present, calculate the **Delta Ratio** to look for the presence of additional disorders.

(Measured AG – 12)/(24 – measured bicarbonate) (30-12)/(24-13) = **1.64**

- If 1-2 = ***pure elevated anion gap metabolic acidosis = final answer*** (probably DKA in this case).

ANSWERS

Case 1: Primary Metabolic Alkalosis with full respiratory compensation (normal pH)

Case 2: Primary Respiratory Acidosis uncompensated (since HCO3 is normal)

Case 3: Normal Gap Metabolic Acidosis with partial respiratory compensation.

Case 4: Primary Metabolic Alkalosis uncompensated (since PCO2 is normal)

Case 5: Primary Respiratory Acidosis with full metabolic compensation (normal pH)

Case 6: Mixed disorder: Primary elevated anion gap acidosis + metabolic alkalosis (delta >2).

Case 7: Primary Respiratory Alkalosis with partial metabolic compensation.

Case 8: Primary high anion gap metabolic acidosis with partial respiratory compensation + concurrent non anion gap acidosis (since delta <1)

RENAL CELL CARCINOMA

- Tumor of the proximal convoluted renal tubule cells (they are very metabolically active cells so they are the most prone to dysplasia).
- **95% of primary tumors originating in the kidney (clear cell most common** histological pattern).
- Characterized by lack of warning signs, variable presentations, & resistance to chemo & radiation.

RISK FACTORS
- **Smoking, hypertension, obesity, men, dialysis,** cadmium or industrial exposure.

CLINICAL MANIFESTATIONS
- **Classic triad of hematuria, flank or abdominal pain, & palpable abdominal mass.** The triad is classically seen in locally advanced disease.
- Hypertension & hypercalcemia common.
- **Left-sided varicocele** if the tumor blocks left testicular vein drainage. Malaise, weight loss.
- METS: **cannon ball metastases to the lungs** (most common site of metastasis); Bone.

DIAGNOSIS
- **CT scan usually the initial test.** Renal ultrasound, MRI. Erythrocytosis often present.

MANAGEMENT
- Stage I-III: **radical nephrectomy.** Immune-mediated therapy (eg, interleukin-2 and monoclonal antibody molecular targeted treatment). Usually resistant to chemo and radiation therapy.
- Partial nephrectomy patients with bilateral involvement of solitary kidney or an option in early disease.
- Molecularly targeted agents and debulking nephrectomy may be used in advanced disease.

NEPHROBLASTOMA (WILMS TUMOR)

- **Most commonly seen in children within the first 5 years of life.**
- Most common renal malignancy in children (**most common abdominal mass in children**).

RISK FACTORS
- May be associated with other GU abnormalities (eg, cryptorchidism, hypospadias, horseshoe kidney). WAGR (**W**ilms tumor, **A**niridia, **G**enitourinary malformations & mental **R**etardation) associated with chromosome 11 abnormalities.
- Beckwith-Wiedemann syndrome (Wilms tumor, adrenal cytomegaly, hemihypertrophy).

CLINICAL MANIFESTATIONS
- **Palpable abdominal mass most common manifestation.** The mass **doesn't cross the midline** (unlike Neuroblastoma).
- **Hematuria, constipation,** abdominal pain, nausea, vomiting, hypertension, anemia, anorexia, fever.

DIAGNOSIS
- **Abdominal ultrasound best initial test.**
- CT with contrast or MRI most accurate imaging tests.
- Lung is the common site for METS so chest imaging usually required.

MANAGEMENT
- **Total nephrectomy followed by chemotherapy.** 80-90% cure rate. Partial nephrectomy if bilateral involvement.
- Post-surgery radiation therapy if it extends beyond renal capsule, pulmonary METS, or large tumor.

CHAPTER 9 - GENITOURINARY SYSTEM (MALE AND FEMALE)

URGE INCONTINENCE

- Involuntary urine leakage preceded by or accompanied by sudden urge to urinate.
- **Most common in older women.**

PATHOPHYSIOLOGY
- **Detrusor muscle overactivity:** detrusor muscle is stimulated by muscarinic acetylcholine receptors. Detrusor overactivity leads to uninhibited (involuntary) detrusor muscle contractions during bladder filling.
- Etiologies: increased age, idiopathic & bladder infection (eg, cystitis).
- Clinical manifestations: increased urgency, frequency, small volume voids, **nocturia.** The patient has a strong urge to void with an inability to make it to the bathroom in time.

MANAGEMENT
- **Bladder training:** (75% improvement). Timed frequent voiding, using a voiding diary to identify the shortest voiding intervals, decreased fluid intake. Diet: avoidance of spicy foods, citrus fruit, chocolate, alcohol, & caffeine. Lifestyle modifications & Kegel exercises.
- **Antimuscarinics: first-line medical therapy (eg, Tolterodine, Oxybutynin).** Mechanism: **anticholinergics**, antispasmodics that also increase bladder capacity.
- **Mirabegron:** beta-3 agonist that causes bladder relaxation.
- Tricyclic antidepressants: Imipramine. Mechanism: central & peripheral anticholinergic effect & alpha-adrenergic agonist (bladder muscle relaxation, increased bladder outlet resistance, antispasmodic effect on detrusor muscle, & increased urethral sphincter tone.
- Surgical: increases bladder compliance: injection of Botox, bladder augmentation.

OVERFLOW INCONTINENCE

- Urinary retention & incomplete bladder emptying leads to involuntary urine leakage once the bladder is full (it overflows).

PATHOPHYSIOLOGY
- **Bladder detrusor muscle underactivity** (impaired contractility) or bladder outlet obstruction.

ETIOLOGIES
- **Most common in neurological disorders or autonomic dysfunction** - Diabetes Mellitus, Multiple Sclerosis, spinal injuries, spinal stenosis, peripheral neuropathy associated with vitamin B12 deficiency.
- Also common with bladder outlet obstruction - **Benign prostatic hypertrophy,** uterine fibroids, pelvic organ prolapse, or overcorrection of the urethra from prior pelvic floor surgery.

CLINICAL MANIFESTATION
- Loss of urine with no warning (as in urge) or triggers (as in stress).
- Leakage or dribbling in the setting of incomplete bladder emptying, weak or intermittent urinary stream, hesitancy, frequency & nocturia. Leakage often occurs with changes in position.

DIAGNOSIS:
- Clinical. **Post void residual >200ml.**

MANAGEMENT OF BLADDER ATONY
- **Intermittent or indwelling catheterization first-line treatment.**
- **Cholinergics** (eg, **Bethanechol**) - increases detrusor muscle activity.

MANAGEMENT OF BPH: alpha-blockers for rapid symptom relief. 5-alpha reductase inhibitors.

STRESS INCONTINENCE

- Involuntary leakage of urine that occurs once **increased abdominal pressure** (eg, exertion, coughing, laughing, sneezing) **> than urethral pressure** & resistance to urine flow.

- Most common type of incontinence in younger women (highest incidence 45 – 49 years).

ETIOLOGIES

- **Laxity of the pelvic floor muscles** (eg, childbirth, surgery, postmenopausal estrogen loss). Although rare in men, post prostatectomy may be associated with stress incontinence.

- **Urethral hypermobility** - insufficient support from the pelvic floor musculature and the vaginal connective tissue to the urethra & the bladder neck.

CLINICAL MANIFESTATIONS

- Urine leakage during times of increased intra-abdominal pressure (eg, coughing, laughing, sneezing, lifting heavy objects). There is no urge to urinate prior to leakage.

MANAGEMENT

- **Pelvic floor muscle (Kegel) exercises: initial treatment of choice.** Kegel supportive therapy includes supervised therapy, vaginal weighted cones or biofeedback. Bladder training (eg, timed voidings), topical estrogen for postmenopausal women with vaginal atrophy.

- **Lifestyle modifications: used in conjunction with pelvic floor exercises** - protective garments & pads, weight loss, smoking cessation, & drinking smaller amounts of water throughout the day.

- **Pessaries:** used if incomplete efficacy with lifestyle changes & muscle strengthening or situational stress incontinence.

- **Surgery: midurethral sling – higher success rates than conservative therapy.** More rapid & definitive treatment.

- Alpha-agonists: Midodrine & Pseudoephedrine. Only mildly efficacious.

UTERINE PROLAPSE

- Uterine herniation into the vagina.

RISK FACTORS

- **Weakness of pelvic support structures: most common after childbirth** (especially traumatic), increased pelvic floor pressure: multiple vaginal births, obesity, repeated heavy lifting. Loss of estrogen (postmenopause).

CLINICAL MANIFESTATIONS

- Vaginal fullness, heaviness or "falling out" sensation. Low back pain, abdominal pain.
- Symptoms may be worse with prolonged standing and relieved with lying down.
- Urinary urgency, frequency, or stress incontinence.

PHYSICAL EXAMINATION

Bulging mass especially with increased intrabdominal pressure (eg, Valsalva).

- Grades: 0 (no descent) to 4 (through the hymen).
- Grade 0: no descent
- Grade 1: uterus descent into the upper 2/3 of the vagina
- Grade 2: the cervix approaches the introitus
- Grade 3: the cervix is outside the introitus
- Grade 4: entire uterus is outside of the vagina -complete rupture
- May be accompanied by **cystocele** (posterior bladder herniating into the **anterior vagina**), **enterocele** (pouch of Douglas – small bowel herniating into the **upper vagina**) or **rectocele** (distal sigmoid colon or rectum herniating into the **posterior distal vagina)**.

MANAGEMENT

- Mechanical: pessaries elevate & support the uterus. Estrogen treatment may improve atrophy.

- Surgical: hysterectomy or uterus-sparing techniques including uterosacral or sacrospinous ligament fixation.

PEYRONIE DISEASE

- Acquired localized fibrotic changes of the tunica albuginea leading to **abnormal penile curvature.**

PATHOPHYSIOLOGY

- Unknown but contributing factors include penile trauma, tissue ischemia & genetic susceptibility. This leads to excessive collagen (fibrous plaque).

CLINICAL MANIFESTATIONS

- Penile pain, curvature, induration, shortening and/or sexual dysfunction.

MANAGEMENT

- Observation: urologist referral. Observation is an option for mild curvature (30 degrees or less) in men with satisfactory function.

- Medical or surgical management: if curvature 30 degrees or more or associated with sexual dysfunction. Oral Pentoxifylline if within 3 months of onset. Intralesional injection with collagenase *Clostridium histolyticum* if > 3 months.

PANCE PREP PEARL OF THE WEEK

PRERENAL VS. ACUTE TUBULAR NECROSIS

	PRERENAL AZOTEMIA	ACUTE TUBULAR NECROSIS (ATN)
Etiologies	**Decreased renal perfusion** – hypovolemia from: • GI loss - diarrhea, vomiting • Renal loss – diuretics • Blood or insensible loss – e.g., hemorrhage, burns	• **Ischemic: prolonged prerenal** • **Nephrotoxic:** **contrast dye, aminoglycosides,** uric acid (tumor lysis syndrome), myoglobinuria (rhabdomyolysis), Bence-jones protein (multiple myeloma), Cyclosporine
Pathophysiology	Because kidney is intact, **water & electrolyte conservation intact** leading to following labs:	Because of tubular damage, **water & electrolyte conservation impaired** leading to following labs:
BUN:Creatinine	**> 20:1**	<20:1
Urine sodium	**Decreased** (<20 mEq/L) if not due to diuretics	>40
FeNa	**<1%** (same as urine sodium)	**>2-3%**
Urine osmolarity	**Increased** (> 500 mOsm/kg)	**Isosthenuria – inability to concentrate the urine** (< 500 mOsm/kg)
Specific gravity	**Increased** (same as Urine osm)	Decreased
UA	Normal urine sediment	**Epithelial or Muddy brown casts**

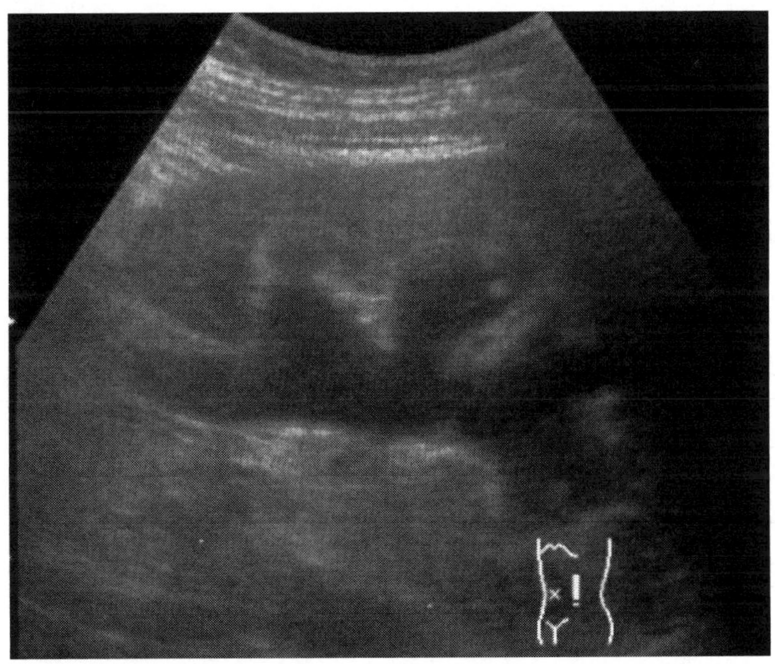

Ultrasound image of Hydronephrosis due to a ureteral stone
morning2k [CC BY-SA 3.0 (http://creativecommons.org/licenses/by-sa/3.0/)]

VESICOURETERAL REFLUX

- Retrograde passage of urine from the bladder into the upper urinary tract.

TYPES

- **Primary VUR: most common type.** Due to inadequate closure of or incompetent ureterovesical junction that contains a segment of the ureter within the bladder wall. Low-grade reflux (grades I and II).

- Secondary VUR: due to abnormally high voiding pressure in the bladder that leads to failure of the closure of the UVJ during bladder contraction.

CLINICAL MANIFESTATIONS

- Prenatal presentation – hydronephrosis on prenatal ultrasound.
- Postnatal – **febrile UTI.**

DIAGNOSIS

- **Renal & bladder ultrasound often the initial imaging ordered** (but may miss significant VUR).

- **Voiding cystourethrogram imaging test of choice to diagnose VUR** (or radionuclide cystogram).

- An initial postnatal renal ultrasound is performed in all patients with prenatal hydronephrosis.

- A VCUG is performed in infants with persistent postnatal abnormal ultrasound findings or who develop a UTI.

MANAGEMENT

- Grades I and II: **observation or antibiotic prophylaxis** to reduce the risk of recurrent UTI (eg, Trimethoprim-sulfamethoxazole, Trimethoprim or Nitrofurantoin).

- Grades III & IV: **surgical correction** definitive treatment.

ACUTE CYSTITIS

- Pathophysiology: usually an ascending infection of the lower urinary tract from the urethra.

RISK FACTORS
- Women: sexual intercourse "honeymoon cystitis", spermicidal use (especially with diaphragm).
- Pregnancy: progesterone & estrogen causes ureter dilation & inhibition of bladder peristalsis.
- Elderly & Postmenopausal, Diabetes mellitus & presence of an indwelling catheter. In children, may indicate vesicourethral reflux.
- Infants (should receive a bladder and renal ultrasound to rule out congenital abnormalities).
- Complicated: **underlying condition with risk of therapeutic failure**: symptoms >7 days, pregnancy, diabetics, immunosuppression, indwelling catheter, anatomic abnormality, elderly, males.

ETIOLOGIES
- ***Escherichia coli*** **most common** (>80%),
- ***Staphylococcus saprophyticus*** 2nd most common in sexually active women.
- Other gram-negative uropathogens - *Klebsiella, Proteus, Enterobacter,* & *Pseudomonas.*
- Enterococci with indwelling catheters.

CLINICAL MANIFESTATIONS
- Irritative symptoms: **dysuria** (burning), **frequency, & urgency.**
- **Hematuria, suprapubic pain, & tenderness** may occur.

DIAGNOSIS
- Urinalysis: **pyuria (>10 WBCs/hpf)**, hematuria, leukocyte esterase; nitrites, cloudy urine, bacteriuria, increased pH with Proteus.

- Urine culture: **definitive diagnosis. Women:** ≥1,000 CFU/ml of uropathogens - **clean catch specimen.** Epithelial (squamous cells) = contamination.
  - Indications: complicated UTI, infants or children, elderly, males, urologic abnormalities, refractory to treatment, or catheterized patients.

MANAGEMENT OF UNCOMPLICATED
- 1st-line: **Nitrofurantoin** or **Trimethoprim-sulfamethoxazole** or Fosfomycin (if resistance pattern < 20%)
- 2nd-line: **Fluoroquinolones** (may be used first line if sulfa allergies or increased resistance patterns). Cephalosporins or Cefpodoxime.

ADJUNCT
- Increase fluid intake, void after intercourse, Hot sitz baths may provide relief of abdominal discomfort.
- **Phenazopyridine is a bladder analgesic** not used more than 48h due to side effects (methemoglobinemia, hemolytic anemia). **Inform the patient Phenazopyridine turns the urine an orange color.**

COMPLICATED
- **Fluoroquinolones PO or IV, Aminoglycosides** x 7-10 or 14 days (depending on the severity).

CYSTITIS DURING PREGNANCY
- Amoxicillin, Amoxicillin-clavulanate, Cephalexin, Cefpodoxime, Nitrofurantoin, & Fosfomycin. Sulfisoxazole is safe except in last days of pregnancy (can lead to kernicterus).
- Avoid Trimethoprim-sulfamethoxazole in the first trimester, Aminoglycosides, Fluoroquinolones, and Doxycycline.

ASYMPTOMATIC BACTERIURIA

- Asymptomatic patient with incidental bacteriuria on urinalysis.
- **No treatment needed:** general population, elderly, diabetics, nonpregnant premenopausal women, spinal cord injury patients or patients with chronic indwelling urinary catheters.
- **Treatment needed:** pregnancy, patients with urologic intervention & hip arthroplasty.
- Pregnancy requires screening & treatment because it can be associated with pre-term birth, perinatal death, & pyelonephritis in the mother.

PYELONEPHRITIS

- Infection of the **upper genitourinary tract** (kidney parenchyma & renal pelvis).

PATHOPHYSIOLOGY
- Usually an ascending infection from the lower urinary tract.

ETIOLOGIES
- ***E. coli* most common (>80%)**, other gram-negative uropathogens (eg, *Proteus, Enterobacter, Klebsiella* & *Pseudomonas). Enterococci* with indwelling catheters.

RISK FACTORS
- Diabetes mellitus, history of recurrent UTIs or kidney stones, pregnancy, congenital urinary tract malformations.

CLINICAL MANIFESTATIONS
- Upper tract symptoms: **fever, chills, back or flank pain. Nausea & vomiting** not common but suggestive.
- Lower tract symptoms: dysuria, urgency, & frequency.

PHYSICAL EXAMINATION
- **⊕ costovertebral angle tenderness, fever, & tachycardia.**

DIAGNOSIS
- UA: **Pyuria [>10 WBCs**/hpf], + leukocyte esterase, +Nitrites (90% bacteria causing UTIs), hematuria, cloudy urine, bacteriuria. **WBC casts hallmark of Pyelonephritis.** Increased pH with Proteus.
- CBC: leukocytosis with left shift.
- **Urine culture definitive diagnosis.**

OUTPATIENT MANAGEMENT
- **Fluoroquinolones first-line** (if resistance rate < 10%).
- If resistance > 10%, initiate either IV Ceftriaxone or Gentamicin followed by an oral Fluoroquinolone.

INPATIENT MANAGEMENT
- **Third- or fourth-generation Cephalosporins, Fluoroquinolones, Aminoglycosides, or extended-spectrum Penicillins** total duration 2 weeks.
  - Indications for admission include older age, signs of obstruction, comorbid conditions, or inability to tolerate oral antibiotics.

PREGNANCY
- **IV Ceftriaxone first-line**. Aztreonam if Penicillin-allergic.
- Avoid Trimethoprim-Sulfamethoxazole, Aminoglycosides, Fluoroquinolones, & Tetracyclines.

URETHRITIS

- **Nongonococcal urethritis (NGU):**
  - ***Chlamydia trachomatis*** **is the most common cause of nongonococcal urethritis.** *Chlamydia trachomatis* is also the most common bacterial STI in the US. 5-8 days incubation period followed by purulent or mucopurulent discharge. May be associated with pruritus, hematuria, or dyspareunia. Up to 40% asymptomatic.

  - Others include *Ureaplasma urealyticum, Trichomonas vaginalis, M. genitalium,* & viruses.

- **Gonococcal urethritis:** abrupt onset of symptoms (especially within 3-4 days). Opaque, yellow, white or clear thick discharge, pruritus. Up to 20% of patients are asymptomatic.

CLINICAL MANIFESTATIONS

- **Urethral discharge** & **penile or vaginal pruritus**.

- **Dysuria** seen in both gonococcal & nongonococcal urethritis.

- Abdominal pain or abnormal vaginal bleeding.

DIAGNOSIS

- **Nucleic acid amplification most sensitive & specific for *C. trachomatis, N. gonorrhoeae*** & *M. genitalium* (recommended over culture). First-void or first-catch urine ideal.

- Gram stain: 2 or more WBCs/hpf. No organisms seen suggestive of NGU. Gram-negative diplococci = *N. gonorrhoeae*. Urethral swab.

- Urinalysis or dipstick: positive leukocyte esterase on dipstick or 10 or more WBCs/hpf (pyuria) on microscopy suggestive.

MANAGEMENT

- 25-30% of patients have co-infection of both **Gonorrhea & Chlamydia** so **empiric treatment of both** is recommended if test results are not available.

Based on testing:

- ***N. gonorrhoeae*:** **Ceftriaxone 250mg** IM x 1 dose **PLUS Azithromycin** 1g x 1 dose (for additional coverage for Gonorrhea due to increased resistance as well as to cover possible Chlamydia).

- **Chlamydia: Azithromycin** 1g orally (single observed dose) or **Doxycycline** 100mg orally bid x 10 days.

PROSTATITIS

- Prostate gland inflammation secondary to an ascending infection.

ETIOLOGIES OF ACUTE PROSTATITIS

- **> 35 years:** ***Escherichia coli* most common,** other gram-negatives - *Proteus*, Enterobacteriaceae (*Klebsiella, Enterobacter* & *Serratia* species), *Pseudomonas.*
- **< 35 years: Chlamydia & Gonorrhea most common,** *E. coli, Treponema, Trichomonas, Gardnerella.*
- Children: viral (Mumps most common cause).

ETIOLOGIES OF CHRONIC PROSTATITIS

- ***Escherichia coli* most common** (~80%), ***Proteus,*** *Enterococci, Trichomonas,* HIV, inflammatory.
- Structural or functional abnormality, recurrent UTIs.
- Acute prostatitis may progress to chronic (> 3 months).

CLINICAL MANIFESTATIONS

- Irritative voiding symptoms: frequency, urgency, & dysuria.
- Obstructive symptoms: hesitancy, poor or interrupted stream, straining to void, & incomplete emptying. Malaise, arthralgias
- **Acute: fever, chills, perineal pain.** Lower back or abdominal pain.
- **Chronic:** usually presents as **recurrent UTIs or intermittent dysfunction**. Malaise, arthralgias. Symptoms are milder. Fever not common.

PHYSICAL EXAMINATION

Boggy prostate = Prostatitis

- Acute: **exquisitely tender,** normal or hot, **boggy prostate.**
- Chronic: **usually nontender, boggy prostate.**

DIAGNOSIS

- Urinalysis & urine culture: pyuria & bacteriuria in Acute prostatitis. UA & culture often negative in chronic so prostatic massage often done in chronic prostatitis to increase bacterial yield on UA/culture. **Avoid prostatic massage in Acute prostatitis** (may cause bacteremia).
- Transrectal ultrasound or CT scan of the pelvis with IV contrast may be helpful for suspected prostatic abscess.

MANAGEMENT

- **Acute > 35 years: Fluoroquinolones or Trimethoprim-sulfamethoxazole** x 4-6 weeks (outpatient). If hospitalized: IV fluoroquinolones with or without Aminoglycoside OR Ampicillin with or without Gentamicin.
- **Acute < 35 years or STI likely:** cover for Gonorrhea & Chlamydia - **Ceftriaxone plus Doxycycline** (Azithromycin an alternative to Doxycycline).
- Chronic: Fluoroquinolones or Trimethoprim-sulfamethoxazole x 6-12 weeks. Alpha blockers (eg, Tamsulosin) can help with chronic pain syndrome.
- Refractory chronic: **Transurethral resection of the prostate (TURP).**

EXAM TIP

- Acute Prostatitis: **exquisitely tender, normal or hot, boggy prostate.**
- Chronic Prostatitis: **usually nontender** (or minimally tender), **boggy prostate.**
- Benign prostatic hypertrophy: symmetrically enlarged, firm, nontender prostate.
- Prostate cancer: rock hard prostate.

EPIDIDYMITIS

- Epididymal pain & swelling thought to be secondary to retrograde infection or reflux of urine. Bacterial infection most common cause.

ETIOLOGIES

- **Males 14 - 35 years:** ***Chlamydia trachomatis*** **(most common) &** ***Neisseria gonorrhoeae***. *Ureaplasma, E. coli, Treponema, Trichomonas & Gardnerella.*
- **Men >35y:** enteric organisms - (***E. coli*** **most common**), *Klebsiella, Pseudomonas, & Proteus.*
- Prepubertal: viruses, bacterial (*E. coli, Mycoplasma pneumoniae*).

CLINICAL MANIFESTATIONS

- **Gradual onset** (over a few hours to days) of **localized testicular pain and swelling** (usually unilateral). Groin, flank, or abdominal pain.
- May be associated with fever, chills, or irritative symptoms (dysuria, urgency, frequency).

PHYSICAL EXAMINATION

- Scrotal swelling and tenderness. Epididymal tenderness & induration (posterior & superior to the testicle). The affected testis is usually in normal (vertical) position.
- **Positive Prehn sign – relief of pain with scrotal elevation** (classic but not reliable).
- **Positive (normal) cremasteric reflex** – elevation of the testicle after stroking the inner thigh.

DIAGNOSIS

- **Scrotal ultrasound best initial test - enlarged epididymis, increased testicular blood flow.** US also done to rule out Testicular torsion.
- UA: pyuria (increased WBCs) or bacteriuria.
- Nucleic acid amplification for *N. Gonorrhoeae* & *Chlamydia.*

MANAGEMENT

- Scrotal elevation, NSAIDs, cool compresses.
- <35 years or STI likely: **cover** ***Chlamydia*** **&** ***N. Gonorrhoeae*** - **Doxycycline** (100mg bid x 10d) **PLUS Ceftriaxone** (250mg IM x 1). Azithromycin 1g x 1 dose is an alternative to Doxycycline.
- **>35 years:** cover enteric organisms (eg, ***E. coli***) - **Fluoroquinolones** (eg, Ciprofloxacin, Ofloxacin, Levofloxacin). Trimethoprim-sulfamethoxazole alternative.
- Bacterial in children: Cephalexin or Amoxicillin.

ORCHITIS

ETIOLOGIES

- **Viral most common** (eg, **Mumps,** Echovirus, coxsackie, rubella).

CLINICAL MANIFESTATIONS

- Scrotal pain, swelling, and tenderness.
- Physical examination: scrotal erythema and tenderness.

MANAGEMENT

- **Symptomatic management first-line –** NSAIDs, bed rest, scrotal support, & cool packs.

TESTICULAR TORSION

- **Spermatic cord twists & cuts off testicular blood supply** due to congenital malformation.
- **Males 10-20 years of age** & neonates at highest risk. **True urologic emergency.**
- Pathophysiology: insufficient fixation of the lower pole of the testis to the tunica vaginalis (bell-clapper deformity), leading to increased mobility of the testicle.

CLINICAL MANIFESTATIONS
- **Abrupt onset of scrotal, inguinal, or lower abdominal pain** (usually <6 hours).
- If nausea or vomiting is present, suspect torsion (usually absent in Epididymitis).

PHYSICAL EXAMINATION
- Swollen, tender, retracted testicle ((high-riding) that may have a horizontal lie.
- **Negative Prehn sign – no pain relief with scrotal elevation.**
- **Negative (absent) cremasteric reflex** on affected side – no elevation of the testicle after stroking the inner thigh.

DIAGNOSIS
- **Clinical diagnosis** – in patients with a history and physical examination suggestive of Torsion, imaging studies should not be performed, rather, these individuals should undergo immediate surgical exploration.
- **Emergency surgical exploration (definitive diagnosis)** - preferred over ultrasound if Torsion is very likely.
- **Testicular Doppler ultrasound** most commonly used imaging modality – decreased or absent testicular blood flow.
- Radionuclide scan – most specific imaging study (not used often).

MANAGEMENT
- **Urgent detorsion & orchiopexy ideally within 6 hours of pain onset** (irreversible damage likely after 12 hours of ischemia).
- Manual detorsion should be performed if surgical intervention is not immediately available.
- Orchiectomy if not salvageable.

TORSION OF APPENDIX TESTIS

- Most cases are seen in children 7- 14 years.

CLINICAL MANIFESTATIONS:
- Abrupt testicular pain (usually more gradual compared to Testicular torsion).

Physical examination:
- Torsed appendage **"blue dot" sign** – bluish discoloration in the scrotal area directly over the torsed appendage (infarction and necrosis).
- May also be associated with a reactive hydrocele.

DIAGNOSIS
- Primary clinical.
- Color doppler US: low echogenicity of the torsed appendage with a central hypoechogenic area.

MANAGEMENT
- Local application of ice & NSAIDs.
- Surgical excision of the appendix testis is usually only performed with persistent pain after initial management.

CRYPTORCHIDISM

- **Testicle that has not descended into the scrotum** by 4 months of age.
- Most descend spontaneously (~70%).
- Most common on the right side. 10% bilateral.
- Most commonly found just outside the *external ring (suprascrotal)*, inguinal canal, or in the abdomen.

INCREASED RISK
- **Prematurity** (30% of premature vs. 5% in full-term infants)
- **Low birth weight**
- Maternal obesity or Diabetes.

CLINICAL MANIFESTATIONS
- Empty, small, poorly rugated scrotum.
- May have inguinal fullness (if located in the inguinal canal).

DIAGNOSIS
- Physical examination in majority of cases.
- Scrotal ultrasound, MRI

MANAGEMENT
- **Orchiopexy** is recommended as **early as <u>4-6 months of age</u>** for congenitally undescended testicles and **definitely should be done before 2 years of age** (ideally before 1 year of age).
  Orchiopexy = testicle fixation in scrotum.
- **<u>Observation</u> can be done only if <6 months of age.** Most descend by 3 months of age (rarely spontaneously descend after 4-6 months of age).
- <u>hCG or gonadotropin releasing hormone</u>: human chorionic gonadotropin stimulates testosterone & hormonal testicular descension. Rarely used (may be used for Cryptorchidism associated with Prader-Willi syndrome.
- Orchiectomy recommended if detected at puberty to reduce testicular cancer risk.

COMPLICATIONS
- **Increased risk of Testicular cancer** (reduced with early orchiopexy), decreased fertility, Testicular torsion, Inguinal hernia.

TESTICULAR CANCER

- Most common solid tumor in young men **15 – 35 years** (average age 32).

RISK FACTORS

- **Cryptorchidism (most significant)** - 4-10 x risk in both the undescended & normal testicle.
- Caucasians, Klinefelter's syndrome, Hypospadias.

MAJOR TYPES

- **Germinal cell tumors most common** (97%) – Nonseminomas (2/3) & Seminomas (1/3).
  - **Nonseminomas:** embryonal cell carcinoma, teratoma, yolk sac (most common in boys 10y or younger), Choriocarcinoma (worst prognosis). Mixed tumors (seminomatous + nonseminomatous components). Mixed tumors are treated like Nonseminomas. **Nonseminomas are associated with increased serum alpha-fetoprotein & beta-hCG and resistance to radiation.**

  - **Seminomas:** The 4 S's of **Seminoma** - **Simple (lacks the tumor marker alpha-fetoprotein)**, **Sensitive (sensitive to radiation), Slower growing** & associated with **Stepwise spread.**

- NonGerminal cell tumors most common (3%).
  - Leydig cell tumors: may be benign. May secrete hormones (ex. androgens or estrogens), which may lead precocious puberty in children or gynecomastia/loss of libido in adults.

  - Sertoli cell tumors: often benign. May secrete hormones (ex. estrogens, androgens).

  - Gonadoblastoma, Testicular lymphoma.

CLINICAL MANIFESTATIONS

- **Testicular mass most common (usually painless)**.
- May have dull pain or testicular heaviness. Acute pain in only 10%.
- Secondary hydrocele present in 10%. Gynecomastia rare.
- Physical examination: firm, hard, fixed mass that does not transilluminate.

DIAGNOSIS

- **Scrotal ultrasound initial test of choice** - Seminoma (hypoechoic mass); Nonseminoma (cystic, nonhomogeneous mass).
- Tumor markers: **Increased alpha-fetoprotein in Nonseminomas**. Increased beta-hCG in Nonseminomas (especially Choriocarcinoma) & < 25% of Seminomas.
- Staging: CT of the abdomen, pelvis, and chest.

MANAGEMENT

- Low-grade (Stage I) Nonseminoma (limited to testes): radical orchiectomy with retroperitoneal lymph node dissection.

- Low-grade Seminoma: radical orchiectomy. May need radiation to paraaortic lymph nodes or Platinum-based chemotherapy.

- High-grade Seminoma: debulking chemotherapy followed by orchiectomy & radiation.

PROGNOSIS

- Generally excellent (5-year survival rate > 95%).

HYDROCELE

- Serous fluid collection within the layers of the tunica vaginalis of the scrotum.
- **Most common cause of painless scrotal swelling.**
- Idiopathic most common. A reactive hydrocele can occur with inflammatory conditions (eg, Epididymitis, Orchitis, Testicular tumor).

TYPES
- Communicating: peritoneal/abdominal fluid enters the scrotum via a patent processus vaginalis that failed to close.
- Noncommunicating: derived from fluid from the mesothelial lining of the tunica vaginalis (no connection to the peritoneum).

CLINICAL MANIFESTATIONS
- **Painless scrotal swelling** (may increase throughout the day).
- May complain of dull ache or heavy sensation with increasing size.

PHYSICAL EXAMINATION
- **Translucency** (transilluminates). Fluid located anterior and lateral to the testis.
- Swelling worse with Valsalva if Communicating.

DIAGNOSIS
- **Testicular ultrasound initial test of choice** - used to rule out testicular tumor & other masses.

MANAGEMENT
- **Usually no treatment needed (watchful waiting)** - often resolves within the first 12 months of life in infants. In adults they are often self-limited.
- Surgical excision may be needed if it persists beyond 1 year of age in infants, older patients with communicating hydroceles (elective) to reduce the risk of hernia, or hydroceles associated with complications.

SPERMATOCELE (EPIDIDYMAL CYST)

- **Epididymal cyst** (scrotal mass) that contains sperm.
- Spermatocele if > 2 cm.

CLINICAL MANIFESTATIONS
- Painless, cystic testicular mass.

PHYSICAL EXAMINATION
- Round, soft mass in the head of the epididymis **superior, posterior & separate from the testicle**, freely movable mass above the testicle that **transilluminates.**

DIAGNOSIS
- Scrotal ultrasound

MANAGEMENT
- **No treatment usually necessary** unless the mass is bothersome.
- Surgical excision for chronic pain (rarely needed).

VARICOCELE

- **Cystic testicular mass of <u>varicose veins:</u>** pampiniform venous plexus & internal spermatic vein.
- **Most common surgically correctable cause of male infertility** (seen in ~30% of infertile men because the increased temperature from the increased venous blood flow inhibits spermatogenesis).
- Most are left-sided (increased left renal vein pressure transmitted to left gonadal vein).

<u>CLINICAL MANIFESTATIONS</u>
- Asymptomatic varicoceles found in 10% of the population. May cause testicular atrophy.
- Usually painless but may cause a dull ache or heavy sensation.

<u>PHYSICAL EXAMINATION</u>
- Soft scrotal mass with a **"bag of worms"** feel **superior to the testicle.**
- **Dilation worsens when patient is upright or with Valsalva.**
- Less apparent when the patient is supine or with testicular elevation.

<u>DIAGNOSIS</u>
- Clinical diagnosis.
- **<u>Ultrasound</u>: initial test of choice** - dilation of the pampiniform plexus > 2 mm.

<u>MANAGEMENT</u>
- Observation in most.
- Surgery in some cases for pain, infertility or delayed testicular growth (spermatic vein ligation, varicocelectomy or percutaneous venous embolization).

<u>ASSOCIATIONS:</u>
- **Right-sided varicocele** may be due to **retroperitoneal or abdominal malignancy** (unilateral right-sided varicoceles are otherwise uncommon).
- Sudden onset of **left-sided varicocele in an older man** may be possibly due to **Renal cell carcinoma**.

URETHRAL STRICTURES

- Narrowing of the urethral lumen.

<u>ETIOLOGIES</u>
- Infection (eg, STI or UTI), trauma or instrumentation of the urethra, idiopathic.

<u>CLINICAL MANIFESTATIONS</u>
- **Chronic obstructive voiding symptoms** (**weak urinary stream** & incomplete bladder emptying), recurrent UTIs, urinary spraying, or dysuria.

<u>DIAGNOSIS</u>
- Patients with symptoms and poor bladder emptying (increased postvoid residual) should undergo cystourethroscopy, retrograde urethrogram, voiding cystourethrogram, or ultrasound urethrography.

<u>MANAGEMENT</u>
- Endoscopic treatment (dilation, cold knife incision, incision with electrocautery or laser), intermittent catheter dilation, or surgical reconstruction.
- Prophylactic antibiotics recommended prior to cystourethroscopy & surgery.
- <u>Complications:</u> urinary fistula

BLADDER CARCINOMA

- Most common malignancy of the genitourinary system.
- **Urothelial (Transitional cell) carcinoma most common type** (90%).
- Squamous cell carcinoma, adenocarcinoma, sarcoma, & small cell.

RISK FACTORS

- **Smoking most common** (>60%)
- Occupational exposure to **dyes, leather, & rubber** (beauticians & auto workers)
- Age > 40y, **Caucasian,** male sex. Schistosomiasis.
- Medications: **Cyclophosphamide,** Pioglitazone.
- Long-term indwelling catheter use & infected bladder stones are associated with squamous cell carcinoma.

CLINICAL MANIFESTATIONS

- **Painless gross hematuria most common** (may be microscopic). Usually intermittent and throughout micturition.
- Irritative symptoms – dysuria (second most common), urgency, & frequency.

DIAGNOSIS

- UA with microscopy and cultures to rule out benign causes (eg, UTI, pyelonephritis).
- Imaging of GU tract: CT urography (preferred) or Intravenous pyelogram.
- **Cystoscopy with biopsy gold standard** (can be both diagnostic and curative). Urine cytology (adjunctive).

MANAGEMENT

- **Localized or superficial: transurethral resection of bladder tumor (electrocautery)** & follow-up every 3 months.
- Invasive disease (advanced or muscular invasion): **radical cystectomy**, Chemotherapy, radiation therapy.

RECURRENT

- **Intravesicular BCG** (Bacillus Calmette-Guérin) **vaccine** if electrocautery is unsuccessful - immune reaction stimulates cross reaction with tumor antigens. Do not use BCG if immunosuppressed or if gross hematuria is persistent.

PARAPHIMOSIS

- **Retracted foreskin that cannot be returned to the normal position** (the foreskin cannot be pulled forward).
- **Urological emergency.**
- Pathophysiology: retracted foreskin becomes trapped behind the corona of the glans & forms a tight band, constricting penile tissues, which can lead to gangrene.

ETIOLOGIES
- Forceful retraction of phimotic foreskin.
- Infants and young boys: usually physiologic or iatrogenic (retraction by the caretaker).
- Adolescents & adults: can occur after balanoposthitis or penile inflammation (eg, Diabetes mellitus) or after sexual activity.

CLINICAL MANIFESTATIONS
- Severe penile pain & swelling of the penis.

PHYSICAL EXAMINATION
- Enlarged, painful glans with constricting band of foreskin behind the glans.

MANAGEMENT
- **Manual reduction:** restore original position of the foreskin. Reduce edema with cool compresses or pressure dressing then gentle pressure to restore the foreskin to its normal position.
- Pharmacologic therapy: granulated sugar, injection of hyaluronidase.
- Definitive management: incision (eg, dorsal slit) or circumcision.

PHIMOSIS

- **Inability to retract the foreskin over the glans.**
- Phimosis is not a urological emergency (unlike Paraphimosis).

PATHOPHYSIOLOGY
- Distal scarring of the foreskin (eg, after trauma, inflammation or infection).

MANAGEMENT
- Proper hygiene, stretching exercises (many spontaneously resolve).
- 4-8 weeks of topical corticosteroids can increase foreskin retractility (may be an adjunct to stretching).
- Circumcision definitive management.

BENIGN PROSTATIC HYPERPLASIA (BPH)

- Prostate hyperplasia (periurethral or transitional zone) leading to **bladder outlet obstruction.**
- Common in older men (discrete nodules in the periurethral zone). Hyperplasia is part of the normal aging process & is hormonally dependent on increased dihydrotestosterone production.

CLINICAL MANIFESTATIONS
- **Irritative symptoms**: increased frequency, urgency, nocturia.
- **Obstructive symptoms:** hesitancy, weak or intermittent stream force, incomplete emptying, & terminal dribbling.
- Sympathomimetics (eg, Pseudoephedrine) and anticholinergics may worsen the symptoms.

DIAGNOSIS
- Digital Rectal Exam (DRE): **uniformly enlarged, firm, nontender, rubbery prostate.**
- Prostate Specific Antigen (PSA): correlated with risk of symptom progression. Normal <4 ng/mL.
- UA: to look for hematuria or other causes of symptoms.
- Urine cytology: if increased risk of bladder cancer (history of tobacco use, irritative bladder symptoms or hematuria).

MANAGEMENT
- Observation: mild symptoms (monitored annually).
- **Alpha blockers: best initial therapy to rapidly relieve symptoms** but they do not change prostate size (eg, **Tamsulosin,** Terazosin, Doxazosin). Hypotension most common adverse effect.
- **5-alpha reductase inhibitors: reduce the size of the prostate** over time (6 -12 months). **Finasteride,** Dutasteride.

Surgical management:
- Option if persistent, progressive or refractory despite combination therapy for 12-24 months.
- **Transurethral resection of prostate (TURP)** – removes excess prostate tissue, relieving the obstruction. May cause sexual dysfunction, urinary incontinence.
- Laser prostatectomy.

Alpha-1 blockers

Tamsulosin most uroselective, Alfuzosin, Doxazosin, Terazosin.
- Indications: **provides rapid symptom relief but no effect on the clinical course of BPH.**
- Mechanism of action: **smooth muscle relaxation of prostate & bladder neck, leading to decreased urethral resistance, obstruction relief, & increased urinary outflow.** Alpha-1a activation in the prostate & urethra normally causes bladder neck contraction & decreased flow.
- Adverse effects: nonselective - **dizziness & orthostatic hypotension** (due to alpha-1b antagonism). Retrograde ejaculation.

5-alpha reductase inhibitors

Finasteride & Dutasteride
- Mechanism of action: **androgen inhibitor** - inhibits the conversion of testosterone to dihydrotestosterone **suppressing prostate growth, reduces bladder outlet obstruction.** Doesn't provide immediate relief but **has positive effect on clinical course of BPH (size reduction & decreases need for surgery)** unlike alpha-blockers. Reduction of size in 6-12 months.
- Indications: BPH & male pattern baldness.
- Adverse effects: sexual or ejaculatory dysfunction, decreased libido, breast tenderness, & enlargement.

PROSTATE CANCER

- Slow growing tumor usually.
- After skin cancer, Prostate cancer is the most common cancer in men in the US.
- Prostate cancer is the second most common cause of cancer deaths in men (behind lung cancer). However, most men die with Prostate cancer than from it.
- **Adenocarcinoma most common type** (95%).

RISK FACTORS

- **Increasing age** > 40 years (strongest risk factor) & **genetics.**
- **African-Americans have a higher incidence.**
- Diet (eg, high in animal fat, decreased vegetable intake).

CLINICAL MANIFESTATIONS

- **Most are asymptomatic** and are diagnosed either via an abnormal digital rectal exam or via workup after an abnormal PSA or until invasion of bladder, urethral obstruction or bone involvement.
- Urethral obstruction: urinary frequency, urgency, urinary retention, decreased urinary stream.
- **Back or bone pain: increased incidence of METS to bone,** weight loss.

DIAGNOSIS

- Digital rectal exam (DRE): **hard, indurated, nodular, enlarged, asymmetrical prostate.**
- Prostate Specific Antigen (PSA): can be seen in other prostate disorders. Abnormal values may be based on general number (> 4 ng/mL) or based on age-related normal values.
- Transrectal ultrasound-guided needle biopsy: **most accurate test.** Indications include PSA > 4 ng/mL in patients with suspicion (eg, palpable mass). If >10, order bone scan to rule out METS.
- **Gleason grading system** determines aggressiveness or malignant potential of Prostate cancer (higher grade suggests more benefit from surgical removal).

MANAGEMENT

- Appropriate management controversial because many cases are latent and do not progress while others metastasize.
- Local disease: options include observation/active surveillance (eg, very low risk, clinically localized or life expectancy < 10 years) vs. definitive treatment (eg, external beam radiation therapy, brachytherapy, or radical prostatectomy). **Adverse effects of prostatectomy include incontinence & erectile dysfunction** (more likely compared to radiation).

ADVANCED DISEASE

- External beam radiation therapy.
- **Hormonal therapy: androgen deprivation** (orchiectomy/Flutamide + GnRH agonists). Abiraterone is a 17-hydroxylase inhibitor that decreases progression of metastatic prostate cancer.
- Chemotherapy if hormonal therapy is ineffective.

HEMATURIA

ETIOLOGIES

- Causes vary with age, with the **most common in <40 years being inflammation or infection of the prostate or bladder, or Nephrolithiasis.**
- In >40 years, a kidney or urinary tract malignancy or benign prostatic hyperplasia may be the cause.
- Upper GU tract: Nephrolithiasis, kidney disease, renal cell carcinoma, trauma, Diabetes mellitus, sickle cell trait or disease.
- Lower GU tract: **BPH (Most common cause of microscopic hematuria in men),** urothelial cell cancer (in the absence of infection). Sexual or physical activity & illness.
- Pseudo hematuria: Rhabdomyolysis, beets, rhubarb, myoglobinuria (contains heme), hemoglobinuria.
- Medications: Ibuprofen, Phenazopyridine, Rifampin. **Cyclophosphamide (hemorrhagic cystitis).**

TIMING OF HEMATURIA

- **Terminal:** bladder irritation (eg, stone or infection) or prostate.
- Throughout micturition: bladder, ureter, or kidneys.
- **Initial** urethral in origin.

DIAGNOSIS

- **Urinalysis: usually initial test of choice** to rule out benign causes (eg, UTI or Pyelonephritis). Urine culture performed if UA suggestive for UTI. Repeat UA after 6 weeks of treatment for resolution of hematuria.
- **CT urography & cystoscopy:** recommended if UA negative for infection + gross hematuria with visible clots. **Workup of choice after noninfectious UA in patients > 40 years old,** especially if initial imaging is negative.
- Nephrology referral: if gross hematuria + no visible blood clots. The nephrologist can determine which tests needs to be done.
- Intravenous pyelogram: useful to evaluate the kidney, ureters etc. but uses contrast dye.
- Ultrasound: to evaluate the kidney & to rule out kidney stones. **Ultrasound may be the initial test of choice after UA in pregnant patients or patients unable to receive contrast.**
- Cytology: may be an adjunct test to rule out Bladder cancer.

NEPHROLITHIASIS

TYPES
- **Calcium: calcium oxalate most common.** Calcium phosphate.
- Uric acid: 5-8%. Increased uric acid due to high protein foods, gout, chemotherapy (tumor lysis). Acidic urine promotes uric acid stone formation.
- **Struvite:** composed of **Magnesium ammonium phosphate.** May form **staghorn calculi** in the renal pelvis due to urea-splitting organisms (eg, **Proteus,** Klebsiella, Pseudomonas, Serratia, & Enterobacter) or be a complication of a UTI with these organisms.
- Cystine: Rare (1-3%). Congenital defect in reabsorption of the amino acid cysteine.

CLINICAL MANIFESTATIONS:
- **Renal colic: sudden, constant upper lateral back or flank pain** over the costovertebral angle **radiating to the groin or anteriorly** (testicle in men, labia in women). May be difficult to find a comfortable position.
- Nausea, vomiting, frequency, urgency or **hematuria**.
- Pain varies with stone location: flank, CVA tenderness with proximal ureteral stones, midabdominal pain with midureteral & groin pain with distal ureteral stones.

PHYSICAL EXAMINATION:
- **Costovertebral angle tenderness.** Usually afebrile.

DIAGNOSIS
- UA: microscopic or gross **hematuria** (85%). Nitrites if infectious. **Acidic urine (pH < 5.0): uric acid & cystine. Alkaline urine (pH > 7.2) associated with struvite stones.**
- **Noncontrast CT abdomen & pelvis: imaging test of choice.**
- Renal ultrasound: detects stones or complications (eg, hydronephrosis). Used in children or if CT contraindicated (eg, pregnancy).
- KUB radiographs: **only calcium & struvite stones are radiopaque** (visible on radiographs). May miss small stones even if radiopaque.
- Intravenous pyelography – not used as often. Less sensitive & specific than CT scan.

MANAGEMENT

Stones < 5-mm in diameter:

80% chance of spontaneous passage.
- **IV fluids & analgesics,** antiemetics (if nauseous).
- **Tamsulosin** (alpha blocker) that may facilitate passage.
- Stones at the **ureterovesicular junction (narrowest point of the urinary tract)** & ureteropelvic junction may make passage of small stones difficult.

Stones 5 - 10 mm in diameter:

20% chance of spontaneous passage. If uric acid stones presents, alkalinization of the urine to pH to >6.5 helps to dissolve uric acid stones.
- **Extracorporeal shock wave lithotripsy:** may be used to break up larger stones that are less likely to pass spontaneously. May need multiple treatments to reduce the size of the stones.
- **Ureteroscopy with or without stent: used to provide immediate relief to an obstructed or at-risk kidney.**
- **Percutaneous nephrolithotomy:** most invasive. Used for **large stones (>10 mm), struvite**, or if other less invasive modalities fail. Incision made in the back & the stone is removed via a tube.

NEPHROLITHIASIS PREVENTION

Calcium:

- **Calcium oxalate most common. Calcium phosphate.**
- Calcium stones make up about 80% of all stones.
- Risk factors: **decreased fluid intake most common**, alkaline urinary pH, higher urinary calcium, high urine oxalate, lower urine citrate. Males, medications (loop diuretics, acetazolamide, antacids, chemotherapeutic drugs, indinavir & topiramate), high animal protein intake, hypercalcemia, polycystic kidney disease & increased vitamin C intake in men.
- Prevention: **increased fluid intake, Thiazide diuretics**, Citrate, low sodium diet, decreased animal protein diet.

Uric acid:

- 5-8%. Increased uric acid due to high protein foods, gout, chemotherapy (tumor lysis). Acidic urine promotes uric acid stone formation.
- Not usually visualized on a KUB.
- Prevention: increased fluids, Allopurinol or potassium citrate. Urine alkalinization. Adequate hydration prior to chemotherapy.

Struvite:

- Composed of **Magnesium ammonium phosphate.** May form **staghorn calculi** in the renal pelvis due to urea-splitting organisms (eg, **Proteus,** Klebsiella, Pseudomonas, Serratia & Enterobacter) or be a complication of a UTI with these organisms.
- Prevention: control the source of infection.

Cystine:

- Rare (1-3%). Congenital defect in reabsorption of the amino acid cysteine from the urine. Not usually visualized on a KUB.
- Prevention: dietary modification, low sodium, **urine alkalinization**. Chelating agents in refractory cases.

PENILE CANCER

- Rare in the US, Europe and other industrialized countries.
- Mean age at diagnosis is 60.
- **Squamous cell carcinoma: most common type.** Commonly associated with **HPV 16,** 6, & 18, **smoking, lack of circumcision,** HIV.
- Bowen's disease: leukoplakia on the shaft of the penis or scrotum. Peak incidence > 50 years. Associated with HPV 16. Minority progresses to Squamous cell carcinoma.

CLINICAL PRESENTATION
- Mass, palpable lesion, or ulcer on the penis. Most common on the glans, coronal sulcus or prepuce. May have inguinal lymphadenopathy.
- Rare presentations include rash, bleeding or balanitis.

DIAGNOSIS
- Biopsy. May seed to inguinal lymph nodes followed by pelvic and retroperitoneal lymph nodes.

MANAGEMENT
- Early disease: limited excision.
- Later disease: penile amputation with therapeutic lymph node dissection.

ERECTILE DYSFUNCTION

- Consistent or recurrent inability to generate or maintain an erection.

Etiologies:
- **Vascular most common** (eg, atherosclerosis, diabetes), neurologic, psychogenic, prolactinoma, trauma, surgery.
- Medications: beta-blockers, thiazide diuretics, spironolactone, calcium channel blockers, SSRIs, TCAs.
- Abrupt onset most likely psychological whereas gradual worsening indicates systemic causes.

Diagnosis:
- History & physical exam, testosterone level, other hormone testing.
- Nocturnal penile tumescence used to evaluate sleep erections.
- Duplex ultrasound to evaluate penile blood flow.

MANAGEMENT

Phosphodiesterase-5 inhibitors:
- **Sildenafil, Tadalafil** & Vardenafil.
- Indications: **first-line therapy.**
- Mechanism: phosphodiesterase-5 inhibition increases cyclic GMP & potentiates **nitric oxide – mediated** penile smooth muscle relaxation, leading to the ability to generate & maintain an erection.
- Adverse effects: headache, flushing, rhinitis, visual disturbances, hearing loss.
- Contraindications: **not used with nitrates or patients with cardiovascular disease** (may cause severe hypotension – synergistic nitric oxide).

Second-line therapy:
- Intracavernosal injection therapy: prostaglandin E1 (Alprostadil), Papaverine or combination of Papaverine plus Phentolamine (causes vasodilation – increased arterial inflow). Vacuum pump.

Third-line therapy:
- Penile prosthesis or corrective penile revascularization.

Testosterone:
- hormone replacement if testosterone is low (eg, androgen deficiency).

HYPOSPADIAS

- Congenital anomaly of the male urethra that results in **abnormal ventral placement of the urethral opening,** penile curvature, and abnormal foreskin development.
- The urethral opening an be within the glans, shaft, the scrotum, or perineum.
- Second most common congenital in males after Cryptorchidism.

Pathophysiology:
- **Failure of urogenital folds to fuse** during development - abnormal development of the urethral fold and the ventral foreskin of the penis.
- Proximal hypospadias is usually associated with additional genitourinary malformation.

Clinical manifestations
- Increased risk of UTIs, deflection of the urinary stream, erectile dysfunction.

Physical examination:
- Ventral placement of the urethra.
- Abnormal foreskin with incomplete closure around the glans (dorsal hooded prepuce).
- Abnormal penile curvature (chordee).

MANAGEMENT:
- These patients should NOT be circumcised in the neonatal period because the **foreskin may be used to repair the defect**.
- Elective surgical correction (arthroplasty) may include penile straightening. **Hypospadias repair usually performed in healthy full-term infants most commonly between 6 months and one year of age.**

EPISPADIAS

- Congenital anomaly of the male urethra that results in **abnormal dorsal placement of the urethral opening.**
- **Often associated with bladder exstrophy** (protrusion of the bladder wall through a defect in the abdominal wall).

PATHOPHYSIOLOGY
- Epispadias: **failure of midline penile fusion.**
- Bladder exstrophy: in utero rupture of an overdeveloped cloacal membrane, leading to herniation of the lower abdominal contents.

CLINICAL MANIFESTATIONS
- Males: opening of the urethral meatus on the dorsal (top) surface of the penis, dorsal (upward) curvature of the penis, absent dorsal foreskin.
- Females: bifid clitoris and small, laterally displaced labia minora.

DIAGNOSIS:
- Bladder exstrophy often made via prenatal ultrasound.

MANAGEMENT:
- Surgical correction

URETHRAL INJURIES

- More common in men.

ETIOLOGIES

- **Blunt trauma most common** (80%) – anterior urethral injury (**straddle-type falls** or direct blows), posterior urethral injury (pelvic fractures, MVA).
- Physical or sexual assault.

CLINICAL MANIFESTATIONS

- **Gross hematuria,** difficulty urinating, urinary retention or lower abdominal pain.

PHYSICAL EXAMINATION

- **Blood at the urethral meatus, swelling or ecchymosis** of the scrotum, penis or perineum.
- **High-riding prostate.**

DIAGNOSIS

- Assess for injuries & fractures.
- **Retrograde urethrogram is the diagnostic test of choice (must be done prior to transurethral catheterization).** UA: hematuria.
- Hallmark triad of urethral injury = blood at the urethral meatus, inability to void & distended bladder.

MANAGEMENT

- Non-operative management: catheter placement & monitoring for healing.

- Surgical repair: indicated in severe injuries. May involve **temporary suprapubic catheter placement prior to repair.**

TUMOR MARKER	MAIN ASSOCIATIONS
ALPHA FETOPROTEIN	• **Hepatocellular carcinoma** • **Nonseminomatous germ cell testicular cancer** • Decreased in Down syndrome (Trisomy 21) "AFP is down in Down syndrome"
Beta-hCG	• **Nonseminomatous germ cell testicular cancer** • **Choriocarcinomas,** Teratomas • **Trophoblastic tumors** (eg, hydatidiform molar pregnancy)
CA-125	• **Ovarian cancer**
CA 19-9	• **Pancreatic cancer** • GI – Colorectal, Esophageal & Hepatocellular cancers
CALCITONIN	• **Medullary thyroid cancer**
CEA	• **Colorectal cancer** • Medullary thyroid, pancreatic, gastric, lung & breast cancers
PROSTATE SPECIFIC ANTIGEN	• **Prostate cancer** • Can also be elevated in BPH & Prostatitis

PRIAPISM

- Prolonged, painful erections without sexual stimulation.
- **Ischemic (low-flow): decreased venous outflow** may lead to a compartment syndrome, increasing acidosis, & hypoxia in the cavernous tissues. Painful & rigid erection. **Most common type.**
- **Nonischemic (high-flow): increased arterial inflow** due to a fistula between the cavernosal artery & corpus cavernosum. Commonly related to **perineal or penile trauma.** Less painful & not fully rigid compared to ischemic.

ETIOLOGIES
- **Idiopathic most common** (50%), **sickle cell disease** (10%), injection of erectile agent for erectile dysfunction, drugs (eg, cocaine, marijuana), alcohol. Trauma (high flow) may cause rupture of the cavernosal artery.
- Medications: PDE-5 inhibitors, **Trazodone**, antipsychotics, anticonvulsants, alpha blockers.
- Neurologic: head trauma, meningitis, subarachnoid hemorrhage & postoperative.

DIAGNOSIS
- Primarily based on history and physical examination. Blood gas may be performed in erections > 4 hours.
- **Cavernosal blood gas**: high-flow results similar to ABG & normal glucose. Low-flow shows hypoglycemia, hypoxemia, hypercarbia, & acidemia.
- Doppler ultrasound: normal or high blood flow in nonischemic, minimal or absent blood flow in ischemic.

MANAGEMENT OF ISCHEMIC (LOW-FLOW)
- **Phenylephrine: first-line medication (intracavernosal injection).** Mechanism: alpha-agonists cause contraction of the cavernous smooth muscle, which increases venous outflow. Contraindications: cardiac or cerebrovascular history.
- **Needle aspiration** of corpus cavernosum & irrigation to remove blood especially if >4 hours duration with or without Phenylephrine (Combo therapy). Combination therapy is more effective than corporal aspiration alone. Ice packs.
- Terbutaline: orally or SQ (constricts cavernosal artery, reducing arterial inflow) may be used if <4 hours. Not as effective
- Shunt surgery may be performed if not responsive to medical & aspiration therapy.

MANAGEMENT OF NONISCHEMIC (HIGH-FLOW)
- **Observation** - most resolve within hours to days.
- Refractory: nonpermanent arterial embolization or surgical ligation may be used if refractory.

ENURESIS

- Distinct episodes of urinary incontinence (bedwetting) while sleeping in children 5 years of age or older.

- Evaluation: complete history, physical examination, voiding diary, & urinalysis.

- Monosymptomatic: enuresis in the absence of lower urinary tract infection symptoms & without bladder dysfunction. High rate of spontaneous resolution.

PRIMARY ENURESIS:
- Absence of any period of nighttime dryness. Most common type. May have a family history.

SECONDARY ENURESIS:
- Enuresis after a dry period of at least 6 months. Usually due to an unusually stressful event (birth of a sibling, parental divorce).

MANAGEMENT
- **Behavioral: first-line therapy** - motivational therapy (especially in children 5-7y), education & reassurance. Use of washable products & room deodorizers. Bladder training: regular voiding schedule, deliberate voiding prior to sleeping, waking the child up to urinate intermittently. Avoidance of caffeine-based & drinks with high sugar content. Fluid restriction.

- **Enuresis alarm: most effective long-term therapy.** Usually **used if children fail to respond to behavioral therapy**. Often attempted before medical therapy. A sensor is placed on a bed pad or in the undergarments and goes off when wet. Usually continued until there is a minimum of 2 weeks of consecutive dry nights.

- **Desmopressin** (DDAVP): used in nocturnal polyuria with normal bladder function capacity. Better for short-term use.
  Mechanism: **synthetic antidiuretic hormone (ADH),** which reduces urination. May cause hyponatremia so patients may use liberal amounts of salt to reduce the incidence.

- **Imipramine**: a **Tricyclic antidepressant** that may be used in refractory cases.
  Mechanism: stimulates ADH secretion, detrusor muscle relaxation & decreases time spent in REM sleep.

CHAPTER 10 – NEUROLOGIC SYSTEM

TRAUMATIC BRAIN (INTRACRANIAL) INJURY

- Sequelae from an external force injuring the brain (head trauma).
- Can result in cognitive, physical, social, emotional, and behavioral symptoms.

ETIOLOGIES
- **Falls (especially in the elderly) most common,** MVAs

CLASSIFICATION OF SEVERITY
- The GCS is scored between 3 and 15, 3 being the worst and 15 the best.
- It is composed of three parameters: best eye response (E), best verbal response (V), and best motor response (M). The components of the GCS should be recorded individually; for example, E4V2M2 results in a GCS score of 8.
  - Mild: score of 13 or higher
  - Moderate: score of 9 to 12
  - Severe: score of 8 or less

	SCORE
Eye opening	**4**
Spontaneous	4
Response to verbal commands	3
Response to pain	2
No eye opening	1
Best Verbal Response	**5**
Oriented	5
Confused	4
Inappropriate words	3
Incomprehensible sounds	2
No verbal response	1
Best Motor Response	**6**
Obeys commands	6
Localizing response to pain	5
Withdrawal response to pain	4
Flexion to pain	3
Extension to pain	2
No motor response	1

PATHOPHYSIOLOGY
- Primary: intra- and extraparenchymal hemorrhages and diffuse axonal injury.
- Secondary: multitude of molecular damage, which can be worsened by fever, seizures, hypoxia, and hypotension. Cushing's triad: hypertension, bradycardia, and irregular respiration.

MANAGEMENT OF SEVERE TRAUMATIC BRAIN INJURY (TBI)
- Managed in a neurosurgical ICU with frequent clinical & neurological assessments.
- Prevention of hypoxia (PaO2 < 60 mmHg), hypotension (SBP < 100 mmHg). Endotracheal intubation.
- Surgical evaluation of hematomas based on hematoma size, mass effect, and neurological status.
- Reduction of intracranial pressure: head of bed, hyperventilation, mannitol.
  - Hyperventilation should be avoided in the first 24 to 48 hours and should not exceed $PaCO_2$ <30 mmHg except as a temporizing measure in a patient with impending cerebral herniation.
  - Positive end-expiratory pressure (PEEP) up to 15 to 20 cm H_2O may be utilized to manage acute respiratory distress syndrome (ARDS) following TBI while ICP is monitored.
- For patients with severe TBI and an abnormal CT scan revealing evidence of mass effect from lesions such as contusions, hematomas, or swelling, ventriculostomy and ICP monitoring along with treatment of elevated ICP to target pressures below 22 mmHg is recommended.
- Short-term (one-week) use of antiseizure drugs for the prevention of early seizures (eg, Levetiracetam), Fosphenytoin.
- Fever and hyperglycemia should be avoided (may exacerbate secondary injury).

CONCUSSION SYNDROME

- **Mild traumatic brain injury** leading to **alteration in mental status**, with or without loss of consciousness.
- May result after blunt force or an acceleration/deceleration head injury.

CLINICAL MANIFESTATIONS
- Headache, dizziness, psychological symptoms, and cognitive impairment.
- **Confusion:** confused or blank expression, blunted affect.
- **Amnesia:** pretraumatic (retrograde) or posttraumatic (antegrade) amnesia. The duration of retrograde amnesia is usually brief. Headache, dizziness, visual disturbances: blurred or double vision.
- Delayed responses & emotional changes: emotional instability.
- Signs of increased intracranial pressure: persistent vomiting, worsening headache, increasing disorientation, changing levels of consciousness.
- **CT head without contrast** is the **study of choice for evaluating most acute head injuries.**
- MRI study of choice if prolonged symptoms >7-14 days or with worsening of symptoms not explained by concussion syndrome.
- CT angiography of the head or neck if vascular injury is suspected.

MANAGEMENT
- **Cognitive & physical rest is the main management of patients with concussion.**
- Some form of observation is recommended for a minimum of 24 hours (outpatient or inpatient).
- **Patients may resume strenuous activity after resolution of symptoms & recovery of memory as well as cognitive functions.**
- Neurosurgical or neurologic consult if CT scan shows mass effect, substantial hematomas (epidural, subdural, cerebral), subarachnoid hemorrhage, pneumocephalus, depressed skull fracture, cerebral edema.

PANCE PREP PEARL OF THE WEEK

LOWER MOTOR NEURON

Muscles are **FLABBY**
- **Fasciculations** in advanced stage
- **Flaccid paralysis** (flabby muscle)
- **Loss of muscle tone & strength**
- **Areflexia** (decreased DTR)
- **Babinski** towards the **Basement downwards**
- **Young** (infantile poliomyelitis known as infantile paralysis)

Conditions: Bs:
- Guillain-**B**arré Syndrome,
- **B**otulism,
- Poliomyelitis (**B**aby),
- Cauda Equina Syndrome (**B**ack)
- **B**ell palsy

UPPER MOTOR NEURON

Muscles are **SPASTIC**
- **S**light muscle loss **(no atrophy)**
- **Positive Babinski (toe up),** Posturing
- **A**bsence of fasciculations
- **Strong Tone (Spastic paralysis)**
- **Tone increased** (Spastic paralysis)
- **I**ncreased deep tendon reflexes
- **C**lonus

- **Conditions: S: S**troke (CVA), Multiple **S**clerosis, Cerebral pal**S**y **S**pinal cord or brain damage (ex traumatic brain injury)

CRANIAL NERVES

EYELID
- CN III opens eyelid (damage causes ptosis)
- CN VII closes the eyelid

PUPILLARY REFLEX
- CN II afferent (sensory)
- CN III efferent (motor)

CORNEAL REFLEX
- CN V (afferent) sensory
- CN VII (efferent) motor

CRANIAL NERVE (CN)		PHYSICAL EXAMINATION	ABNORMALITIES
I. OLFACTORY	S	Smell	
II. OPTIC	S	***Visual acuity, visual fields, pupillary light reflex (swinging light test)***	***Optic neuritis, Marcus Gunn***
III. OCULOMOTOR	M	Inferior rectus, ciliary body	***Oculomotor, Dilated pupil***
IV. TROCHLEAR	M	Superior oblique rectus	
V. TRIGEMINAL	B	**Motor:** ***muscles of mastication,*** closing jaw, moves chin side to side. **Sensory:** ***light touch (with cotton wisp)*** to test the 3 divisions of the nerve (ophthalmic, maxillary & mandibular branches)	***Trigeminal Neuralgia***
VI. ABDUCENS	M	Lateral rectus (lateral gaze). III, IV & VI help with extraocular movements.	
VII. FACIAL	B	**Motor**: Muscles of ***facial expression*** (including blinking of the eyelid, raising eyebrows, frown smile, close eyes tightly, puff cheeks), tear glands. **Sensory:** ***taste (anterior $^2/_3$ of tongue). Somatic fibers to external ear.***	***Bell's Palsy*** ***CN 7 Palsy*** ***Ramsay Hunt syndrome***
VIII. ACOUSTIC (Vestibulocochlear)	S	***Hearing:*** speech, Weber & Rinne test ***Vestibular Function: balance & proprioception***	***Acoustic neuroma***
IX. GLOSSOPHARYNGEAL	B	**Motor:** Swallow, gag reflex **Sensory:** taste (posterior $^1/_3$ of tongue)	
X. VAGUS	B	**Motor:** Voice, soft palate, gag reflex **Sensory:** relays to the brain sensory information about organs (ex GI, pulmonary heart)	
XI. ACCESSORY	M	Shoulder shrug, turning head from side to side	
XII. HYPOGLOSSAL	M	Tongue: inspect for fasciculations & asymmetry	

M = Motor, S = Sensory, B = both sensory & motor. "Some Say Money Matters But My Brother Says Big Bucks Matters More"

	MOTOR	MUSCLES	SENSORY	REFLEXES
C5	• Shoulder abduction • Elbow Flexion (palm up)	• Deltoid • Biceps	• Lateral arm (below deltoid & above elbow) • Axillary nerve	• Loss of bicep jerk reflex
C6	• Elbow flexion (thumb up) • Wrist extension	• Brachioradialis • Extensor carpi radialis	• Thumb • Radial side of the hand	• Brachioradialis
C7	• Elbow extension • Wrist Flexion	• Triceps • Flexor carpi radialis	• Radial side of the fingers • Fingers 2, 3, 4	• Triceps jerk reflex
C8	• Finger flexion	• Flexor digitorum superficialis	• Median nerve • ±Horner's syndrome	
T1	• Finger abduction	• Interossei	• Medial elbow, Ulnar nerve	

S1-S2 Loss of Ankle Jerk **L3-L4** Loss of Knee Jerk **C5-C6** Loss of Biceps Jerk **C7-C8** Loss of Triceps Jerk.

PERONEAL NERVE: innervates the peroneus longus, peroneus brevis, and the short head of the biceps femoris muscles. Injuries lead to a ***FOOT DROP****

HEADACHES

PRIMARY (90%): migraine, tension, cluster or rebound.
- Primary = idiopathic in nature. Tension & migraine MC in women.

SECONDARY (4%):
- Meningitis, subarachnoid hemorrhage, intracranial hypertension, hypertensive crisis, acute glaucoma. Suspect 2ry if abrupt or progression of severity.

TENSION-TYPE HEADACHE

- **Most common overall cause of Primary headache**. Mean age of onset ~30y.
- Risk factors: mental stress, sleep deprivation, & eye strain.

CLINICAL MANIFESTATIONS
- **Bilateral, pressing, tightening "band-like", nonthrobbing (nonpulastile)** steady or aching headache (often worsens throughout the day).
- Worsened with stress, fatigue, noise, or glare.
- **Not worsened with routine activity** (as in Migraines).
- Usually **not pulsatile** & **not associated with nausea, vomiting, photophobia, phonophobia, or focal neurological symptoms** (auras).

PHYSICAL EXAMINATION
- Usually normal but may have pericranial muscle tenderness (tenderness to the head, neck, or shoulders).

DIAGNOSIS
- Clinical – diagnosis of exclusion (there are no specific tests).

MANAGEMENT
- **First-line: NSAIDs & other analgesics** (eg, Acetaminophen or Aspirin). Local heat.
- Anti-migraine medications.

TRIGEMINAL NEURALGIA (TIC DOULOUREUX)

- Pathophysiology: compression of the trigeminal nerve (cranial nerve V) root by the superior cerebellar artery or vein (90%). Idiopathic (10%).
- **Most common in middle-aged women.**
- In younger patients, suspect Multiple sclerosis.

CLINICAL MANIFESTATIONS
- Headache: paroxysmal, **brief, episodic, stabbing, lancinating or shock-like pain** in the 2nd or 3rd division of the Trigeminal nerve, lasting seconds-minutes.
- **Worse with touch, chewing, brushing teeth, drafts of wind, & movements (often unilateral).**
- Pain starts near mouth & shoots to the eye, ear & nostril on the ipsilateral side and often occurs many times throughout the day.

PHYSICAL EXAMINATION
- Usually normal but light palpation of "trigger zones" may trigger attack.

DIAGNOSIS
- Usually a clinical diagnosis in the absence of history or physical findings suggestive of a serious underlying cause.

MANAGEMENT
- **Carbamazepine first-line. Oxcarbazepine.**
- Gabapentin, Baclofen, Lamotrigine.
- Surgical decompression or gamma knife surgery may be needed in severe or recalcitrant cases.

MIGRAINE HEADACHE

- More common in women. Family history (80%).

2 MAJOR TYPES
- **Migraine without aura (most common)**
- Rarer **Migraine with aura (classic).**

CLINICAL MANIFESTATIONS
- Usually **lateralized, pulsatile (throbbing) headache** often associated with **nausea, vomiting, photophobia, & phonophobia**, usually 4-72 hours in duration, and moderate to severe in intensity.

- **Worsened with routine physical activity**, stress, lack or excessive sleep, alcohol, specific foods (eg, chocolate, red wine), hormonal (eg, oral contraception & menstruation), dehydration etc.

- **Auras: focal neurologic symptoms** that **usually last <60 minutes** (5-20 minutes common). Auras accompany or follow the headache within 60 minutes. **Visual (most common type),** auditory, somatosensory, or loss of function (eg, aphasia, hearing etc.).

PHYSICAL EXAMINATION
- Usually normal. May have aphasia, dysarthria, paresthesias, or weakness.

DIAGNOSIS: clinical.

SYMPTOMATIC (ABORTIVE) MANAGEMENT
- **NSAIDs, Acetaminophen or Aspirin first-line if mild.** Some migraine medications have caffeine added to improve symptoms.
- IV fluids & placing the patient in a dark & quiet room are helpful.
- **Triptans or Ergotamines if moderate to severe or no response to analgesics** (Ergotamines have more adverse effects compared to Triptans).
- **Antiemetics** (eg, **Metoclopramide, Prochlorperazine**).

PROPHYLACTIC (PREVENTATIVE)
- **Anti-hypertensives: Beta-blockers** (eg, Propranolol) & **Calcium channel blockers**.
- Tricyclic antidepressants, anticonvulsants (eg, Valproate, Topiramate), NSAIDs.

TRIPTANS

- **Sumatriptan** (oral, subcutaneous or nasal spray), **Zolmitriptan** (nasal, oral).
  Oral: Rizatriptan, Eletriptan, Almotriptan.
- Mechanism of action: **serotonin (5HT-1b/d) agonists** cause vasoconstriction & block pain pathways in the brainstem.
- Indications: **moderate to severe migraines or no response to analgesics in mild disease.** Can be combined with analgesics.
- Adverse effects: **chest tightness from vasoconstriction,** nausea, vomiting, abdominal cramps, flushing, malaise.
- Contraindications: **ischemic stroke or ischemic heart disease,** uncontrolled hypertension, pregnancy, hemiplegic or basilar migraines. Triptans should not be used within 24 hours of the use of Ergotamines.

ERGOTAMINES

- **Ergotamine** (oral), **Dihydroergotamine** (IM, IV, SQ, and intranasal)

Mechanism of action:
- **Serotonin (5HT-1b/d) agonists** cause vasoconstriction & block pain pathways in the brainstem.

Indications:
- Reserved use due to its adverse effects & contraindications (Triptans are associated with lower occurrence of adverse effects compared to Ergotamines).

Adverse effects:
- Rebound headache

Contraindications:
- **Coronary artery disease** (may cause coronary artery vasoconstriction), **hypertension, cerebrovascular or peripheral arterial disease**, hepatic or renal disease, Migraines with prolonged aura.

ABORTIVE MIGRAINE THERAPY - ANTIEMETICS

- IV **Metoclopramide, Chlorpromazine** (IV or IM), **Prochlorperazine** (IV or IM).

Mechanism of action:
- **Dopamine receptor antagonists.** May also reduce headache pain intensity.

Indications:
- **Nausea &/or vomiting** in patients with Migraine.

Adverse effects:
- **Extrapyramidal symptoms - acute dystonic reactions** (dyskinesias characterized by intermittent spasmodic or sustained contractions of muscles in the face, neck, trunk, etc.).
  - **IV Diphenhydramine can be given to prevent or treat dystonic reactions**.
- QT interval prolongation.

PROPHYLACTIC (PREVENTATIVE) MIGRAINE THERAPY

Indications:
- Frequent & long lasting migraine headaches, especially if associated with disability or affects the quality of life.
- Lifestyle changes: good sleep hygiene, regular exercise, avoidance of triggers.
- **Antihypertensives: Beta-blockers** (eg, **Propranolol).** Calcium channel blockers (eg, Verapamil).
- Antidepressants: Tricyclic antidepressants (eg, Amitriptyline). Other – Venlafaxine
- Anticonvulsants: eg, Valproate, Topiramate
- NSAIDs.

CLUSTER HEADACHE

- Predominantly young & middle-aged **males** (10 times more common than women).
- Associated with multiple frequent headaches with high intensity and brief duration.

TRIGGERS
- **worse at night, alcohol,** stress, or ingestion of specific foods.

CLINICAL MANIFESTATIONS
- Headache: **severe, unilateral periorbital or temporal pain (sharp, lancinating). Bouts last <2 hours with** spontaneous remission.

- Bouts occur several times a day. May have one or two cluster periods per year (each lasting weeks to months).

PHYSICAL EXAMINATION
- **Ipsilateral findings: Horner's syndrome** (ptosis, miosis, anhidrosis), **nasal congestion, rhinorrhea, conjunctivitis, & lacrimation.**

DIAGNOSIS
- Clinical

ACUTE MANAGEMENT
- **100% Oxygen first-line** (6-10L).

- Anti-migraine medications help during attack - SQ **Sumatriptan** or Ergotamines (vasoconstriction).

PROPHYLAXIS
- **Verapamil first-line.** Corticosteroids, Ergotamines, Valproic acid, Lithium.

IDIOPATHIC INTRACRANIAL HTN (PSEUDOTUMOR CEREBRI)

- **Idiopathic increased intracranial (CSF) pressure** with no clear cause evident on neuroimaging (eg, CT or MRI).

- **AKA Pseudotumor cerebri** (mimics a brain tumor with nausea, vomiting, and visual disturbances).

RISK FACTORS
- **Obese women** of childbearing age.
- Meds: corticosteroid withdrawal, growth hormone, thyroid replacement, oral contraceptives, long-term tetracycline use, & **vitamin A toxicity**.
- Venous sinus thrombosis.

CLINICAL MANIFESTATIONS
Signs & symptoms of increased intracranial pressure
- **Headache: pulsatile, worse with straining** or changes in posture.
- Retrobulbar pain that may be worse with eye movements.
- **Nausea, vomiting**, tinnitus.
- **Visual changes** may lead to blindness if not treated.

OCULAR EXAMINATION
- Funduscopic exam: **papilledema** (usually bilateral & symmetric).
- May have visual field loss.
- May have **diplopia** due to a **cranial nerve VI (abducens) palsy**.

DIAGNOSIS
- CT scan: performed prior to LP to rule out intracranial mass.
- **Lumbar puncture: increased CSF pressure** (250 mmH_2O or greater) **+ otherwise normal CSF.**
- MRI with MR venography ideal neuroimaging.

MANAGEMENT
- **Acetazolamide first-line** (decreases CSF production) & weight loss recommended.
- Furosemide may be adjunct.
- Short-course of systemic corticosteroids may be indicated if acute visual loss as a temporizing measure prior to surgical intervention. Repeat lumbar puncture reduces intracranial pressure.
- Refractory: ventriculoperitoneal shunt or optic nerve sheath fenestration.

CLASSIC CSF FINDINGS

1. MULTIPLE SCLEROSIS	High IgG (oligoclonal bands)
2. GUILLAIN BARRÉ SYNDROME	High protein with normal WBC/cell count
3. BACTERIAL MENINGITIS	High protein with increased WBC (primarily polymorphonuclear neutrophils), decreased glucose
4. VIRAL (ASEPTIC) MENINGITIS	Normal glucose, increased WBCs (lymphocytes)
5. FUNGAL or TB MENGITIS	Decreased glucose, increased WBCs (lymphocytes)
6. IDIOPATHIC INTRACRANIAL HTN	Increased CSF pressure otherwise normal
7. SUBARACHNOID HEMORRHAGE	Xanthochromia, blood in the CSF

ACUTE BACTERIAL MENINGITIS

- Bacterial infection of the meninges.
- 25% have a recent history of otitis or sinusitis.

ETIOLOGIES

***Streptococcus pneumoniae*:**
- **Most common cause in adults** of all ages & children ages > 3 months – 10 years.

***Neisseria menigitidis*:**
- **Most common in older children** (10y – 19y).
- Second most common cause in adults.
- May be associated with a **petechial rash** on the trunk, legs, and conjunctivae.

Group B *Streptococcus* (*S. agalactiae*):
- **Most common cause** in **neonates < 1 month** (part of the vaginal flora) & infants <3 months.

***Listeria monocytogenes*:**
- Increased incidence **neonates, >50 years, immunocompromised states** (eg, history of glucocorticoid use, alcoholism, pregnant, AIDS or HIV, chemotherapy).

Neonates:
- Group B *Streptococcus*, *Escherichia coli,* & gram-negative rods are common causes of neonatal meningitis. *Listeria monocytogenes* an important pathogen.
- *Haemophilus influenzae* (reduced incidence due to Hib vaccine)

CLINICAL MANIFESTATIONS
- Meningeal symptoms: **headache, neck stiffness, photosensitivity, fever,** chills, nausea, vomiting.
- May develop altered mental status changes and seizures.

PHYSICAL EXAMINATION
- **Meningeal signs**: **nuchal rigidity, positive Brudzinski** (neck flexion produces knee and/or hip flexion), **positive Kernig sign** (inability to extend the knee/leg with hip flexion).
- Focal neurologic findings (30%).

DIAGNOSIS
- **Lumbar puncture + CSF examination best initial test & definitive diagnosis - decreased glucose** <45, **increased neutrophils,** increased protein, & increased pressure.
- **Head CT scan best initial test prior to LP ONLY** if you need to rule out mass effect if any of these are present - **papilledema, seizures**, confusion, focal neurologic findings, >60 years, immunocompromised, or history of CNS disease.

	NORMAL	BACTERIAL	VIRAL (ASEPTIC)	FUNGAL/TB
Opening pressure (cm H_2O)	5-20 cm	Increased	Normal or mildly increased	Normal or Mildly increased
Appearance	Normal	Turbid	Clear	Fibrin web
Protein (g/L)	0.18 – 0.45	Increased	Normal or mildly increased	Increased
Glucose (mg/100mL)	50-80	**Decreased** (<45)	**Normal**	**Decreased**
WBC Count	0-5 (no RBC's)	100-100,000 (pleocytosis) **>80% Neutrophils (PMN's)**	10-300 **Lymphocytes**	10-200 **Lymphocytes**
Gram Stain	Normal	60-90% positive	Normal	

MANAGEMENT

- **Antibiotics**, along with Dexamethasone when indicated, **should be started as quickly as possible after lumbar puncture** is performed, if LP is contraindicated, or **prior to head CT** if a head CT is to be performed prior to LP (as quickly as possible after blood cultures are obtained).
- In adults, **Dexamethasone has been shown to reduce mortality and sequelae of *S. pneumo,*** *H. flu* & *N. meningitidis*. Also recommended in children if *H. influenzae* type B is suspected (reduces incidence of CN VIII-related hearing loss).

Empiric for >1 month - 50y:

- **Vancomycin + Ceftriaxone** (or Cefotaxime).

Empiric for >50y:

- **Vancomycin + Ceftriaxone + Ampicillin** (for Listeria).

Empiric for neonates (up to 1 month):

- Ampicillin + either Gentamicin and/or Cefotaxime.

Additional management for *N. meningitidis*:

- **Droplet precautions** - should be continued for 24 hours after the initiation of antibiotics with suspected or confirmed *N. meningitidis* infection.
- **Post-exposure prophylaxis: Ciprofloxacin** (500mg oral x 1 dose) or **Rifampin** (600mg orally every 12 hours for 2 days). **Prophylaxis only needed for "close contacts" with prolonged exposure (>8 hours) or direct exposure to respiratory secretions** (eg, household contacts, roommates, kissing, sharing utensils, performing mouth to mouth resuscitation etc.).
- Prophylaxis is not recommended for healthcare workers who have not had direct exposure to respiratory secretions.

NORMAL PRESSURE HYDROCEPHALUS

- Dilation of the cerebral ventricles with normal opening pressures on lumbar puncture.

PATHOPHYSIOLOGY

- Unknown but thought to be due to impaired CSF absorption after a CNS injury (eg, Subarachnoid hemorrhage, chronic meningitis, tumors, inflammatory disease, head injury etc.).

CLINICAL MANIFESTATIONS

- **Triad ❶ dementia/cognitive dysfunction ❷ gait disturbance** & **❸ urinary incontinence** - "wet, wobbly, & wacky".
- **Gait disturbances: wide-based, shuffling gait** – described as gait apraxia or *"magnetic"* gait (as if the feet are stuck to the floor). May be associated with postural instability, especially when attempting to turn. Most prominent feature.
- **Dementia:** includes impaired executive function, psychomotor depression, & apathy.
- **Urinary incontinence** may present as **urinary urgency early in the disease**.
- Other: weakness, lethargy, malaise, rigidity, hyperreflexia, & spasticity.

DIAGNOSIS

- Neuroimaging: **enlarged ventricles** in the absence of or out of proportion to sulcal dilation. **MRI is superior to CT scan.**
- Lumbar puncture: CSF pressure is usually normal. Removing fluid during LP may cause improvement of symptoms.

MANAGEMENT

- **Ventriculoperitoneal shunt treatment of choice.** Gait abnormalities usually the most improved.

ASEPTIC MENINGITIS

- Clinical and laboratory evidence of meningitis with negative routine bacterial cultures.

ETIOLOGIES
- **Enteroviruses most common cause** (eg, **Coxsackievirus & Echovirus**).
- Other viruses, mycobacteria, fungi, spirochetes, medications, and malignancies.

CLINICAL MANIFESTATIONS
- Classic symptoms of meningitis but may be milder.
- Meningeal symptoms: **headache, neck stiffness, photosensitivity, fever,** chills, nausea, vomiting.

PHYSICAL EXAMINATION
- **Meningeal signs: nuchal rigidity,** positive **Brudzinski** (neck flexion produces knee and/or hip flexion), positive **Kernig sign** (inability to straighten the knee with hip flexion).
- **No focal deficits in aseptic meningitis** helps to distinguish it from encephalitis.

DIAGNOSIS
- **Diagnosis of exclusion** after ruling out bacterial meningitis.
- **Lumbar puncture best initial test and most accurate** if no symptoms of mass effect.
  CSF: classic findings are **normal glucose, lymphocyte predominance**, protein count usually <200.

MANAGEMENT
- **Supportive** eg, antipyretics, IV fluids, & analgesics.
- Most patients have a self-limited course with resolution even without specific therapy.

ENCEPHALITIS

- **Infection of the brain parenchyma.**

ETIOLOGIES
- **Herpes simplex virus-1 most common cause.**
- Varicella zoster virus, Epstein-Barr virus, measles, mumps, rubella, HIV, St. Louis virus.

CLINICAL MANIFESTATIONS
- Meningeal symptoms: **headache, neck stiffness, photosensitivity, fever,** chills, nausea, vomiting, **seizures.**
- **The presence of altered mental status, changes in personality, speech, & movement** distinguishes encephalitis from aseptic meningitis.

PHYSICAL EXAMINATION
- **Focal neurologic deficits** (eg, hemiparesis, sensory deficits, cranial nerve palsies).

DIAGNOSIS
- **CT scan of the head must be performed first to rule out space-occupying lesions** (these patients often have altered mental status, requiring imaging before LP).
- **Lumbar puncture** performed after CT – normal glucose, increased lymphocytes (similar to Aseptic meningitis).
- MRI: preferred modality for encephalitis - **temporal involvement characteristic of HSV**.
- PCR testing of CSF fluid is the most accurate test for herpes encephalitis.

MANAGEMENT
- **IV Acyclovir: early empiric treatment for HSV encephalitis** should be initiated as soon as possible if the patient has encephalitis with no obvious cause. Supportive management

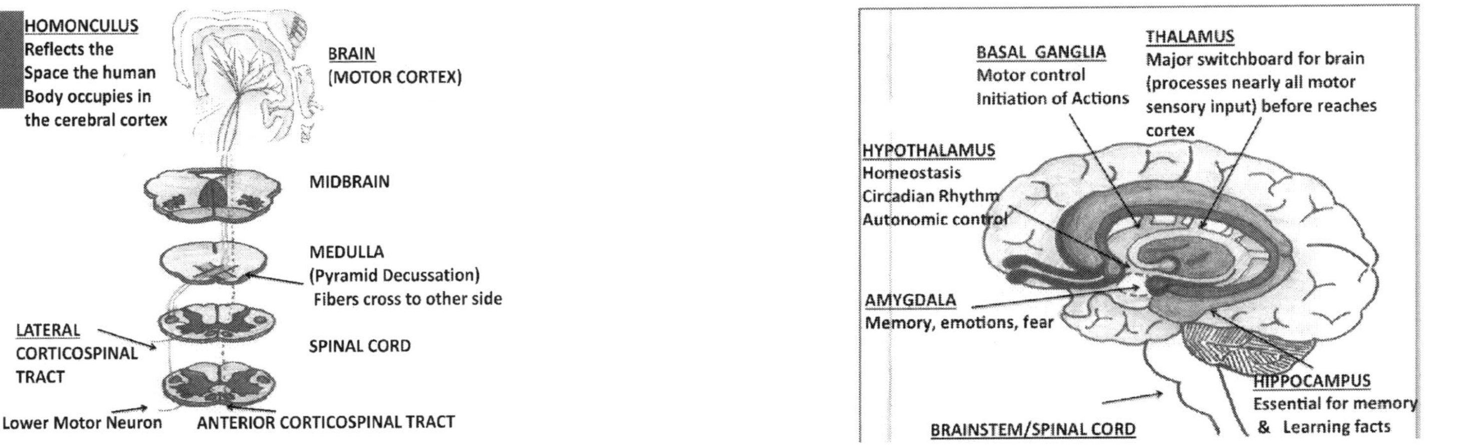

BASAL GANGLIA DISORDERS: since the basal ganglia is involved in coordinated movement, emotion & cognition, problems can lead to movement disorders (***dyskinesias, dystonias, Parkinsonism, Huntington's disease)*** *or behavior control* ***(Tourette's, obsessive compulsive).***

"EXTRAPYRAMIDAL SYMPTOMS"	
DYSKINESIA	***Involuntary spasms, repetitive motions or abnormal voluntary movement.***
DYSTONIA	***Sustained contraction*** (muscle spasm) especially of antagonistic muscles (ex simultaneous biceps & triceps contraction) ⇨ ***twisting of the body, abnormal posturing*** (ex. torticollis, writer's cramp).
MYOCLONUS	Sudden ***brief, sporadic involuntary jerking/twitching*** of 1 muscle or muscle group (not suppressible).
TICS	Sudden, ***repetitive nonrhythmic movements or vocals*** using specific muscle groups. Tics are ***suppressible*** *(unlike myoclonus which is not suppressible).* Ex. Tourette syndrome.
CHOREA	***Rapid involuntary jerky, uncontrolled, purposeless movements.*** Ex. ***Huntington chorea*** (due to caudate nucleus atrophy in the basal ganglia), Sydenham's chorea (rheumatic fever)
MUSCLE SPASMS	Muscle contractions. **Tonic: *prolonged sustained contraction/rigidity;* Clonic: *repetitive rapid movements***
TREMORS	Rhythmic movement of a body part. - **Resting tremor:** tremor at rest (ex Parkinson disease) - **Postural tremor:** tremor occurs while holding position against gravity. - **Intentional tremor:** tremor occurs during movement or when approaching nearer to a target.

PARKINSONISM: disorders associated with tremor, bradykinesia, rigidity, and postural instability. Includes:

❶ ***Parkinson disease:*** loss of the dopamine producing cells of the substantia nigra (in the basal ganglia).

❷ ***Dopamine antagonists: medications that block dopamine include the typical antipsychotics*** *(Haloperidol, Droperidol, Fluphenazine, Chlorpromazine)* > ***atypical antipsychotics*** *(ex. Olanzapine, Clozapine, Risperidone).* Antiemetics: *Prochlorperazine, Promethazine, Metoclopramide.*

❸ ***Lewy body disease:*** loss of dopaminergic neurons leads to motor features similar to Parkinson disease. Loss of anticholinergic neurons lead to dementia (similar to Alzheimer's), visuospatial dysfunction & recurrent visual hallucinations.

❹ Other: head trauma, HIV, carbon monoxide or mercury poisoning, CNS dysfunction (ex stroke, meningitis).

MOVEMENT DISORDERS

HUNTINGTON DISEASE

- **Autosomal dominant** neurodegenerative disorder.

PATHOPHYSIOLOGY
- Inheritance of trinucleotide repeats (CAG/glutamine) on the Huntingtin gene (chromosome 4).
- Huntingtin gene leads to neurotoxicity as well as cerebral, putamen, & caudate nucleus atrophy.

CLINICAL MANIFESTATIONS:
- Symptoms usually appear **30-50y** of age.
- 3 hallmark manifestations: 3 Ms: mood, movement, & memory - **behavioral & mood changes, chorea** (rapid involuntary movements), & **dementia.**
- **Behavioral changes:** personality, cognitive, intellectual, & psychiatric including irritability.
- **Chorea**: rapid, involuntary or arrhythmic movement of the face, neck, trunk, & limbs initially. Chorea worsened with voluntary movements & stress (usually disappears with sleep).
- **Dementia**: most develop dementia before 50y (primarily executive dysfunction).
- Gait abnormalities, ataxia (often irregular & unsteady), incontinence, & facial grimacing.

PHYSICAL EXAMINATION
- Restlessness, fragility. Quick, involuntary hand movements. Brisk deep tendon reflexes.

DIAGNOSIS:
- Clinical symptoms + **family history** (if known) + **genetic confirmation**.
- Neuroimaging: **cerebral & striatal (caudate nucleus & putamen) atrophy** (CT, MRI). PET scan: decreased glucose metabolism in the caudate nucleus & putamen.

MANAGEMENT
- No cure. **Usually fatal within 15-20 years after presentation** (due to disease progression).
- No medication stops the disease progression.
- **Tetrabenazine for dyskinesia or chorea.**
- Antidopaminergics: typical & atypical antipsychotics.
- Benzodiazepine use intermittently may help with chorea & sleep, especially during stressful situations.

ESSENTIAL FAMILIAL TREMOR (BENIGN)

- **Autosomal dominant** inherited disorder of unknown etiology.
- Incidence increases with age.

CLINICAL MANIFESTATIONS
- **Intentional tremor – postural bilateral action tremor most commonly affecting the upper extremities & head** (hands, forearms, head, neck, or voice).
- **Tremor worsened** with **intentional movement** & adrenergic activity (eg, **emotional stress, anxiety**).
- **Tremor improved with alcohol ingestion.** Slight improvement with rest.

PHYSICAL EXAMINATION
- On finger to nose testing, the tremor increases at the end of approaching the target or holding a position against gravity.
- Besides the tremor, there are no other significant neurologic findings (cogwheel phenomenon may be seen in some).

DIAGNOSIS
- Diagnosis of exclusion based on history, **family history**, physical after ruling out other causes.

MANAGEMENT
- Treatment not usually needed.
- **Propranolol may help if severe or situational.**
- **Primidone** (barbiturate) if no relief with Propranolol, instead of Propranolol or with it.
- Alprazolam (benzodiazepine) third-line.
- Thalamotomy in refractory cases.

ESSENTIAL TREMOR VS PARKINSON

ESSENTIAL TREMOR	PARKINSON DISEASE
Tremor affects **head & voice**	
•**INTENTIONAL POSTURAL** • Worse with movement, stress	•**RESTING** tremor •Worse at rest & stress
•**Relieved with alcohol Propranolol**	•**Relieved with voluntary activity, intentional movement & sleep.**
•Usually **BILATERAL & SYMMETRICAL**	•Usually starts on **ONE SIDE of the body**

PARKINSON DISEASE

- Movement disorder due to **idiopathic loss of dopaminergic neurons in the substantia nigra.**

PATHOPHYSIOLOGY

- Loss of dopaminergic neurons leads to failure of acetylcholine inhibition in the **basal ganglia** (acetylcholine is an excitatory CNS neurotransmitter, dopamine is inhibitory).
- Also affects dopamine's ability to initiate movement.
- Onset of symptoms 45-65y most common.

CLINICAL MANIFESTATIONS

- **Triad: resting tremor, bradykinesia, & muscle rigidity.**
- Normal deep tendon reflexes, relatively immobile face. Dementia is a late finding.

- **Resting tremor:** often the first symptom. **"Pill-rolling"** tremor of the hand.
  - **Worse at rest** and with emotional stress.
  - **Improves with voluntary activity**, intentional movement, and sleep.
  - Usually confined to one limb or one side for years before it becomes generalized.

- **Bradykinesia: slowness of voluntary movement & decreased automatic movements** (eg, lack of swinging of the arms while walking & shuffling gait).

- **Rigidity:** increased resistance to passive movement (**cogwheel,** flexed posture). Festination = increasing speed while walking.

- Normal deep tendon reflexes. Usually no muscle weakness.

- **Face involvement:** relatively immobile face **(fixed facial expressions),** widened palpebral fissure, **Myerson's sign:** tapping the bridge of nose repetitively causes a sustained blink. Decreased blinking. Seborrhea of the skin common.

- **Postural instability**: usually a late finding. Pull test – standing behind the patient & pulling the shoulders causes the patient to fall or take steps backwards.

- Dementia in 50% (usually a late finding). Many develop depression.

DIAGNOSIS

- Clinical diagnosis.
- Post-mortem histology: cytoplasmic inclusions **(Lewy bodies)** & loss of pigment cells seen **in the substantia nigra.**

MANAGEMENT

- **Levodopa-carbidopa - most effective treatment.**
- **Dopamine agonists** (eg, Bromocriptine, Pramipexole, Ropinirole) may be used as initial treatment.
- Anticholinergics (eg, Trihexyphenidyl, Benztropine)
- Amantadine – increases dopamine
- MAO-B inhibitors (eg, Selegiline, Rasagiline)
- COMT inhibitors (eg, Entacapone, Tolcapone).
- Deep brain stimulation is extremely effective for rigidity and tremors in select patients.

Levodopa

Mechanism of action:

- Levodopa is converted to dopamine once it crosses the blood brain barrier.
- **Carbidopa reduces amount of Levodopa needed** & also reduces the peripheral conversion of levodopa into dopamine, reducing the adverse effects of Levodopa.

Indications:

- **Most effective treatment for symptoms of PD.**

Adverse effects:

- Nausea, vomiting, orthostatic hypotension, somnolence, headache.
- Psychosis & hallucinations upon initiation of therapy.
- Dyskinesia (involuntary movements especially the lower extremities) & akinesia.
- **Long-term use associated with "wearing off"** (decreased efficacy).
- Levodopa should be used at the minimum dose of clinical efficacy to reduce wearing off effect. If Levodopa is stopped abruptly, a syndrome similar to neuroleptic malignant syndrome can occur.

Dopamine agonists - Bromocriptine, Pramipexole, Ropinirole

Mechanism of action:

- Directly stimulates dopamine receptors.
- Less motor adverse effects than Levodopa but not as effective as Levodopa.

Indications:

- **Can be used as first-line agents in younger patients (<65y) to delay the use of Levodopa**. If patient is not sensitive to Levodopa, they will often be insensitive to dopamine agonists.

Adverse effects:

- Similar to Levodopa - orthostatic hypotension, headache, dizziness, hallucinations, confusion, anorexia.
- More frequent nonmotor side effects compared to Levodopa (eg, sleep disturbances, somnolence, dizziness, impulse control such as compulsive shopping or gambling, hypersexuality from dopamine reward effect)

Anticholinergics - Trihexyphenidyl, Benztropine

Mechanism of action:

- Anticholinergic (antimuscarinic) that blocks the excitatory effects of acetylcholine.

Indications:

- Most useful as **monotherapy in younger patients (<70y) with <u>tremor as the predominant symptom</u>** (without significant bradykinesia or gait disturbance).
- **Does not improve bradykinesia.**
- Adjunctive treatment for severe tremor despite Levodopa or dopamine agonists.

Adverse effects:

- Anticholinergic – constipation, dry mouth, blurred vision, tachycardia, urinary retention.
- **May worsen glaucoma and benign prostatic hypertrophy.**

Amantadine

Mechanism of action:

- Increases presynaptic dopamine release & inhibits dopamine reuptake.

Indications:

- **Low-potency** antiparkinsonian therapy that can help early on with **mild symptoms.**
- Improves long-term levodopa-induced dyskinesia.

Adverse effects:

- Livedo reticularis and ankle edema.
- Rare – confusion and hallucinations (more likely in older patients).

Selective MAO-B Inhibitors - Selegiline, Rasagiline

Mechanism of action:

- **Increases dopamine in the striatum** (MAO-B normally breaks down dopamine).

Indications:

- Can be used as early therapy in patients with very mild sign and symptoms.
- May have neuroprotective properties in PD.

Adverse effects:

- Nausea, headache, confusion, hallucinations.

COMT inhibitors - Entacapone, Tolcapone.

Mechanism of action:

- Catechol-O-methyltransferase inhibition prevents dopamine breakdown

Indications:

- **Adjunctive treatment with Levodopa** (prolongs the therapeutic dose of Levodopa) in patients experiencing wearing "off" periods.
- Not used as monotherapy.

Adverse effects:

- Nausea, orthostatic hypotension, hallucination, orthostatic hypotension, GI symptoms, brown discoloration of the urine.
- Tolcapone associated with **hepatotoxicity**.

AMYOTROPHIC LATERAL SCLEROSIS (ALS) LOU GEHRIG'S DISEASE

- Neurodegenerative disorder due to necrosis of BOTH upper & lower motor neurons, leading to **progressive motor degeneration**. Idiopathic etiology.
- **Sensation, voluntary eye movement, sphincter function (bowel & bladder), and sexual function are spared.**

CLINICAL MANIFESTATIONS

- **Asymmetric limb weakness is the most common presenting symptom,** muscle weakness, loss of ability to initiate & control motor movements.
- Bulbar symptoms: dysphagia, dysarthria, speech problems, **difficulty in chewing, aspiration**.
- Cognitive impairment (frontotemporal dysfunction).

PHYSICAL EXAMINATION

Mixed upper & lower motor neuron signs & symptoms hallmark.

- Upper motor neuron: spasticity, stiffness, hyperreflexia, weakness.
- Lower motor neuron: progressive bilateral fasciculations, muscle atrophy, hyporeflexia, weakness.

DIAGNOSIS

- Electromyography: loss of neural innervation & reinnervation in muscle groups. Elevated CPK levels.

MANAGEMENT

- **Riluzole** reduces glutamate buildup in neurons. Only drug known to impact ALS (reduces the progression for up to 6 months). Edaravone.
- CPAP, BiPAP, and ventilator may be needed as the disease advances.

PROGNOSIS

- Usually fatal within 3-5 years after onset – **Respiratory failure most common cause of death.**

TOURETTE DISORDER

- Idiopathic movement disorder characterized by vocal tics, motor tics, and Obsessive-compulsive disorder.
- **Onset usually in childhood** (onset 4-6 years) with peak severity 10-12 years of age with decreased symptoms in adolescence & significant decrease in adulthood. Most common in boys.

PATHOPHYSIOLOGY
- Idiopathic. May be due to excess dopamine + GABA deficiency in the caudate nucleus.

CLINICAL MANIFESTATIONS
- **Motor tics: most common initial symptom** – usually involves the face, head or neck (eg, **blinking,** shrugging, head thrusting, sniffling).
- **Verbal or phonetic tics:** eg, grunts, throat-clearing, obscene words (coprolalia), repetitive phrases, repeating the phrases of others (echolalia).
- Self-mutilating tics: hair pulling, nail biting, biting of the lips etc.

Diagnostic criteria
- **Multiple motor & 1 or more vocal tics** (not required to occur concurrently) for **> 1 year** since the first tic (frequency may wax and wane).
- **Onset prior to age 18 years**. Not caused by a substance or medical condition.

Management
- **Habit reversal therapy first-line** (most don't need medical management).

MEDICAL MANAGEMENT
- Dopamine blocking agents: eg, **Tetrabenazine**, Risperidone, Haloperidol, Fluphenazine, Pimozide.
- Alpha-2 adrenergics: eg, **Clonidine** (more sedating) or **Guanfacine**.
- Clonazepam may also be used as adjunct.

CEREBRAL PALSY

- CNS disorder associated with **muscle tone, movement, & postural abnormalities** due to brain injury during perinatal or prenatal period.
- Types include spastic, dyskinetic, & ataxic.

CLINICAL MANIFESTATIONS
- **Spasticity is hallmark.**
- Varying degrees of motor deficits. May develop seizures.
- Often associated with intellectual or learning disabilities & development abnormalities.

PHYSICAL EXAMINATION
- Hyperreflexia, limb-length discrepancies, congenital defects, & persistent primitive reflexes.

DIAGNOSIS
- **Primarily clinical but MRI required in all patients.**
- Workup includes screening for commonly associated conditions.

MANAGEMENT
- Multidisciplinary approach. Pain management.
- Spasticity: Baclofen, Diazepam. Antiepileptics for seizures.

RESTLESS LEG SYNDROME (Willis-Ekbom disease)

- Sleep-related movement disorder.
- Etiologies: usually primary (idiopathic) but may occur secondary to **CNS iron deficiency**, pregnancy, peripheral neuropathy, uremia, & chronic alcohol use.

CLINICAL MANIFESTATIONS

- **Uncomfortable or unpleasant sensation** (itching, burning, paresthesias, etc.) in the **legs that creates an urge to move the legs.**
- Symptoms **worsen at night** & **with prolonged periods of rest or inactivity**.
- During sleep, periodic limb movements may disturb sleep or cause the patient to awake from sleep.
- **Symptoms improve with leg movement.**

DIAGNOSIS

- Primarily a clinical diagnosis.
- Iron workup usually performed as part of workup for underlying causes.

MANAGEMENT

- **Dopamine agonists**: **treatment of choice** (eg, **Pramipexole, Ropinirole).**
- **Iron supplementation** recommended in patients with a serum ferritin levels lower than 75 mcg/L because of the association with iron deficiency in the central nervous system.
- Alpha-2-delta calcium channel ligands: eg, **Gabapentin**, Pregabalin.
- Benzodiazepines: may be used as adjunctive treatment. (eg Clonazepam).
- Opioids may be used in disease resistant to the aforementioned medications.

BELL PALSY

- **Idiopathic, unilateral CN VII/facial nerve palsy** leading to **hemifacial weakness & paralysis** due to inflammation or compression.
- Lower motor neuron disorder.
- Although idiopathic may be related to **Herpes simplex virus reactivation.**
- Risk factors: Diabetes mellitus, pregnancy (especially the 3rd trimester), post URI, dental nerve block.

CLINICAL MANIFESTATIONS:

- sudden onset of **ipsilateral hyperacusis (ear pain)** 24-48 hours followed by **unilateral facial weakness or paralysis involving the forehead**: **unable to lift the affected eyebrow,** wrinkle forehead, smile, loss of the nasolabial fold, drooping of the corner of mouth, **taste disturbance (anterior $^2/_3$)**, biting the inner cheek, eye irritation (due to decreased lacrimation & **inability to fully close eyelid**). Bell phenomenon: eye on the affected side moves laterally & superiorly when eye closure is attempted. The **weakness & paralysis ONLY affects the face**.

- DIAGNOSIS: diagnosis of exclusion.

MANAGEMENT:

- **No treatment is required** (>85% of cases resolve within 1 month) – **supportive: artificial tears** (replaces lacrimation, reduces vision problems). Eye patches worn during sleep if severe to prevent corneal ulceration.
- **Prednisone (especially if started within the first 72 hours of symptom onset) reduces the time to full recovery & increases the likelihood of complete recuperation.**
- Acyclovir in combination with glucocorticoids in severe cases has been shown to improve symptoms & timing of recovery.

GUILLAIN BARRÉ SYNDROME

- Acquired autoimmune **demyelinating polyradiculopathy** of the **peripheral nervous system.**
- Pathophysiology: autoantibody attacks the myelin sheath of the peripheral nerves (molecular mimicry) after an infection.

ETIOLOGIES

- **Increased incidence with *Campylobacter jejuni* (most common)** or other **antecedent GI or respiratory infections,** CMV, Epstein-Barr virus, HIV, Mycoplasma infections, immunizations & postsurgical.

CLINICAL MANIFESTATIONS

- **Symmetric ascending weakness & sensory changes (paresthesias, pain)** - distal lower extremities first.
- May develop **weakness of the respiratory muscles** & bulbar muscles (swallowing abnormalities).

PHYSICAL EXAMINATION

- Lower motor neuron signs: **decreased deep tendon reflexes**, flaccid paralysis, weakness.
- **Sensory deficits.** Cranial nerve palsies (eg, CN VII).
- **Autonomic dysfunction:** tachycardia, arrhythmias, hypotension or hypertension, **breathing difficulties.**

DIAGNOSIS

- **Electrophysiologic studies:** Nerve conduction studies and needle electromyography - decreased motor nerve conduction velocities & amplitude – **most specific tests**.
- **CSF analysis: high protein with a normal WBC count** (usually seen 1-3 weeks after symptom onset).
- Pulmonary function test: important to assess peak inspiratory pressure and forced vital capacity (FVC) - both decrease with GBS. Most important to determine the need for intubation.

MANAGEMENT

- **Plasmapheresis or IV immune globulin (IVIG) are first-line** (for antibody removal and neutralization).
- Mechanical ventilation if respiratory failure or decreased FVC on PFTs.
- **Prednisone not indicated** in the management of GBS.
- Prognosis: 60% full recovery in 1 year (10-20% left with permanent disability).

MYASTHENIA GRAVIS

- Autoimmune peripheral nerve disorder due to autoantibodies against the acetylcholine receptor on the muscles, leading to weakness.

- **Most common in young women** <40 and older men >50y.

- Strong association with an **abnormal thymus gland** (eg, hyperplasia or thymoma) 75%, HLA B8 & DR3.

PATHOPHYSIOLOGY
- **Autoantibodies against acetylcholine (nicotinic) postsynaptic receptor at the neuromuscular junction** cause decreased skeletal muscle neuromuscular transmission with muscle recovery after a period of rest.

CLINICAL MANIFESTATIONS
- 2 main clinical manifestations: ❶ Ocular weakness & ❷ Generalized weakness. The **weakness is worsened with repeated muscle use** & throughout the day.

- Ocular weakness: **diplopia & ptosis** usually first presenting symptoms. **Pupils are spared.**

- Generalized muscle weakness: **Bulbar (oropharyngeal) weakness** - weakness with prolonged chewing, dysphagia, dysphonia, & dysarthria. **Respiratory muscle weakness**: may lead to **respiratory failure = Myasthenic crisis.**

DIAGNOSIS IN OUTPATIENT SETTING
- **Acetylcholine receptor antibodies initial test of choice.**

- MuSK antibodies should be obtained if ACR antibodies negative.

- Electrophysiology testing: repetitive nerve stimulation or electromyography (most accurate test for MG).

- Chest imaging: (eg, CXR, CT, or MRI) done in all patients to detect thymus gland abnormalities.

DIAGNOSIS IN EMERGENT SETTING
- **Edrophonium (Tensilon) test:** brief improvement of symptoms after administration.

- **Ice pack test:** application of ice for 10 minutes improve ocular symptoms.

MANAGEMENT
- **Myasthenic crisis or severe: Plasmapheresis or IV immunoglobulin.**

- Long-term: acetylcholinesterase inhibitors (eg, **Pyridostigmine or Neostigmine) first-line treatment** of symptoms. Glucocorticoid. Azathioprine, or Cyclosporine are steroid alternatives.

- **Thymectomy,** even if thymus gland is normal, can improve symptoms and removes the source of antibodies. Useful if no improvement with medical management. Glucocorticoids if > 60 years.

- Avoid medications known to exacerbate MG (eg, fluoroquinolones, aminoglycosides, beta blockers).

ACETYLCHOLINESTERASE INHIBITORS

Pyridostigmine, Neostigmine

Mechanism of action:

- Acetylcholinesterase inhibitors (prevent acetylcholine breakdown in the synapse).

Indications:

- **First-line medical management of Myasthenia gravis.**
- **Edrophonium** short-acting drug that is **used for diagnostic purposes**.

Adverse effects:

- **Cholinergic: abdominal cramps, diarrhea, sweating, nausea, vomiting,** increased salivation, increased bronchial secretions, bradycardia. Acetylcholine causes SLUDD-C (salivation, lacrimation, urination, digestion, defecation and pupillary constriction).
- Glycopyrrolate and Hyoscyamine are anticholinergic drugs with little to no effect on the nicotinic receptors. They are used to help control some of the adverse effects of acetylcholinesterase inhibitor therapy.
- Cholinergic crisis: excess medication leading to weakness, nausea, vomiting, pallor, sweating, salivation, diarrhea, miosis, bradycardia, & respiratory failure.

LAMBERT-EATON MYASTHENIC SYNDROME

- **Antibodies against presynaptic voltage-gated calcium channels** prevent acetylcholine release, leading to muscle weakness.
- **Most commonly associated with Small cell lung cancer** & other malignancies.

CLINICAL MANIFESTATIONS

- **Proximal muscle weakness that improves with repeated muscle use** (unlike Myasthenia gravis). The weakness may cause difficulty arising from a chair, gait alteration or managing stairs.
- **Autonomic symptoms: dry mouth most common,** postural hypotension, & erectile dysfunction.
- Physical examination: **Hyporeflexia.** Sluggish pupillary response. No muscle atrophy.

DIAGNOSIS

- Voltage-gated calcium channel antibody assay.
- Electrophysiology: reproducible post exercise increase in compound muscle activation on repetitive nerve stimulation testing.
- CT scan to assess for underlying malignancy.

MANAGEMENT

- **Treat the underlying malignancy.**
- Initial medical management: **Pyridostigmine**. 3,4-diaminopyridine.
- Second-line: Plasmapheresis, IVIG, oral immunosuppressants.

MULTIPLE SCLEROSIS

- **Autoimmune, inflammatory demyelinating disease of the CNS** of idiopathic origin.
- Associated with axon degeneration of **white matter (brain & spinal cord)**.
- Most common in **women & young adults 20-40y,** colder climates. Associated with HLA-DR2

3 main types:
- **Relapsing-remitting disease most common** - episodic exacerbations.
- Progressive disease: progressive decline without acute exacerbations.
- Secondary progressive: relapsing-remitting pattern that becomes progressive.

CLINICAL MANIFESTATIONS
- **Sensory disturbances followed by weakness & visual disturbances are the most common presenting symptoms.** Sensory deficits (pain, paresthesias), motor deficits (weakness, gait, and balance problems). Visual disturbances **(diplopia, Optic neuritis),** fatigue. **Trigeminal neuralgia**.
- Uhthoff's phenomenon: worsening of symptoms with heat (eg, exercise, fever, hot tubs, weather etc.).
- Spinal cord symptoms: bladder or bowel dysfunction.

PHYSICAL EXAMINATION
- **Upper motor neuron signs: spasticity, upward Babinski, hyperreflexia,** muscle rigidity.
- Lhermitte's sign: neck flexion causes lightning-shock type pain radiating from the spine down the leg.
- Marcus-Gunn pupil with Optic neuritis – during swinging-flashlight test *from the unaffected eye into the affected eye, the pupils appear to dilate* (due to less than normal pupillary constriction). This response is due to the brain perceiving the delayed conduction of affected optic nerve as if light was reduced.
- Internuclear ophthalmoplegia - inability to adduct the eye on the side of the lesion with nystagmus in the other eye.
- Cerebellar: Charcot's neurologic triad (nystagmus, staccato speech, and intentional tremor). Ataxia.
- Spinal cord symptoms: bladder, bowel, or sexual dysfunction.

DIAGNOSIS
- Mainly clinical (at least 2 distinct episode of CNS deficits).
- **MRI with gadolinium best initial & most accurate test - hyperintense white matter plaques** hallmark finding. There should be proof at least 2 areas of white matter involvement before the diagnosis is made.
- Lumbar puncture indicated if negative MRI - **increased IgG & oligoclonal bands –** small discrete bands in the gamma globulin region seen on electrophoresis, which reflects inflammatory cells penetrating the blood brain barrier.

MANAGEMENT – ACUTE EXACERBATION
- **IV Glucocorticoids first-line treatment** (high-dose).
- Plasmapheresis if not responsive to glucocorticoids.

PREVENTION OF RELAPSE & PROGRESSION
- **Beta-interferon or Glatiramer first-line**.
- Natalizumab (may cause progressive multifocal leukoencephalopathy), Teriflunomide.
- Amantadine helpful for fatigue symptoms. Baclofen & Diazepam for spasticity.

ASTROCYTOMA

- Derived from astrocytes (astrocytes are star-shaped glial cells of the brain & spinal cord that support the endothelial cells of the blood-brain barrier, provide nutrients for cells, maintain extracellular ion balance, and also repair the brain after injury).
- Can appear in any part of the brain. *Most often infratentorial in children (supratentorial in adults).*

TYPES OF ASTROCYTOMAS

- **PILOCYTIC ASTROCYTOMA (GRADE I):** (Juvenile Astrocytoma) - typically localized. Considered the **"most benign"** (noncancerous) of all the Astrocytomas. **Most common in children & young adults.** Other grade I Astrocytomas include cerebellar Astrocytoma & desmoplastic infantile.

- **DIFFUSE ASTROCYTOMA** (**Grade II** or Low-grade) Types: Fibrillary, Gemistocytic & Protoplasmic. They tend to invade surrounding tissues but grow at a relatively slow pace.

- **ANAPLASTIC ASTROCYTOMA**: **(Grade III).** Rare but aggressive.

- **GRADE IV: Glioblastoma multiforme is the most common primary CNS tumors in adults.**

- Subependymal Giant cell Astrocytoma - ventricular tumors associated with tuberculous sclerosis.

CLINICAL MANIFESTATIONS

1. Focal deficits: most common. Depends on the location of the lesion. MC in frontal & temporal areas of the cerebral hemisphere.
   - General symptoms: **headaches** (may be worse in the morning, **may wake patients up at night**, may be positional), cranial nerve deficits, altered mental status changes, neurological deficits, ataxia, vision changes, weakness.
2. Increased intracranial pressure*:* due to mass effect ⇨ headache, nausea, vomiting, papilledema, ataxia, drowsiness, stupor.

DIAGNOSIS

1. CT scan or MRI with contrast: Grade I & II non-enhancing. Grade III & IV are enhancing.
2. Brain biopsy: usually guided by imaging studies. Histologic appearance includes:
   - **Pilocytic Astrocytomas (Grade I)** generally form sacs of fluid (**cystic**), or may be enclosed within a cyst. Although they are usually slow-growing, these tumors can become very large. **Rosenthal fibers** (eosinophilic corkscrew fibers).

   - **Diffuse Astrocytomas** tend to contain microcysts and mucus-like fluid. They are grouped by the appearance and behavior of the cells for which they are named.

   - **Anaplastic Astrocytomas** tend to have tentacle-like projections that grow into surrounding tissue, making them difficult to completely remove during surgery.

   - **Astrocytoma Grade IV (glioblastoma)** may contain cystic material, calcium deposits, blood vessels, and/or a mixed grade of cells.

MANAGEMENT

1. Pilocytic Astrocytoma: Surgical excision. In adults and older children, radiation may follow surgery if the tumor cannot be completely removed.
2. Diffuse Astrocytoma: Surgery if the tumor is accessible & can be completely removed. Radiation may be adjunctive to surgery or for unresectable tumors.
3. Anaplastic Astrocytoma: Surgery ⇨ XRT. ±Chemotherapy after radiation or for tumor recurrence.
4. Astrocytoma Grade IV: Surgery ⇨ XRT (radiation therapy) + Chemotherapy.

GLIOBLASTOMA MUTLIFORME

- **Most common & most aggressive primary malignant CNS tumors in adults**
- Glioblastoma = Grade IV Astrocytoma (heterogenous mixture of poorly differentiated astrocytes).
- Risk factors: Males, >50y, HHV-6 & cytomegalovirus infections, ionizing radiation.

TYPES
- **PRIMARY: most common** (60%). **Seen in adults >50y.** Arises de novo (new). Most common type & most aggressive.
- **SECONDARY:** (40%). Most common <45y. Due to malignant progression from a low-grade Astrocytoma (grade II) or anaplastic Astrocytoma (grade III). May transform as early as 1 year or >10y.

VARIANTS
- "Classic": 97%. Presence of extra copies of the epidermal growth factor receptor gene (EGFR). TP53 is rarely mutated in this type (note that the others are associated with TP53 mutation).
- Mesenchymal: high rates of mutations & alterations including the gene encoding for neurofibromatosis type I. TP53 often mutated. An alteration of MGMT (a DNA repair enzyme)

CLINICAL MANIFESTATIONS
- Focal deficits depend on the location of the tumor. Most common in the frontal & temporal areas of the cerebral hemisphere.
- General: **headache** (may be worse in the morning, **may wake patients up at night**, may be positional), cranial nerve deficits (eg, fixed, dilated pupil from a CN III palsy), altered mental status, neurological deficits, ataxia, vision changes, weakness.

DIAGNOSIS
- **Brain MRI with contrast initial study of choice**: classic finding is heterogenous lesion with **variable ring of enhancement** with central necrosis, surrounded by edema & irregular (**serpiginous**) **margins**. Mass effect may cause hydrocephalus. May **cross the corpus callosum ("butterfly" glioma).**
- Histology (usually post-surgical): malignant astrocytes + necrotizing, hemorrhagic center surrounded by **pseudo palisading** (tumor cells lining the area of necrosis).

MANAGEMENT
- Surgical excision when possible, radiotherapy & adjuvant chemotherapy with Temozolomide (alkylating agent).

MENINGIOMA

- Usually **benign, slow-growing tumors** arising from arachnoid meningothelial cells of the meninges (covering the brain & spinal cord).
- **Most commonly arises from the dura** or sites of dura reflection (eg, venous sinuses, falx cerebri).
- Risk factors: females (estrogen receptors on tumor cells), radiation exposure.

CLINICAL MANIFESTATIONS

- Often asymptomatic (incidental finding) or causes **symptoms due to compression & displacement of the brain** (usually does not invade the brain parenchyma). Seizures or focal neurologic signs (depending on the location of the tumor). Fixed dilated pupil (CN III) common.

DIAGNOSIS

- **MRI with contrast** preferred: extra-axial **intensely enhancing, well-defined lesion often attached to the dura** (resembling a snowball). May have increased calcifications.
- Histology: **spindle-cells** concentrically arranged in a **whorled pattern. Psammoma bodies** (concentric round calcifications).

MANAGEMENT

- Asymptomatic: observation if small.
- **Symptomatic: surgical excision when possible** (transarterial embolization may be performed prior to surgery). Radiation therapy may be used if not a surgical candidate or as adjuvant treatment in some.

CNS LYMPHOMA

- Primary: seen without evidence of systemic disease. **Variant of extranodal Non-Hodgkin lymphoma (NHL).** Secondary is more common.
- Secondary: METS from another site (eg, NHL in the neck, chest, groin, abdomen) **especially diffuse large B cell lymphoma (90%).** Burkitt's lymphoma (10%).

RISK FACTORS

- **Epstein-Barr virus** positive in 90% of these patients, immunosuppression (eg, AIDS, post-transplant, receiving immunosuppressant treatment).

CLINICAL MANIFESTATIONS

- Focal deficits: depends on the location of the lesion.
- Ocular symptoms: visual changes, steroid-refractory posterior uveitis.

DIAGNOSIS

- CT scan or MRI with contrast: hypointense **ring-enhancing lesion** in the deep white matter on CT.
- Biopsy: usually guided by imaging study.
- Workup includes CT of abdomen/pelvis, PET scan, bone marrow biopsy, slit lamp examination.

MANAGEMENT

- **Chemotherapy: Methotrexate most effective chemotherapy** (given with folinic acid/leucovorin). Chemotherapy not usually given at the same time as radiation therapy (due to increased risk of leukoencephalopathy).
- Radiation therapy. Corticosteroids: partial response. Surgical resection usually ineffective.

OLIGODENDROGLIOMA

- Oligodendrocyte – a type of cell that makes up the supportive (glial) tissue of the brain. These tumors can be found anywhere within the cerebral hemispheres (especially the frontal & temporal lobes).

CLINICAL MANIFESTATIONS
- May be asymptomatic. May be incidental finding (tumor grows slowly).
- Focal deficits: includes seizures, headaches & personality changes (depends on the tumor location).

DIAGNOSIS
- CT scan or MRI with contrast.
- Brain biopsy: usually guided by imaging studies.
- Histologic appearance: soft, grayish-pink *calcified* tumors, areas of hemorrhage &/or cystic. *Chicken-wire capillary pattern* with *"fried-egg shaped"* tumor cells seen with microscope.

MANAGEMENT
- Surgical resection standard treatment. ± Radiation and/or chemotherapy (eg, anaplastic).

EPENDYMOMA

- Ependymal cells line the ventricles & parts of the spinal column.
- **Most common in children** (mean age at diagnosis is 5 years of age).
- **Most commonly seen in 4th ventricle, spinal cord** & medulla. May cause Cauda equina in adults.

CLINICAL MANIFESTATIONS
- Infants: increased in head size, irritability, sleeplessness & vomiting.
- Older children & adults: nausea, vomiting, headache.

DIAGNOSIS
- CT scan or MRI with contrast: hypointense T1, hyperintense T2. Enhances with gadolinium.
- Brain biopsy: **perivascular pseudo rosettes** (tumor cells surrounding a blood vessel).

MANAGEMENT
- Surgical resection ⇨ adjuvant radiation therapy. Chemotherapy not as helpful usually.

HEMANGIOMAS

- **Hemangioma:** abnormal buildup of blood vessels in the skin or internal organs. 2% of all 1ry brain tumors. Von Hippel-Lindau syndrome 10% - (hemangiomas, tumors of the liver, pancreas & kidney).
- **Hemangioblastoma:** arises from the blood vessel lining. Benign, slow growing well-defined tumors. MC found in the posterior fossa (**brainstem & cerebellum**). Often >40y. May occur in the cerebral hemispheres or spinal cord. **Retinal hemangiomas associated with von Hippel-Lindau syndrome.**
- Hemangiopericytoma: originate from the cells surrounding the blood vessels & the meninges. May spread to the lung & liver.

CLINICAL MANIFESTATIONS
- Hemangioblastoma: headache, nausea, vomiting, gait abnormalities, poor coordination of the limbs. May produce erythropoietin (secondary polycythemia). Hemangiopericytoma: depends on tumor location.

DIAGNOSIS
- CT scan or MRI. Biopsy: well-defined borders, usually does not invade surrounding healthy tissue. **Foam cells with high vascularity.**

MANAGEMENT: surgical resection. Radiation may be used in tumors attached to the brainstem.

NEUROCOGNITIVE DISORDERS

DELIRIUM

- **Acute, abrupt transient confused state** due to an **identifiable cause** (eg, medications, infections, electrolyte abnormalities, CNS injury, uremia, organ failure, illicit drugs intoxication or withdrawal etc.).
- Rapid onset associated with fluctuating mental status changes & marked deficit in short-term memory.
- Usually associated with full recovery within 1 week in most cases.

ALZHEIMER DEMENTIA

- **Most common type of dementia.**

RISK FACTORS

- Increasing age, genetics, family history.

PATHOPHYSIOLOGY

- Unknown – 3 hypotheses: 1. Amyloid hypothesis: **extracellular amyloid-beta protein deposition (senile plaques)** in the brain are neurotoxic. Tau hypothesis: **neurofibrillary tangles (hyperphosphorylated tau proteins)** are neurotoxic. 3. Cholinergic hypothesis: **acetylcholine deficiency** leads to memory, language, & visuospatial changes.

CLINICAL MANIFESTATIONS

- **Short-term memory loss (often first symptom).** Progresses to **long-term memory loss and cognitive deficits**: disorientation, behavioral & personality changes, language difficulties, loss of motor skills etc. Usually gradual in nature.

DIAGNOSIS

- **Clinical diagnosis (no specific test)**. Workup to rule out other causes include MRI of the brain, CBC, renal and liver tests, VDRL or RPR to rule out Syphilis, B12, and thyroid function studies.
- **MRI preferred neuroimaging test – cortex atrophy (eg, medial temporal lobe atrophy),** reduced hippocampal volume, white matter lesions.
- Histologic findings: **amyloid-beta protein deposition(senile plaques)** in the brain. Amyloid precursor proteins (APP) are normally degraded by alpha-cleavage. Beta cleavage of APP results in Amyloid-beta accumulation. **Neurofibrillary tangles** = intracellular aggregations of **tau protein** (an insoluble cytoskeletal microtubule element).

MEDICAL MANAGEMENT

- **Acetylcholinesterase inhibitors: Donepezil, Tacrine, Rivastigmine, Galantamine**. Used to improve memory function & symptom relief (does not slow down the disease progression).

- NMDA antagonist: **Memantine** – can be adjunctive or used as monotherapy in moderate to severe disease.
  Mechanism: *blocks NMDA* receptor, slowing calcium influx & nerve damage. Glutamate is an excitatory neurotransmitter of the NDMA receptor. Excitotoxicity causes cell death. NMDA antagonists reduce glutamate excitotoxicity. May be adjunctive.

VASCULAR DEMENTIA

- Brain disease due to chronic ischemia & multiple infarctions (eg, **lacunar infarcts**).
- **Hypertension most important risk factor.** Diabetes mellitus, history of CVA, Atrial fibrillation.

CLINICAL MANIFESTATIONS
- **Sudden decline in functions with a stepwise progression of symptoms** (random infarct then decline ⇨ stable then another infarct ⇨ decline etc.).
- **Cortical manifestations:** depends on areas affected. Medial frontal: executive dysfunction, apathy, abulia. Left parietal: apraxia aphasia or agnosia. Right parietal: hemineglect, confusion, visuospatial abnormalities.
- **Subcortical manifestations:** focal motor deficits, gait abnormalities, urinary difficulties, personality changes.

DIAGNOSIS
- Clinical diagnosis. Workup similar to Alzheimer disease - rule out other causes of symptoms (eg, B12 and folate levels, RPR, etc.).
- MRI: white matter lesions, cortical or subcortical infarcts. CT scan may show lacunar infarcts.

PREVENTION: strict blood pressure control

FRONTOTEMPORAL DEMENTIA (PICK'S DISEASE)

- **Localized brain degeneration of the frontotemporal lobes.** May progress globally.

CLINICAL MANIFESTATIONS
- **Marked changes in social behavior, personality, and language (aphasia) are early signs of FTD** with eventual executive and memory dysfunction (dementia with advanced disease). The onset of dementia is earlier than Alzheimer disease (usually presents in the 6th decade).
- **Behavioral changes: disinhibition or socially inappropriate behaviors**, apathy, **hyperorality** (binge-eating, changes in food preferences, putting large amounts of food in their mouth), compulsive ritualistic behaviors, loss of sympathy & empathy.

PHYSICAL EXAMINATION
- Preserved visuospatial. In advanced disease, they may have positive primitive reflexes (palmomental & palmar grasp). May have Parkinsonism.
- Histology: **Pick bodies:** round or oval aggregates of Tau protein seen on silver-staining of the cortex

DIFFUSE LEWY BODY DISEASE

- Progressive dementia characterized by the diffuse presence of Lewy bodies (abnormal neuronal protein deposits) in comparison to Parkinson disease, where the Lewy bodies are localized.

CLINICAL MANIFESTATIONS
- Core features that occur early: **visual hallucinations,** episodic delirium (**cognitive fluctuations**), **Parkinsonism** & rapid eye movement (REM) sleep disorder. Dementia late finding. Delusions, sensitivity to antipsychotic drugs, **autonomic dysfunction** (eg, orthostatic hypotension).

HISTOLOGY
- Cortical Lewy bodies (abnormal deposition of alpha-synuclein proteins).

MANAGEMENT
- Treatment of the Parkinsonian symptoms may worsen the neuropsychiatric symptoms and vice versa.

FOCAL (PARTIAL) SEIZURE

- Abnormal neuronal discharge from one discrete section of one hemisphere.
- **With retained awareness** (simple): consciousness fully maintained.
- **With impaired awareness** (complex): consciousness impaired.

CLINICAL MANIFESTATIONS

- **Focal sensory, motor or autonomic symptoms** depending on the lobe affected. May be followed by a neurologic deficit (**Todd's paralysis**) lasting up to 24 hours.
- Motor: jerky rhythmic movements. May start in one area (focal) and then spread to other parts of the affected limb or body (**Jacksonian march**). May be tonic (muscular rigidity) or tonic (rhythmic jerking).
- Sensory: paresthesias, numbness, pain, heat, cold, sensation of movement, olfactory, flashing lights (photopsia).
- Autonomic: abdominal (pain, nausea, vomiting, hunger), cardiovascular (sinus tachycardia), blood pressure changes, bronchoconstriction. Psychologic: fear, déjà vu, hallucinations.
- Auras: may precede, accompany of follow the seizure onset.
- **Automatisms: repetitive behaviors** (eg, lip smacking, facial grimacing, chewing, manual picking, patting, coordinated movements or repeating words or phrases) that **may accompany complex partial seizures.**

DIAGNOSIS

- **Initial workup is to rule out reversible causes** (CBC, electrolytes, liver and renal function, & RPR). MRI to rule out focal mass.

Electroencephalogram

- Simple partial - **focal discharge** at the onset of the seizure.
- Complex partial - **interictal spikes or with slow waves in the temporal or frontotemporal area.**

ABSENCE (PETIT MAL) SEIZURE

- Generalized seizure (involving both hemispheres).
- **Most commonly seen in childhood** - age at onset usually 4 – 10 years (often ceases by early puberty or 20 years of age in most patients).

CLINICAL MANIFESTATIONS

- **Pause/stare: sudden, marked impairment of consciousness without loss of body tone** (patient remains upright), **staring episodes** with **pauses (behavioral arrest)**.
- **Episodes typically last between 5-10 seconds.** If >10 seconds, it can be associated with **eyelid twitching & lip smacking.**
- No postictal phase. May occur tens of times daily.
- May be associated with automatisms (predominantly oral), or myoclonus.
- May be provoked by hyperventilation.

DIAGNOSIS

- EEG: **bilateral symmetric 3 Hertz spike and wave activity** (2.5 – 5 Hz).

MANAGEMENT

- **Ethosuximide first-line medical management.** Valproic acid second-line. Lamotrigine.
- Carbamazepine or Gabapentin can exacerbate Absence seizures.

GENERALIZED (GRAND MAL) SEIZURE

- Simultaneous neuronal discharge of both hemispheres (diffuse brain involvement).
- Generalized tonic clonic (Grand mal) most common type.

CLINICAL MANIFESTATIONS

- **Tonic-clonic (Grand Mal):** sudden loss of consciousness with **tonic** activity (contraction & **rigidity**) that may be associated with respiratory arrest **followed by 1-2 minutes of clonic** activity (repetitive, rhythmic, symmetric jerking usually lasting <3 minutes) followed by **postictal confusion phase. Cyanosis & urinary incontinence can occur.**
- Clonic: repetitive rhythmic jerking (usually lasting < 2-3 minutes) often associated with a postictal state.
- Myoclonic: sudden, brief, sporadic involuntary twitching. May be one muscle or a group of muscles. No loss of consciousness.
- Tonic: loss of consciousness followed by **rigidity.**
- Atonic: sudden partial or complete loss of muscle and postural tone ("drop attacks").
- Absence: nonconvulsive brief lapse of consciousness with brief staring episodes or without loss of postural tone.

DIAGNOSIS

- **Initial workup is to rule out reversible causes** (CBC, electrolytes, liver and renal function, and RPR).
- **Increased prolactin & lactic acid immediately after seizures** may be helpful to rule out pseudo seizures. MRI to rule out focal mass.
- EEG: generalized high-amplitude rapid spiking during active episodes of tonic-clonic seizures.

MANAGEMENT

- Treat the underlying cause if known.
- Long-term options for epilepsy include Levetiracetam, Phenytoin, Valproic acid, Carbamazepine, Lamotrigine, Phenobarbital, Topiramate. Levetiracetam & Lamotrigine safest in pregnancy.
- Ethosuximide first-line for Absence. Valproic acid second-line.

STATUS EPILEPTICUS

- A single, continuous epileptic seizure lasting 5 minutes or greater, or more than 1 seizure within a 5 minute period without recovery in between the episodes. Considered a neurologic emergency

ETIOLOGIES

- Structural abnormalities, infections (eg, meningitis, encephalitis), metabolic abnormalities, medications, toxins.

DIAGNOSIS: Neuroimaging: once stabilized to determine if intracranial mass or hemorrhage is present.

MANAGEMENT

- **Benzodiazepines are the preferred initial agents (Lorazepam** usually preferred). They are associated with rapid control of seizure. Additional doses can be given. Midazolam can be used as initial IM therapy if an IV access cannot be established.
- Second-line: **Phenytoin or Fosphenytoin if no response to benzodiazepines.** They can also be used to prevent recurrence. Valproate and Levetiracetam alternatives.
- Third-line: **Phenobarbital if no response to Phenytoin** (refractory).
- General anesthesia: Midazolam and Propofol can be used.

COMPLICATIONS

- Hypoxia, aspiration, respiratory failure, cardiac arrhythmias.

PANCE PREP PEARL OF THE WEEK

PHENYTOIN

- **Mechanism:** stabilizes neuronal membranes by **blocking voltage-gated sodium channels**.
- Indications: generalized tonic-clonic & focal seizures (simple & complex), seizure prophylaxis. **Status epilepticus after benzodiazepines**

SLOW·DOWN
YIELD TO
Slow to prevent low BP & arrhythmias

SIDE EFFECTS

P-450 inducer & **induces lupus-like syndrome**
H yperplasia of the gums & **Hirsutism**
E rythema multiforme, Stevens-Johnson syndrome
N europathies: vertigo, ataxia, headache
Yield: if you don't give it slow, it can cause **hypotension & arrhythmias**
T eratogenicity (cleft lip & palate, microcephaly)
O steopenia
I nhibits folic acid absorption (megaloblastic anemia)
N ystagmus

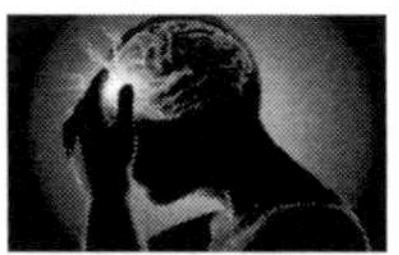

CARBAMAZEPINE

Mechanism of action:
- **Blocks sodium channels,** decreasing seizure spread by increasing the refractory period of the channels.
- Exact mechanism in Trigeminal neuralgia & Bipolar disorder is unknown.

Indications:
- Generalized tonic-clonic & focal seizures (simple & complex)
- **Drug of choice for Trigeminal neuralgia,** bipolar disorder (2nd -line)
- Central diabetes insipidus (2nd line after Desmopressin).

Adverse effects:
- **Hyponatremia (causes SIADH)**
- **Stevens-Johnson syndrome (test for HLA-B*1502** - genetic susceptibility marker in Asians associated with an increased risk of developing Stevens-Johnson syndrome).
- Dizziness, diplopia, ataxia, drowsiness, nausea, vomiting, **hepatotoxicity (increased LFTs),** arrhythmias
- **Blood dyscrasias** (agranulocytosis, aplastic anemia, thrombocytopenia),
- Teratogenic (cleft lip & palate, spina bifida).
- Inducer of the P450 & **drug-induced lupus**

Contraindications:
- **Not used in Absence (petit mal) seizures** – can worsen absence seizures.

ETHOSUXIMIDE

Mechanism of action:

- **Blocks calcium channels,** leading to motor cortex depression. Elevates the stimulation threshold, decreasing neuronal firing.

Indications:

- **Drug of choice for Absence (Petit mal) seizures.** Can only be used in Absence seizures.

Adverse effects:

- **Drowsiness**, ataxia, dizziness, headache, rash (**Stevens-Johnson syndrome)**, **GI upset** (nausea, vomiting & diarrhea), weight gain.
- Caution: renal or hepatic failure
- Monitoring: UA, CBC, LFTs

PHENOBARBITAL

Mechanism of action:

- Barbiturate that binds to GABA receptors & **potentiates GABA-mediated CNS inhibition.**

Indications:

- Partial (simplex & complex) or generalized (tonic-clonic) seizures.
- **Status epilepticus after Phenytoin administration.**

Adverse effects:

- Inducer of CP450, sedation, permanent neurologic deficit if injected into or near peripheral nerves, alteration of sleep wake cycle, suicidality, **depression,** Stevens-Johnson syndrome, dependence, & hyperactivity in pediatric patients.

BENZODIAZEPINES

- **Lorazepam,** Diazepam

Mechanism of action:

- **Potentiates GABA-mediated CNS inhibition. Lorazepam is most effective** & has a shorter half-life than Diazepam. Functions as an anxiolytic, sedative-hypnotic, anticonvulsant and muscle relaxant.

Indications:

- Generalized and absence seizures, anxiety, sedation, muscle spasm.
- **First-line for acute generalized (tonic-clonic) seizures & status epilepticus** (usually followed by phenytoin loading to prevent seizure recurrence), alcohol withdrawal, delirium tremens, & eclampsia (recurrent seizures after magnesium sulfate administration).

Adverse effects:

- **Sedation**, ataxia, paradoxical reaction.
- Monitor blood pressure after IV administration.
- Contraindications or caution: suicide risk.

VALPROIC ACID, DIVALPROEX SODIUM

Mechanism of action:

- Multiple mechanisms - potentiates GABA-mediated CNS inhibition, inhibits glutamate & NMDA receptors, increases refractory period of voltage-gated sodium channels.

Indications:

- Partial (simple and complex), generalized (tonic-clonic & absence).
- **First-line for myoclonic seizures.**
- Migraine prophylaxis, Bipolar disorder.

Adverse effects:

- GI: **Pancreatitis, hepatotoxicity,** nausea, vomiting.
- Sedation, thrombocytopenia.
- **Teratogenic (neural tube defects) – Valproate has the highest risk of birth defects** of any of the commonly used antiepileptic drugs. **Valproate should be avoided if patient is not already on it prior to pregnancy.**
- **Tremor,** weight gain, reversible hair loss.
- Inhibitor of the CP450 system.

TOPIRAMATE

Mechanism of action:

- Multiple actions: blocks sodium channels, increases GABA activity, glutamate receptor antagonist.

Indications:

- Generalized (tonic-clonic) seizures, partial (simple & complex) seizures.
- Migraine prophylaxis.

Adverse effects:

- **Renal stones**
- CNS symptoms (sedation headache, dizziness)
- Weight loss, paresthesias, glaucoma, hyperthermia.

GABAPENTIN

Mechanism of action:

- Inhibits voltage-gated calcium channels.
- **Structurally similar to GABA**

Indications:

- Partial (simple & complex) seizures.
- Peripheral neuropathy & neuropathic pain.
- Fibromyalgia, post-herpetic neuralgia.

Adverse effects:

- Sedation, ataxia.
- **Can worsen absence seizures.**

SEIZURE CLASSIFICATION	MANIFESTATIONS	MISCELLANEOUS
PARTIAL (FOCAL) SEIZURES	*Confined to small area of brain (focal part of one hemisphere).* May become generalized.	
SIMPLE PARTIAL	*CONSCIOUSNESS FULLY MAINTAINED** EEG: focal discharge at the onset of the seizures.	May have focal sensory, autonomic, motor sx^ May be followed by transient neurologic deficit (Todd's paralysis) lasting up to 24 hours.
COMPLEX PARTIAL (TEMPORAL LOBE)	*CONSCIOUSNESS IMPAIRED.* Starts focally. EEG: interictal spikes with slow waves in the temporal area. Aura (seconds – minutes) ⇨ impaired consciousness.	*AURAS:* sensory/autonomic/motor symptoms of which the patient is aware of. May precede/accompany or follow. Complex partial includes: *AUTOMATISMS:* ***ex: lip smacking, manual picking, patting, coordinated motor movement*** (ex. walking).
GENERALIZED SEIZURES	*Diffuse brain involvement (both hemispheres)*	
❶ ABSENCE (PETIT MAL) Nonconvulsive	***Brief lapse of consciousness***; patient usually unaware of attacks. ***Brief staring episodes, eyelid twitching.**** ***NO post-ictal phase.***	May be clonic (jerking), tonic (stiffness) or atonic (loss of postural tone). ***MC in childhood ⇨ usually ceases by 20y*** **EEG:** bilateral symmetric 3Hz *spike & wave* action or may be normal.
❷ TONIC-CLONIC (GRAND MAL)	**Tonic Phase:** ***loss of consciousness ⇨ rigidity,*** sudden arrest of respiration (usually <60sec) ⇨ clonic phase. **Clonic Phase:** ***repetitive, rhythmic jerking* (lasts <2-3 minutes)*** ⇨ postictal phase. **Postictal phase:** ***flaccid coma/sleep: variable duration.***	May be accompanied by incontinence, tongue biting or aspiration with postictal confusion. ***Auras are prewarnings to seizures*** **EEG:** generalize high-amplitude rapid spiking. May be normal in between seizures.
❸ Myoclonus	***Sudden, brief, sporadic involuntary twitching** No LOC***	*May be 1 muscle or groups of muscles*
❹ Atonic	***"Drop attacks" – sudden loss of postural tone****	
Status Epilepticus	Repeated, generalized seizures without recovery >30mins	

^motor: jerky, rhythmic, movements one area (focal) or spread to other parts of the affected limb or body (spread = "Jacksonian March"). Tonic or clonic.
^sensory: paresthesias, numbness, pain, heat, cold, sensation of movement, olfactory, flashing lights (photopsia).
^autonomic: abdominal (nausea, vomiting, pain, hunger); cardiovascular (sinus tachycardia).

MANAGEMENT OF SEIZURES

1. **Absence (Petit Mal):** ***Ethosuximide 1st line**** (only works for absence); *Valproic acid* 2nd line (S/E: hepatitis, pancreatitis); Lamotrigine.
2. **Grand Mal:** ***Valproic acid, Phenytoin, Carbamazepine, Lamotrigine,*** Topiramate, Primidone, Levetiracetam, Gabapentin, Phenobarbital, Midazolam
3. **Status Epilepticus:** ***Lorazepam or Diazepam ⇨ Phenytoin ⇨ Phenobarbital.*** Thiamine + Ampule of D50. Place in lateral decubitus position with all possible harmful objects cleared away from the area.
4. **Myoclonus:** Valproic acid, Clonazepam. Febrile: Phenobarbital.

Benzodiazepines (Lorazepam, Diazepam): increases GABA (GABA is an inhibitory neurotransmitter in the CNS).
Phenytoin: blocks Na^+ channels in the CNS (takes longer to work). ***S/E: gingival hyperplasia, Steven Johnson Syndrome, hirsutism***
Barbiturates: (Phenobarbital): binds to GABA receptors to ↑GABA-mediated CNS inhibition.

- ***Prolactin levels are increased in seizures**** (helps to differentiate it from pseudoseizures).
- ***EEG helps to establish the diagnosis & localize the lesions*.***

ANTICONVULSANT MEDICATIONS

SEIZURE MEDICATION	MECHANISM OF ACTION	INDICATIONS	SIDE EFFECTS
ETHOSUXIMIDE (Zarontin)	Blocks Ca^{+2} channels ⇨ motor cortex depression (elevates stimulation threshold, decreases neuronal firing).	Ind: ***drug of choice for absence**** ***(only used in absence)***	S/E: drowsiness, ataxia, dizziness, headache, rash, GI upset (diarrhea), weight gain **Caution:** patient with renal or hepatic failure. **Monitoring:** CBC, UA, ↑LFTs
VALPROIC ACID (Depakene) **DIVALPROEX SODIUM** (Depakote)	Multiple mechanisms of action: - ↑'es GABA's effects (↑CNS inhibition) - inhibits glutamate/NMDA receptor-mediated neuronal excitation.	Ind: absence sz, complex-partial sz, epileptic seizures (Grand Mal). Acute mania in bipolar disorders.	S/E: ***pancreatitis, hepatotoxicity****, GI problems, thrombocytopenia, monitor levels **CI/Cautions:** hepatic disorders
LAMOTRIGINE (Lamictal)	Blocks Na & Ca channels, decreasing presynaptic glutamate & aspartate release. Also inhibits glutamate's effects on NMDA receptor ⇨ decreased neuronal activity.	Ind: absence, grand mal & partial complex seizures.	*Rash, Steven Johnson Syndrome (SJS),* headache, diplopia
PHENYTOIN (Dilantin)	**MOA:** stabilizes neuronal membranes (limits firing of action potentials by blocking Na-dependent channels) – related to barbiturates. ***Does not cause CNS depression***	Ind: generalized tonic-clonic seizures, complex partial seizures, ***seizure prophylaxis****, - ***status epilepticus: started after benzodiazepine.***	**Monitoring:** ***drug levels,*** CBC, UA, significant drug-drug interactions. S/E: ***rash (erythema multiforme/SJS), gingival hyperplasia****, nystagmus, slurred speech, hematologic cx, ***hirsutism***, dizziness, teratogenic, ***hypotension, arrhythmias (esp with rapid administration*** >50mcg/min).
CARBAMAZEPINE (Tegretol)	Blocks Na+ channels, decreases seizure spread. Exact mechanism in trigeminal neuralgia & bipolar disorder is unknown.	Ind: ***seizure disorders, bipolar d/o. trigeminal neuralgia (drug of choice),* central diabetes insipidus.***	S/E: ***Hyponatremia (causes SIADH)*, SJS*** dizziness, drowsiness, N/V, ↑LFT's, arrhythmias ***blood dyscrasias (rare).***
TOPIRAMATE (Topamax)	Blocks Na channels, ↑'es GABA activity, glutamate receptor antagonist.	Grand Mal, partial seizures	Weight loss, nephrolithiasis, paresthesias, headache, hyperthermia
BENZODIAZEPINES **LORAZEPAM** (Ativan) **DIAZEPAM** (Valium)	**MOA:** ***potentiates GABA-mediated CNS inhibition*** ***Lorazepam most effective* (has shorter ½ life than diazepam).***	Generalized sz, absence sz, anxiety, chemo-related N/V, sedation, muscle spasms. **Status epilepticus, *benzodiazepine 1st line for status epilepticus**** (usually followed by phenytoin "loading" to prevent seizure recurrence).	S/E: sedation, ataxia, paradoxical reaction. ***Flumazenil reverses sedation.**** **CI/Cautions:** Suicide risk, ***monitor BP after dose.***
PHENOBARBITAL	Barbiturate: binds to GABA receptor potentiating GABA-mediated CNS inhibition	***Status epilepticus after phenytoin if status epilepticus persistent*** Febrile seizures in children	S/E: permanent neurologic deficit if injected into or near peripheral nerves. ***Depression, osteoporosis, irritability.***

LACUNAR INFARCTS

- **Small vessel disease of the penetrating branches** of the cerebral arteries in the pons and basal ganglia.

- Risk factors: **80% have a history of Hypertension.** Diabetes mellitus

5 CLASSIC PRESENTATIONS

- **Pure motor: most common presentation.** Hemiparesis or hemiplegia in the absence of sensory or "cortical signs" (aphasia, agnosia, neglect, apraxia, or hemianopsia).

- **Ataxic hemiparesis:** ipsilateral weakness and clumsiness in the leg > arm.

- **Pure sensory deficits** – numbness, paresthesias of the arm, face, and leg on one side of the body in the absence of motor or "cortical" signs.

- **Sensorimotor:** weakness and numbness of the face, arm, and leg on one side of the body in the absence of the aforementioned "cortical" signs.

- **Dysarthria (clumsy hand syndrome):** dysarthria, facial weakness, dysphagia and slight weakness and clumsiness of one hand in the absence of "cortical" signs.

- Diagnosis: **CT scan – small punched-out hypodense areas** (lacunar infarcts) usually in the **central & noncortical** areas (eg, basal ganglia).

MANAGEMENT

- Aspirin, control risk factors (hypertension, diabetes mellitus).

- Good prognosis – partial or complete deficit resolution ranging from hours up to 6 weeks.

TRANSIENT ISCHEMIC ATTACK

- **Transient episode of neurologic deficits** caused by focal brain, spinal cord, or retinal ischemia **without acute infarction.**

3 MAIN TYPES:
- Embolic: eg, Atrial fibrillation, left ventricular thrombus
- Lacunar: penetrating small vessels.
- Large artery: ischemia due to atherosclerosis.

CLINICAL MANIFESTATIONS
- Neurologic deficits lasting <24 hours, depending on the artery involved (resembles stroke pattern). **Most last for a few minutes with complete resolution within 1 hour**.
- **Amaurosis fugax** – transient monocular vision loss - *"temporary shade down on one eye"*.

PHYSICAL EXAMINATION: **carotid bruits** may be heard.

DIAGNOSIS
- **Neuroimaging + neurovascular imaging + rule out cardioembolic source.**
- Neuroimaging **CT scan performed initially** to rule out hemorrhage but **MRI more sensitive**.
- Neurovascular imaging **CT or MR angiography, carotid Doppler.**
- Conventional angiography definitive diagnosis (invasive).
- Ancillary testing: rule out cardioembolic source (ECG, telemetry, and echocardiogram). Rule out metabolic or hematologic cause of neurologic symptoms (eg, hypoglycemia, CBC).

MANAGEMENT
- Place patient in the supine position to increase cerebral perfusion, **avoid lowering blood pressure unless >220/120 mmHg.** Thrombolytics contraindicated.

NONCARDIOGENIC TIA
- **Antiplatelet-therapy: first-line medical management - Aspirin, Clopidogrel,** Aspirin + Dipyridamole, Ticlopidine.
- **Carotid endarterectomy recommended if internal carotid artery stenosis 50-99%** with a life expectancy of at least 5 years.
- Long-term: reduce modifiable risk factors (diabetes, hyperlipidemia and hypertension control), exercise regimen.

CARDIOGENIC (ATRIAL FIBRILLATION): oral anticoagulation.

ABCD2 SCORE ASSESSMENT IN TIA

The risk of stroke after a TIA is significantly increased, and the risk is highest during the days immediately following the TIA. The ABCD2 tool is designed to predict the risk of stroke in the 3 to 90 days after a TIA. Patients receive one point each for:
- **A**ge>60
- **B**lood pressure>140/90
- **C**linical symptoms (one point for slurred speech or two points for unilateral weakness)
- **D**uration (one point for > 10 minutes or two points for >60 minutes)
- **D**iabetes

ABCD2 SCORE
- 0-3 points = 3.1% 90 day stroke risk
- 4-5 points = 9.8% 90 day stroke risk
- 6-7 points = 17.8% 90 day stroke risk

ISCHEMIC STROKES

- Acute onset of neurological deficits due to death of brain tissue from ischemia.
- **Ischemic most common type of stroke** (80%). Causes include thrombotic and embolic.
- **Thrombotic most common** (2/3).
- Embolic 1/3. Embolic commonly come from the heart, aortic arch or large cerebral arteries. Sources include: atrial fibrillation, valvular disease, or patent foramen ovale (paradoxical venous emboli).

RISK FACTORS
- **Hypertension is the most significant and modifiable risk factor.**
- Dyslipidemia, diabetes, atrial fibrillation, cigarette smoking.
- Nonmodifiable risk factors: males, increasing age, ethnicity, and family history.

Anterior circulation symptoms (eg, Anterior cerebral artery, Middle cerebral)
- **Contralateral arm/leg weakness** and **contralateral sensory deficits**.
- Visual changes: **contralateral homonymous hemianopsia** (loss of visual fields on the opposite side of the stroke).

Posterior circulation symptoms:
- **V's: vomiting, visual changes** (eg, diplopia), **vertigo**; Nystagmus, nausea, coma, drop attacks, and/or ataxia.
- Contralateral arm/leg weakness and contralateral sensory deficits.

DIAGNOSIS
- **CT head without contrast best initial test** to rule out hemorrhagic stroke. CT may be normal in the first 6-24 hours. MRI is most accurate to diagnose a stroke.

- Ancillary testing: neurovascular imaging (CT or MR angiography), carotid Doppler ultrasound, ECG, echocardiography, cardiac monitoring.
- Conventional angiography rarely needed.

IMMEDIATE MANAGEMENT
- **Within 3 hours of symptom onset: Alteplase (thrombolytic) if no contraindications**. Contraindications include blood pressure 185/110 or greater, recent bleeding, bleeding disorder, & recent trauma. **Thrombolytics can be used within 4.5 hours in some patients**: < 80 years old + < 25 on NIH stroke scale (not maximally severe) + not a diabetic with a previous stroke.

- **Mechanical thrombectomy can be performed within 24 hours of symptom onset** of large artery occlusion in the anterior circulation. Compared to Alteplase alone, thrombectomy is associated with improved reperfusion, early neurological recovery, and functional outcome.

- > 3 - 4.5 hours of symptom onset: Aspirin and long-term management.

- Blood pressure should only be lowered IF blood pressure ≥ 185/110 mmHg if thrombolytics are to be used or ≥ 220/120 mmHg if no plan to use thrombolytics.

LONG-TERM (OUTPATIENT) MANAGEMENT
- **Antiplatelet therapy: Aspirin, Clopidogrel, or Dipyridamole**. Aspirin therapy should not be initiated until 24 hours after the time of thrombolytic therapy.
  - If patient was already on Aspirin prior to stroke, either add Dipyridamole or switch to Clopidogrel.

- **Statin therapy** should be initiated regardless of LDL level (**St**roke = **St**atin)!

MIDDLE CEREBRAL ARTERY ISCHEMIC STROKE

- **Most common type of ischemic stroke.** Think MCA is the **M**ost **C**ommon **A**rtery involved.

CLINICAL MANIFESTATIONS

- **Contralateral sensory & motor deficits greater in the face & arm >** leg > foot.
- Facial involvement **only involves the lower half of the face** (patient will be able to raise forehead).
- Visual: contralateral homonymous hemianopsia (loss of visual fields on the opposite side of the stroke). This leads to **gaze preference towards the side of the lesion initially.**
- **Dominant (left in 90%) hemisphere: aphasia** (Broca – expressive or Wernicke's – sensory), math comprehension deficits, & agraphia.
- **Nondominant (usually right) hemisphere**: spatial deficits, dysarthria, **neglect of the other side, anosognosia**, apraxia, **flat affect, impaired judgment, & impulsivity**.

ANTERIOR CEREBRAL ARTERY STROKE

CLINICAL MANIFESTATIONS

- **Contralateral sensory** and **motor deficits greater in the leg, foot** > arm. The face is usually spared.
- **Urinary incontinence.**
- Contralateral homonymous hemianopsia (leads to gaze preference towards the side of the lesion initially).
- **Personality/cognitive deficits** (eg, confusion, flat affect, impaired judgment).

POSTERIOR CEREBRAL ARTERY STROKE

Think of the **V**s for **v**ertebral: **v**ertigo (including nystagmus), **v**omiting, **v**isual changes (eg, diplopia)

Posterior cerebral artery:

- Homonymous hemianopsia (may spare the macula); alexia without agraphia (if dominant hemisphere - left PCA); visual hallucinations, sensory loss, coma, limb ataxia, nystagmus, cerebellar signs, nausea, vomiting & drop attacks.

Vertebrobasilar artery:

- **"Crossed symptoms" - ipsilateral cranial nerve deficits with contralateral motor or sensory deficits.**
- Diplopia, dizziness, nausea, vomiting, limb and gait ataxia, coma, cerebellar dysfunction.
- **Asymmetric but bilateral deficits are the rule in basilar infarcts** (eg, hemiparesis with motor or reflex abnormalities on the nonhemiparetic side).

STROKE TYPE	CLINICAL MANIFESTATIONS	DIAGNOSIS	MANAGEMENT
ISCHEMIC STROKE	*MC type (80%). Due to* ❶ ***thrombotic MC**** (49%) ❷ ***emboli*** (31%) ❸ ***cerebrovascular occlusion.***		
LACUNAR INFARCT	***Small vessel disease (penetrating branches** of cerebral arteries in pons, basal ganglia.* ❶ PURE MOTOR *MC* (hemiparesis, hemiplegia) ❷ ATAXIC HEMIPARESIS & clumsiness leg >arm ❸ DYSARTHRIA (CLUMSY HAND SYNDROME) ❹pure sensory loss (numbness, paresthesias). ***History of HTN 80%****	**CT scan:** ***small punched out hypodense areas.*** Lesions usually central & in noncortical areas: ex basal ganglia	Aspirin. Control risk factors (HTN & DM). Good prognosis: partial or complete deficit resolution ranging from hours up to 6 weeks.
ANTERIOR CIRCULATION **Middle Cerebral Artery** *MC type** (70%)	• Contralateral sensory/motor loss/hemiparesis: ***GREATER IN FACE, ARM*** > *leg/foot.* • Visual: contralateral homonymous hemianopsia, ***gaze preference towards side of lesion*** (x1 – 2 days). • **Dominant** (usually L-side): ***aphasia: Broca (expressive), Wernicke (sensory), math comprehension, agraphia.*** • **Nondominant** (usually R-side): ***spatial deficits, dysarthria, left-side neglect, anosognosia, apraxia***	**ISCHEMIC STROKE DIAGNOSIS** ***Noncontrast CT scan to rule out hemorrhage in suspected stroke.*** CT scan may be normal during 1st 6-24 hours.	**ISCHEMIC STROKE MANAGEMENT** •***Thrombolytics within 3 hours*** of onset (4.5 hours in some cases). •Tissue plasminogen activator (rTPA) ***Alteplase**** given if no evidence of hemorrhage. ***Alteplase only rTPA effective in ischemic stroke.**** **CI:** BP ≥185/110, recent bleed/trauma, bleeding d/o.
Anterior Cerebral Artery 2%	• Contralateral sensory/motor loss/hemiparesis: ***GREATER IN LEG/FOOT*** > *upper extremity* ⇨ abnormal gait. • ***Face spared:**** speech preservation. Slow responses • Frontal lobe & mental status impairment: ***impaired judgment, confusion. Personality changes* (flat affect)*** • *URINARY INCONTINENCE**. Upper motor neuron weakness. • Gaze preference towards side of the lesion (early on).		•Antiplatelet therapy: Aspirin, Clopidogrel, Dipyridamole. Aspirin used in the acute setting if after 3 hours & thrombolytics aren't given or at least 24h after thrombolytics. •±Anticoagulation tx if cardioembolic
POSTERIOR CIRCULATION **Posterior Cerebral Artery**	• ***Visual hallucinations, contralateral homonymous hemianopsia. "crossed sx"**** *(ipsilateral cranial nerve deficits + contralateral muscle weakness),* coma, drop attacks.		•Only lower BP if ≥185/110 for thrombolytics or ≥220/120 if no thrombolytic use or if MAP >130
Basilar Artery **Vertebral Artery**	• Cerebellar dysfunction, CN palsies, ↓vision, ↓bilateral sensory • ***Vertigo, nystagmus, N/V, diplopia,*** ipsilateral ataxia.		•**Note:** ***strokes with facial involvement involves the lower half of face**** (patient will still be able to raise both eyebrows)!
HEMORRHAGIC STROKE	*20% of strokes. Headache, vomiting favors ICH or SAH*. Impaired consciousness without focal symptoms favors SAH. ↑mortality*		
Spontaneous ICH	***Commonly caused by HTN**** especially in ***basal ganglia. LOC,*** N/V, hemiplegia, hemiparalysis. Sx usually mins-hrs gradually increasing in intensity.	**Noncontrast CT *(Do not perform LP if ICH is suspected).**** Mass effect ± cause herniation if LP done).	Supportive vs. hematoma evacuation If ↑ intracranial pressure ⇨ Head elevation, ± IV Mannitol, hyperventilation
Subarachnoid Hemorrhage (SAH)	***Sudden "worst h/a of my life"**** ⇨ ***brief LOC, N/V, meningeal irritation**** signs (nuchal rigidity), seizures. MC 2ry to rupture of berry aneurysm* or AVM. No focal neurologic symptoms*	1. CT scan. 2. If CT negative & high suspicion ⇨ Lumbar puncture: xanthochromia (RBC's)* esp if >12h & ↑CSF pressure*	Bedrest, no exertion/straining, anti-anxiety meds, stool softeners; ± cautious lowering of BP (only if >220/120 or MAP >130)
"Berry" Aneurysm	***MC circle of Willis (asymptomatic until SAH)***	***Angiography gold standard***	±Aneurysm clipping or coiling.

4 TYPES OF INTRACRANIAL HEMORRHAGE

EPIDURAL HEMATOMA (HEMORRHAGE)	SUBDURAL HEMATOMA (HEMORRHAGE)	SUBARACHNOID HEMORRHAGE (SAH)	INTRACEREBRAL HEMORRHAGE (ICH)
LOCATION • ***Arterial bleed MC* between skull & dura.***	**LOCATION** • ***Venous bleed MC*.*** Between dura & arachnoid due to ***tearing of cortical bridging veins*. MC in elderly.***	**LOCATION** • ***Arterial bleed**** between arachnoid & pia	**LOCATION** • ***Intraparenchymal***
MECHANISM • ***MC after Temporal bone fracture* ⇨ middle meningeal artery**** disruption.	**MECHANISM** • ***MC blunt trauma**** often causes bleeding on other side of injury "contre-coup". ***Venous bleed.***	**MECHANISM** • ***MC Berry aneurysm rupture, AVM***	**MECHANISM** • ***HTN, AVM,*** trauma, amyloid **A**rterio**V**enous **M**alformation
CLINICAL MANIFESTATIONS • Varies. brief LOC ⇨ lucid interval ⇨ coma; headache, N/V, focal neuro sx, rhinorrhea (CSF fluid). • CN III palsy if tentorial herniation.	**CLINICAL MANIFESTATIONS** • Varies. May have focal neuro sx.	**CLINICAL MANIFESTATIONS** • ***Thunderclap sudden headache "worse h/a of my life"**** ±unilateral, occipital area. ± LOC. N/V, ***Meningeal sx: stiff neck, photophobia, delirium*.*** • ***No focal neurologic deficits*** usually. • Terson syndrome: retinal hemorrhages.	**CLINICAL MANIFESTATIONS** • ***Headache, N/V,*** ± LOC, hemiplegia, hemiparesis. Not associated with lucid intervals
DIAGNOSIS • **CT:** ***convex (lens – shaped)* bleed*** • ***Does NOT cross suture lines. Usually in temporal area****	**DIAGNOSIS** • **CT:** ***concave (crescent-shaped) bleed*.*** • ***Bleeding can cross suture lines****	**DIAGNOSIS** • ***CT scan performed first.*** *If CT negative* ⇨ **LP:** ***xanthochromia (RBC's), ↑CSF (ICP) pressure.*** • ***4-vessel angiography*** after confirmed SAH.	**DIAGNOSIS** • **CT:** intraparenchymal bleed. • ***Do NOT perform LP if suspected because it may cause brain herniation!***
MANAGEMENT • ± herniate if not evacuated early. Observation if small. If ↑ICP: Mannitol, hyperventilation, head elevation, ± shunt	**MANAGEMENT** • Hematoma evacuation vs. supportive Evacuation if massive or ≥ 5mm midline shift.	**MANAGEMENT** • Supportive: bed rest, stool softeners, lower ICP. Surgical coiling or clipping. • ± lower BP gradually (ex. ***Nicardipine*, Nimodipine,*** Labetalol).	**MANAGEMENT** Supportive: gradual BP reduction. ± IV Mannitol if ↑ICP ±Hematoma evacuation if mass effect
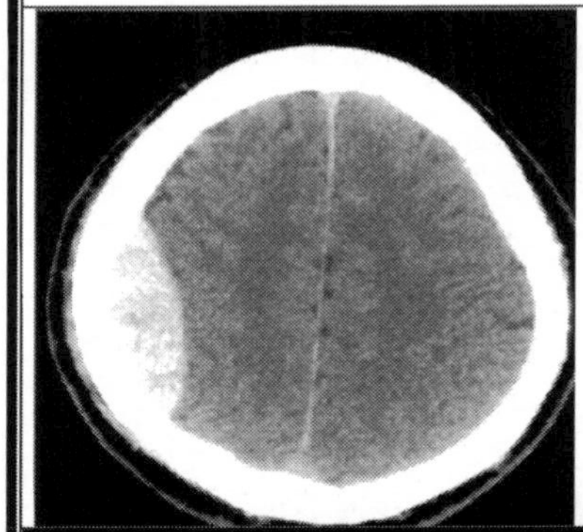 EPIDURAL	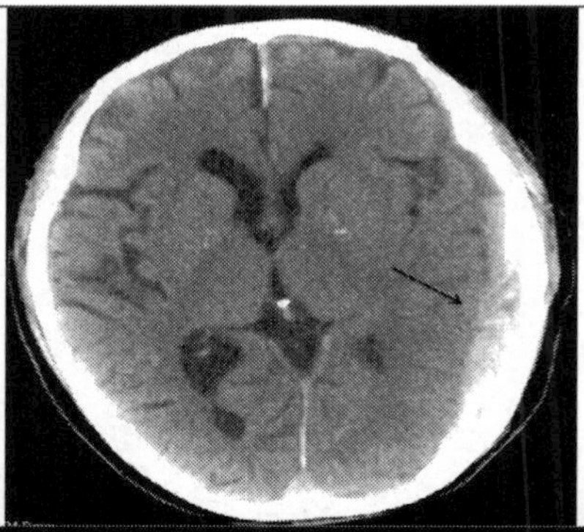 SUBDURAL	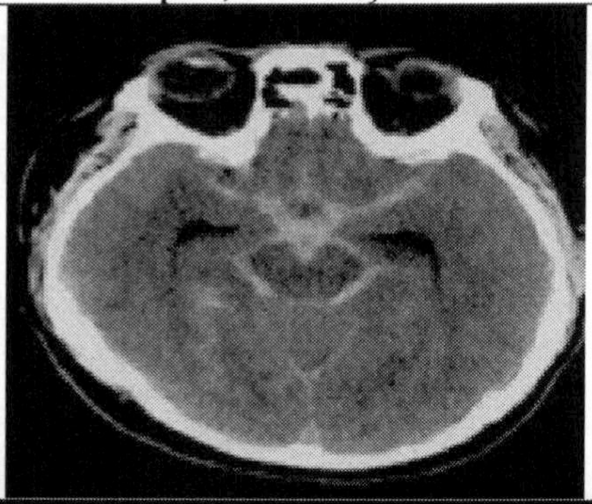 SUBARACHNOID	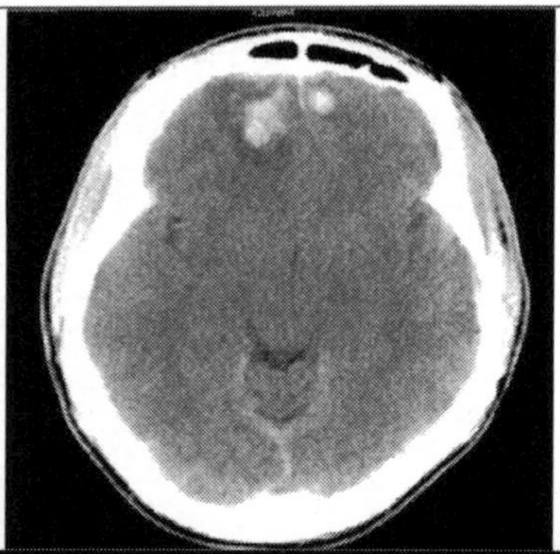 INTRACEREBRAL

EPIDURAL HEMATOMA

- Bleeding in the potential space between the skull and the dura.

PATHOPHYSIOLOGY

- **Most common due to rupture of the <u>middle meningeal artery</u>,** often **associated with a <u>temporal bone fracture</u>.** May lead to hemorrhagic stroke & brain herniation.

CLINICAL MANIFESTATIONS

- **<u>3 classic phases</u> – brief loss of consciousness followed by a lucid interval** (patient regains consciousness and seems fine) followed by **neurologic deterioration** (mental status changes to coma as a result of increased intracranial pressure).
- During the deterioration phase, headache, vomiting, aphasia, hemiparesis, & seizures may occur.
- <u>Uncal herniation:</u> **cranial nerve III palsy – fixed, dilated "blown" pupil** can be seen on the ipsilateral side of the injury (tentorial herniation compressing CN III). **Cushing reflex**: triad of hypertension, bradycardia, & respiratory irregularity.

DIAGNOSIS

- **<u>Head CT without contrast</u>** initial test of choice – **biconvex (lens-shaped)** hyperdensity usually in the temporal area that **does <u>not</u> cross suture lines.**

MANAGEMENT

- **Hematoma evacuation or craniotomy treatment of choice in most** - prevent irreversible brain injury & death.
- May be observed closely with serial imaging if small and the patient is in good condition.
- <u>Increased intracranial pressure:</u> head elevation, short-term hyperventilation, & hyperosmolar therapy (IV Mannitol or hypertonic saline).

SUBDURAL HEMATOMA

- Bleeding between the dura and the arachnoid membranes.
- <u>Etiology:</u> **most commonly due to rupture of the cortical bridging veins** after blunt trauma.

RISK FACTORS

- **Elderly & alcoholics** (brain atrophy puts tension on the bridging veins)
- Anticoagulant use. Shaken baby syndrome or child abuse.

CLINICAL MANIFESTATIONS

- Because the bleeding is venous, it can develop over a longer period of time compared to Epidural hematoma.
- Varies but **usually a gradual increase in generalized neurologic symptoms** (eg, headache, dizziness, nausea, vomiting) or focal neurologic symptoms.
- May be associated with LOC.

DIAGNOSIS

- **<u>Head CT without contrast</u> – concave (crescent-shaped) bleed that can cross the suture lines.** If severe, midline shift may occur due to increased intracranial pressure. CT scan may negative immediately after the injury so serial imaging may be needed.

MANAGEMENT

- <u>Nonoperative management:</u> if clinically stable with a small hematoma or no CT signs of brain herniation (eg, midline shift <5 mm) or no signs of increased intracranial pressure.
- <u>Surgical management:</u> **surgical evacuation may be indicated if ≥5mm or greater midline shift** or severe. Options include burr hole trephination, craniotomy, and decompressive craniectomy.

SUBARACHNOID HEMORRHAGE

- Bleeding between the arachnoid membranes & the pia mater.

ETIOLOGIES
- **Most commonly due to a ruptured berry aneurysm** at the anterior communicating artery (Circle of Willis).
- Arteriovenous malformation, stroke or trauma.

RISK FACTORS
- Cigarette smoking and Hypertension most important.
- Polycystic kidney disease, atherosclerotic disease, smoking, excessive alcohol intake, Ehlers-Danlos syndrome, Marfan syndrome, family history.

CLINICAL MANIFESTATIONS
- **Sudden, intense thunderclap headache** that is often unilateral in the occipital area. Often described as **"the worst headache of my life".**

- May be associated with delirium, seizures, **nausea, vomiting, & meningeal symptoms** (photophobia, neck stiffness, fever).
- May have **loss of consciousness** initially.
- May have a history of a prior, milder headache (sentinel leak).

PHYSICAL EXAMINATION
- May reveal **meningeal signs:** nuchal rigidity, positive Brudzinski and Kernig signs.

- Usually not associated with focal neurologic deficits but may have a CN III palsy (fixed, dilated, "blown" pupil).

- Terson syndrome: retinal hemorrhages.

DIAGNOSIS
- **CT scan without contrast initial study of choice –** subarachnoid bleeding.

- **Lumbar puncture: performed if CT is negative + no papilledema or focal signs – xanthochromia** (yellow to pink color of the CSF fluid due to breakdown of RBCs in the CSF, increased CSF protein from bilirubin, and increased CSF pressure).

- 4-vessel angiography usually performed after confirmed SAH to identify source of bleeding & other aneurysms.

MANAGEMENT
- **Supportive:** bed rest, stool softeners, lower intracranial pressure. **Nimodipine reduces cerebral vasospasms, improving neurologic outcomes** in SAH.

- Lowering blood pressure may decrease the risk of rebleeding but may also increase the risk of infarction. If needed, Labetalol, Nicardipine and Enalapril are preferred antihypertensives.

- Ventriculostomy may be needed if SAH is associated with hydrocephalus.

- Prevention of rebleeding: **endovascular coiling or surgical clipping of aneurysm or AVM used to prevent rebleeding** (coiling often preferred over clipping).

INTRACEREBRAL HEMORRHAGE

- Bleeding within the brain parenchyma.
- May compress the brain, ventricles, and sulci.

RISK FACTORS

- **Hypertension most common overall cause of spontaneous ICH.**
- **Cerebral amyloid angiopathy** is the most common cause of nontraumatic ICH in the elderly.
- **Arteriovenous malformation** is the most common cause in children.
- Trauma, older age, high alcohol intake, and coagulopathy.

CLINICAL MANIFESTATIONS

- Neurologic symptoms usually increase within minutes to hours - **headache, nausea, vomiting, syncope, focal neurologic symptoms** (hemiplegia, hemiparesis, seizures), **altered mental status** (lethargy, obtundation, etc.).

PHYSICAL EXAMINATION

- May have focal motor and sensory deficits.
- Diagnosis:
- CT scan of the head without contrast: initial neuroimaging of choice.

MANAGEMENT

- **Supportive:** gradual blood pressure reduction.
- **Prevention of increased intracranial pressure** - raising the head of the bed 30 degrees, limiting IV fluids, blood pressure management, analgesia & sedation.
- **Reduction of increased intracranial pressure if present - IV mannitol**, temporary hyperventilation.
- Blood pressure reduction: IV Labetalol, Nicardipine, Esmolol, Hydralazine, Nitroprusside and Nitroglycerin. Aggressive reduction only if systolic BP (SBP) >200 mmHg or mean arterial pressure (MAP) >150 mmHg.

BASILAR SKULL FRACTURE

- Most commonly occur after traumatic head injuries. Most involve the temporal bone.

CLINICAL MANIFESTATIONS

- Varies. May have no symptoms.
- Headache, altered mental status, focal cranial nerve, or neurologic deficit.

PHYSICAL EXAMINATION

- **Periorbital ecchymosis** (Raccoon eyes), **mastoid ecchymosis** (Battle's sign), **hemotympanum** (blood behind the tympanic membrane), **rhinorrhea** (CSF leak).

DIAGNOSIS

- Head CT without contrast: in addition to the fracture, pneumocephalus may be seen.

MANAGEMENT

- **Nonoperative in most without underlying brain injury.**
- Surgical management may be indicated if there is mass effect on the brain parenchyma or CSF leak.
- Depressed skull fractures are often considered open fractures and are admitted to neurosurgery.
- Tetanus if needed and prophylactic antibiotics.

BURST (JEFFERSON) FRACTURE OF THE ATLAS (C1)

- **Bilateral fractures of both the anterior & posterior arches of the atlas (C1).**
- Type II atlas fracture.
- Stability is determined by the involvement of the transverse ligament (ligament disruption = unstable). May be associated with a C1/C2 dislocation.

MECHANISM OF INJURY
- **Axial load** on the back of the head or hyperextension of the neck (e.g. caused by diving).

CLINICAL MANIFESTATIONS
- Upper neck pain, decreased range of motion, usually without neurologic symptoms.
- Physical examination: neurologic exam is usually normal.

DIAGNOSIS
- Lateral radiographs: **increase in the predental space between C1 & the odontoid (dens), atlantodens interval** >3mm in adults & >5mm in children.
- Open-mouth (odontoid) view: may also show **step-off of the lateral masses of the atlas** (when the transverse diameter of the atlas is 7 mm greater than that of the axis, suspect transverse ligament rupture).

MANAGEMENT
- Nonoperative management: **external immobilization (hard cervical orthosis vs. halo)** for 6-12 weeks for **stable fractures (intact transverse ligament).**
- Operative: posterior C1-C2 fusion vs. occipitocervical fusion if unstable (controversial).

ODONTOID FRACTURES

- **Fracture of the dens (odontoid process) of the axis (C2).** See attached photo.
- Mechanism: head placed in forced flexion or extension in an anterior-posterior orientation (e.g. forward fall onto the forehead).
- Type I: oblique fracture at the tip of odontoid.
- **Type II:** fracture at the base of the odontoid process (dens) where it attaches to C2. **Most common type. Unstable.** High association with nonunion. Os odontoideum appears like a type II fracture on radiographs.
- Type III: extends into C2.

CLINICAL MANIFESTATIONS
- Neck pain worse with motion. May have dysphagia if large retropharyngeal hematoma is present.
- Physical exam: usually no neurologic deficits because the cervical canal is widest at C2 area.

DIAGNOSIS
- **Best seen on AP odontoid (open mouth) view.** CT best test to delineate fracture pattern. MRI if symptoms of spinal cord injury.

MANAGEMENT:
- Os odontoideum (aplasia or hypoplasia of the odontoid): observation. Posterior C1-C2 fusion if symptoms of myelopathy.
- Type I: cervical orthosis.
- **Type II in young - halo immobilization**. Surgery if risk factors for nonunion. II in elderly - surgery preferred. Cervical orthosis if not surgical candidates (no halo immobilization in the elderly).
- Type III - cervical orthosis.

HANGMAN'S (C2/AXIS PEDICLE) FRACTURE

- **Traumatic bilateral fractures (spondylolysis) of the pedicles or pars interarticularis of the axis vertebra (C2).**
- May lead to **spondylolisthesis between C2 & C3 (anterior dislocation of C2).**
- **Unstable fracture**. 30% are associated with cervical spinal fractures. Usually no cord injury.

MECHANISM
- **Extreme hyperextension** injuries of the skull, atlas & axis (especially in an already extended neck). Most commonly seen in motor vehicle accidents (e.g, chin hitting the steering wheel).

CLINICAL MANIFESTATIONS
- Neck pain. Neurologic exam is usually intact.

DIAGNOSIS
- Cervical radiographs: subluxation of C2 on C3. CT or MRI.

MANAGEMENT
- Nonoperative: Type I (<3mm horizontal displacement) rigid cervical collar 4-6 weeks. Type II (3-5 mm displacement) closed reduction followed by halo immobilization 8-12 weeks.
- Operative: Type II (>5mm displacement with severe angulation), Type III facet dislocations.

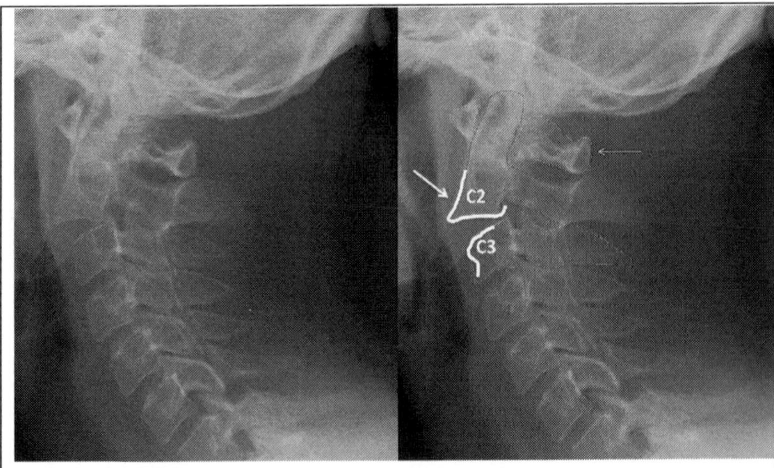

Hangman Fracture
Note slipping of C2 forward compared to C3 (white arrow).

Hangman Fracture
By Lucien Monfils (Own work) [GFDL (http://www.gnu.org/copyleft/fdl.html) or CC BY-SA 3.0 (http://creativecommons.org/licenses/by-sa/3.0)], via Wikimedia Commons

ATLAS FRACTURE & TRANSVERSE LIGAMENTAL INSTABILITY

MECHANISM OF INJURY

Hyperextension & compression injuries.
Low risk of neurologic complications. May be associated with axis fracture.

ATLANTO-OCCIPITAL DISLOCATION

- Extreme flexion injury involving the atlas (C1) & axis (C2). ± associated with odontoid fractures.

ATLANTO-AXIAL JOINT INSTABILITY

- Instability between the atlas (C1) and axis (C2).

MECHANISM

- Traumatic: due to extreme flexion-rotation injuries.
- Non traumatic: degenerative changes: ex Down syndrome, Rheumatoid arthritis, Os odontoideum.

CLINICAL MANIFESTATIONS

- Neck pain, neurologic symptoms or deficits. Myelopathic symptoms: muscle weakness, hyperreflexia, wide gait, bladder dysfunction.

DIAGNOSIS

- Open-mouth (odontoid) view: may see **increase in the atlanto-dens interval (ADI).** ADI > 3.5mm considered unstable. ADI >10mm indicates surgery in RA. CT or MRI.

MANAGEMENT

- Depends on the cause. **Os odontoideum with symptoms of myelopathy and a widened may need a posterior C1-C2 fusion.**

CLAY-SHOVELER'S FRACTURE

- **Spinous process avulsion fracture most common at the lower cervical (C7 most common)** or upper thoracic vertebrae (C6 – T3).

MECHANISM

- **Forced neck flexion** with the muscle pulling off a piece of the spinous process, especially after sudden deceleration injuries (ex. MVA). **Usually a stable injury.**

CLINICAL MANIFESTATIONS

- Neck pain or pain between the shoulder blades.

PHYSICAL EXAM

- May have localized tenderness or crepitus with reduced range of motion of the neck. Usually no neurologic deficits.

DIAGNOSIS

- Cervical radiographs: **lateral view best view** – oblique fracture line with fragment displaced posteroinferiorly. AP view – double spinous process shadow suggestive of displacement. CT scan preferred over radiographs.

MANAGEMENT

- **Nonoperative first-line management:** NSAIDs, rest, immobilization in hard collar for comfort.
- Surgical excision only needed if nonunion or persistent pain.

FLEXION TEARDROP FRACTURES

- **Anterior displacement of a wedge-shaped fracture fragment** (the so-called teardrop shape of the **antero-inferior portion** of the superior vertebra). Often associated with loss of vertebral height.
- Most commonly occurs in the **lower cervical spine**. Often associated with loss of vertebral height.

MECHANISM
- Severe flexion & compression causes the vertebral body to collide with an inferior vertebral body.
- **Highly unstable** (because of disruption of the posterior longitudinal ligament). **May cause anterior cervical cord syndrome.**

CLINICAL MANIFESTATIONS
- Neck pain. **Anterior cord syndrome symptoms.**

MANAGEMENT
- **Surgical decompression** (due to it highly unstable nature).

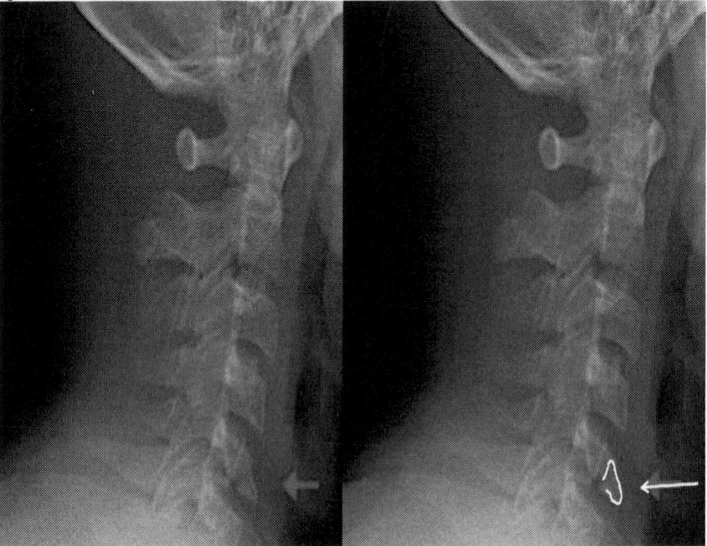

EXTENSION TEARDROP FRACTURE

- Triangular-shaped avulsion fracture of the antero-inferior corner of the vertebral body as a result of rupture of the anterior longitudinal ligament.
- **Most common at C2**. May be seen at C5 – C7. No loss of vertebral height.
- Extension teardrop fractures are unstable in extension & stable in flexion.

MECHANISM
- **Abrupt neck extension**.
- The 'teardrop' appears similar to the flexion teardrop fracture - both can be represented by an anteroinferior vertebral fragment. However, the extension teardrop is not as severe injury, as the vertebral body is not displaced and can cause **central cord syndrome** (not a common occurrence).

MANAGEMENT
- Immobilization in a hard collar in most cases.

BURST FRACTURES

- Burst fracture due to nucleus pulposus of the intervertebral disc being forced into the vertebral body, causing it to shatter or 'burst' outwards. Usually as a result of a vertical compression injury.

MECHANISM OF INJURY
- Axial loading injury causing vertebral compression injuries of the cervical & lumbar spine.
- Stable: all the ligaments are intact and usually no posterior displacement of the fracture segment.
- Unstable: >50% compression of the spinal cord, >50% loss of vertebral height, >20 degrees of spinal angulation or associated neurologic deficits. May cause incomplete or complete spinal cord injury (eg, anterior cord syndrome).

DIAGNOSIS
- Radiographs: comminuted vertebral body and loss of vertebral height (depicted as a vertical fracture on the AP view).

MANAGEMENT
- Unstable - needs surgical correction.

SUBCLAVIAN STEAL SYNDROME

- **Subclavian steal syndrome** refers to **signs and/or symptoms** that occur due to **reversed (retrograde) blood flow from the vertebral artery to the ipsilateral arm as a result of decreased flow in the subclavian artery (stenosis or occlusion).**
- The blood flow to the arm is at the expense of the vertebrobasilar circulation.

ETIOLOGIES
- **Atherosclerosis of the subclavian artery most common**, Takayasu arteritis, dissecting aortic aneurysm, thoracic outlet syndrome.

CLINICAL MANIFESTATIONS
- Most patients are asymptomatic ("subclavian steal" not syndrome).
- **Symptoms of arm arterial insufficiency: arm claudication with exercise, paresthesias.**
- **Symptoms of vertebrobasilar insufficiency:** presyncope or syncope, dizziness, neurologic deficits, vertigo, diplopia, nystagmus, weakness, drop attacks, gait abnormalities.

PHYSICAL EXAM
- **Blood pressure difference between the arms** (reduction of blood pressure in the affected arm **> 15mmHg** compared to the unaffected arm).
- Radial pulse may diminish with arm elevation or arm exercise.

DIAGNOSIS
- Continuous wave Doppler, Duplex US, Transcranial Doppler, CT angiography, angiogram.

MANAGEMENT
- Revascularization or percutaneous transluminal angioplasty in severe cases.

SPINAL CORD SYNDROME - MNEMONICS

ANTERIOR CORD SYNDROME

Because ANT couldn't walk to the bathroom in the TeePee, he peed his pants when his bladder busted into flecks.

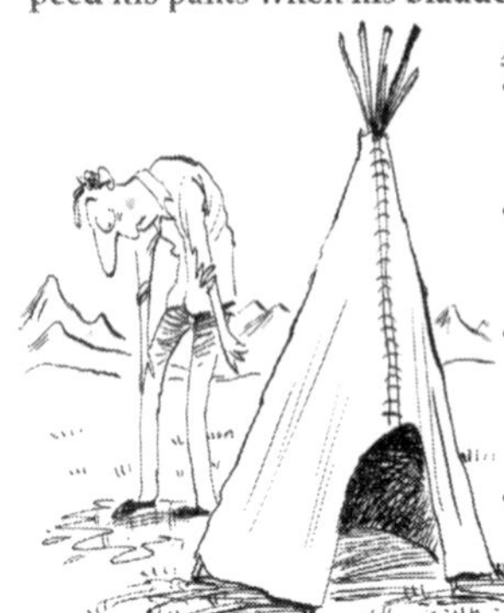

ANT = Anterior Cord Syndrome

- **Couldn't walk:** lower extremity motor deficit
- **TeePee = loss of Temperature & Pain sensation**
- **Peed his pants =** bladder dysfunction, lower extremity involvement
- **Flex =** flexion **compression injuries common mechanism**

CENTRAL CORD SYNDROME

Because Maleficent developed frostbite when she extended her hand to touch the cold window pane, she couldn't put on her shawl with her weak hands.

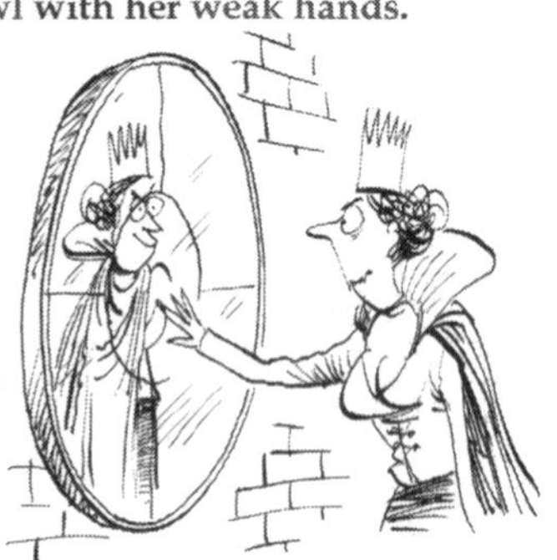

Extension **injuries**

loss of pain & temperature sensation

upper extremity > lower extremity (especially hands)

Shawl = shawl distribution

BROWN SEQUARD SYNDROME

The MVP on the winning side was oblivious 2(to) the stabbing heat of the pain of defeat from the losing side.

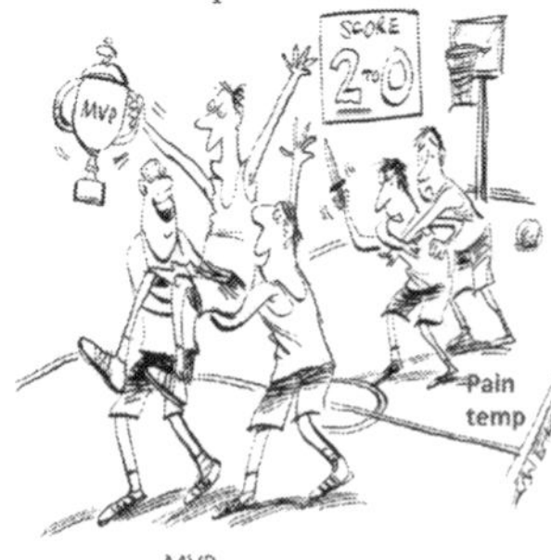

Ipsilateral deficits

- **MVP = Motor, Vibratory and Proprioception deficits**

Contralateral deficits

- pain & temperature **deficits occurring usually** 2 **levels below the level of injury.**

Mechanism

Stabbing: penetration injuries

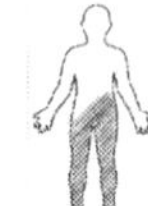

ANTERIOR CORD SYNDROME

Motor & Sensory deficits in lower extremities

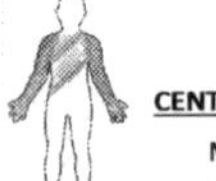

CENTRAL CORD SYNDROME

Motor & Sensory deficits in upper extremities in a "shawl" distribution

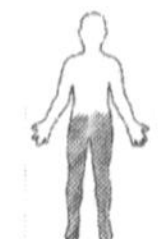

BROWN SEQUARD SYNDROME

Ipsilateral motor, vibratory & propioception deficits.
Contralateral pain & temperature deficits

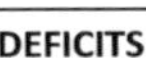

DEFICITS
MOTOR
SENSORY
VIBRATORY PROPRIOCEPTION

	ANTERIOR CORD	CENTRAL CORD	POSTERIOR CORD	BROWN SÉQUARD
MECHANISM OF INJURY	• MC after blowout vertebral body burst fractures (flexion). • Anterior spinal artery injury or occlusion. • Direct anterior cord compression. • Aortic dissection, SLE, AIDS.	• Hyperextension injuries (ex 50% occur c MVA), falls in elderly, gun shot wounds, tumors, cervical spinal stenosis, syringomyelia. • MC incomplete cord syndrome. • It affects primarily the central gray matter (including the spinothalamic tracts).	• Rare • Damage to posterior cord or posterior spinal stenosis.	• Unilateral hemisection of the spinal cord • MC after ***penetrating trauma*** (tumors may cause it) • Rare injury.
DEFICITS	**Motor deficit:** • ***lower extremity > upper**** (corticospinal) **Sensory deficit:** • pain, temperature (spinothalamic tract) • light touch • May develop ***bladder dysfunction*** (retention, incontinence)	**Motor deficit:** • ***upper extremity > lower****. The distal portion of the upper extremity more severe involvement (ex. hands) from corticospinal involvement. **Sensory deficit:** • pain, temperature (spinothalamic tract) deficit greater in the upper extremity > lower extremity. Sometimes described as a ***"shawl" distribution.***	• ***Loss of proprioception & vibratory sense only****	**Ipsilateral deficits:** - ***Motor*** (lateral corticospinal tract) - ***Vibration & proprioception*** (dorsal column) **Contralateral deficits:** - ***pain & temperature*** (lateral spinothalamic tract) usually 2 levels below the injury (where the spinothalamic tract crosses at the spinal cord level)
PRESERVATION	**Preserved:** • Proprioception, vibration, pressure (dorsal column spared) • Light touch preservation.	**Preserved:** Proprioception, vibration, pressure (dorsal column spared)	**Preserved:** • Pain & light touch. • No motor deficits	
	Anterior Cord Syndrome B.	**Central Cord Syndrome** A.	**Posterior Cord Syndrome** CON C.	**BROWN SÉQUARD** IPSILATERAL CONTRALATERAL D.

SELECTED REFERENCES

Jankovic J. Parkinson's disease: clinical features and diagnosis. J Neurol Neurosurg Psychiatr. 2008;79(4):368-76.

Zochodne DW. Autonomic involvement in Guillain-Barré syndrome: a review. Muscle Nerve. 1994;17(10):1145-55.
Conti-fine BM, Milani M, Kaminski HJ. Myasthenia gravis: past, present, and future. J Clin Invest. 2006;116(11):2843-54.
Saidha S, Eckstein C, Calabresi PA. New and emerging disease modifying therapies for multiple sclerosis. Ann N Y Acad Sci. 2012;1247:117-37.

Mackenzie C. Dysarthria in stroke: a narrative review of its description and the outcome of intervention. Int J Speech Lang Pathol. 2011;13(2):125-36.

Abboud H, Ahmed A, Fernandez HH. Essential tremor: choosing the right management plan for your patient. Cleve Clin J Med. 2011;78(12):821-8.

Jankovic J. Parkinson's disease: clinical features and diagnosis. J Neurol Neurosurg Psychiatr. 2008;79(4):368-76.

Walker FO. Huntington's disease. Lancet. 2007;369(9557):218-28.

Hughes RA, Wijdicks EF, Barohn R, et al. Practice parameter: immunotherapy for Guillain-Barré syndrome: report of the Quality Standards Subcommittee of the American Academy of Neurology. Neurology. 2003;61(6):736-40.

Maddison P, Newsom-davis J. Treatment for Lambert-Eaton myasthenic syndrome. Cochrane Database Syst Rev. 2005;(2):CD003279.

Nakahara J, Maeda M, Aiso S, Suzuki N. Current concepts in multiple sclerosis: autoimmunity versus oligodendrogliopathy. Clin Rev Allergy Immunol. 2012;42(1):26-34.

Maher AR, Maglione M, Bagley S, et al. Efficacy and comparative effectiveness of atypical antipsychotic medications for off-label uses in adults: a systematic review and meta-analysis. JAMA. 2011;306(12):1359-69.

Cruccu G, Biasiotta A, Di rezze S, et al. Trigeminal neuralgia and pain related to multiple sclerosis. Pain. 2009;143(3):186-91.

Easton JD, Saver JL, Albers GW, et al. Definition and evaluation of transient ischemic attack: a scientific statement for healthcare professionals from the American Heart Association/American Stroke Association Stroke Council; Council on Cardiovascular Surgery and Anesthesia; Council on Cardiovascular Radiology and Intervention; Council on Cardiovascular Nursing; and the Interdisciplinary Council on Peripheral Vascular Disease. The American Academy of Neurology affirms the value of this statement as an educational tool for neurologists. Stroke. 2009;40(6):2276-93.

Zink BJ. Traumatic brain injury outcome: concepts for emergency care. Ann Emerg Med. 2001;37(3):318-32.
Pelonero AL, Levenson JL, Pandurangi AK. Neuroleptic malignant syndrome: a review. Psychiatr Serv. 1998;49(9):1163-72.

Tyler KL. Herpes simplex virus infections of the central nervous system: encephalitis and meningitis, including Mollaret s. Herpes. 2004;11 Suppl 2:57A-64A.

Rozenberg F, Deback C, Agut H. Herpes simplex encephalitis : from virus to therapy. Infect Disord Drug Targets. 2011;11(3):235-50.

The International Classification of Headache Disorders: 2nd edition. Cephalalgia. 2004;24 Suppl 1:9-160.

Bonte FJ, Harris TS, Hynan LS, Bigio EH, White CL. Tc-99m HMPAO SPECT in the differential diagnosis of the dementias with histopathologic confirmation. Clin Nucl Med. 2006;31(7):376-8.

Singer HS. Tourette syndrome and other tic disorders. Handb Clin Neurol. 2011;100:641-57.

CHAPTER 10 – PSYCHIATRY/ BEHAVIORAL SCIENCE

ABUSE & NEGLECT

INTIMATE PARTNER ABUSE

- According to the CDC, 1 in 4 women and 1 in 7 men will experience physical violence by their intimate partner at some point during their lifetimes. About 1 in 3 women and nearly 1 in 6 men experience some form of sexual violence during their lifetimes.
- **A woman who leaves an abusive partner has a 70% greater risk of being killed by the abuser compared to staying.**
- Abuse during pregnancy can make up about 10% of pregnant pregnancy-related hospital admissions.
- Barriers to screening include lack of privacy, low self-esteem, fear and sensitive nature of intimate partner violence.
- <u>Clues to violence:</u> contusions to breast, chest, abdomen, face, neck, musculoskeletal injuries, and "accidental" injuries. They may have multiple injuries in various stages of healing. Patients may have nonspecific general symptoms, such as fatigue & headache.

<u>MANAGEMENT</u>

- All healthcare facilities should have a plan that includes screening, assessing and referring patients for intimate partner violence.
- Once suspected, patients should be addressed directly with a nonthreatening question to confirm if intimate partner abuse has occurred. If it has occurred, then alternatives should be discussed with referral if the patient accepts as it is the patient's right to accept or refuse help.

SEXUAL ABUSE

- According to the National sexual Violence Resource Center 2015 report, more than one-quarter to one-third of female children have experienced sexual abuse before 18 years of age.
- Common ages of sexual abuse is between ages 9-12 years.
- **Perpetrators are most commonly males and most are relatives to the child or known by the child** (have access)**.**
- ~33% of sexual offenders were once themselves victims of sexual abuse.
- Any of the following should increase the index of suspicion for child abuse - children that exhibit sexual knowledge, initiate sex acts with peers, show knowledge of sexual acts, bruises, pain, or pruritus in the genital or anal area or evidence of a sexually transmitted infection.

PHYSICAL ABUSE

- Abuser often female and usually the primary caregiver.
- Signs may include cigarette burns, burns in a stocking glove pattern, lacerations, healed fractures on radiographs, subdural hematoma, multiple bruises, or retinal hemorrhages.
- Hyphema or retinal hemorrhages seen in shaken baby syndrome

CHILD NEGLECT

- Failure to provide the basic needs of a child (ex. supervision, food, shelter, affection, education) etc.
- Signs include malnutrition, withdrawal, poor hygiene, and failure to thrive.

ANXIETY DISORDERS

PANIC ATTACKS

- Sudden, abrupt, discrete episode of intense fear or discomfort that **usually peaks within 10 minutes** & rarely last more than 1 hour (most end in 20-30 minutes).
- Patients may feel anxious for hours after the attack.

CLINICAL MANIFESTATIONS

- **At least 4 of the following symptoms of sympathetic system overdrive - sense of impending doom or dread (hallmark)**

PANIC ATTACK SYMPTOMS: sympathetic overdrive

1. Dizziness	6. Shortness of breath	11. Palpitations, increased heart rate
2. Trembling	7. Chest pain/discomfort	12. Nausea or abdominal distress
3. Choking feeling	8. Chills or hot flashes	13. Depersonalization (being detached from oneself) or derealization (feelings of unreality)
4. Paresthesias	9. Fear of losing control	
5. Sweating	10. Fear of dying	

MANAGEMENT OF ACUTE ATTACK

- **Benzodiazepines first-line medical management** (eg, **Alprazolam,** Lorazepam, Diazepam etc.). Watch for dependence or abuse.
- With a panic attack (even in patients with Panic disorder), **one must rule out potentially life-threating conditions** (eg, **heart attack, thyrotoxicosis etc.**).
- Panic attacks are a feature of many different anxiety disorders but is not a disorder in & of itself.

PANIC DISORDER

- Average age of onset in early – mid 20s. Greater risk if 1st-degree relative is affected.
- >60% may also have major depression.
- More common in females.

DIAGNOSTIC CRITERIA:

- **Recurrent, unexpected panic attacks** (at least 2 attacks) may or may not be related to a trigger.
- At least one of the following must occur for at least 1 month: ❶ **Panic attacks often followed by persistent concern about future attacks,** ❷ persistent worry about the implication of the attacks (eg, losing control) or ❸ significant maladaptive behavior related to the attacks.
- Symptoms are not due to substance use, medical condition (eg, thyroid, hypoglycemia, cardiac), or other mental disorder.
- **Agoraphobia: anxiety about being in places or situations from which escape may be difficult** (eg, open spaces, enclosed spaces, crowds, public transportation, or outside of the home alone). Agoraphobia now seen as a separate entity from panic disorders & can occur with other psychiatric disorders.

MANAGEMENT

- Long-term: **SSRIs first-line medical treatment** (eg, Sertraline, Citalopram, Fluoxetine). May initiate therapy with SSRIs + benzodiazepines, then taper and discontinue the benzodiazepine. SNRIs also used (eg, Venlafaxine). TCAs option if SSRIs are ineffective.
- Cognitive Behavioral Therapy (CBT): adjunctive treatment that focuses on thinking & behavior (eg, relaxation, desensitization, examining behavior consequences etc.). Psychotherapy may be used in mild cases as initial therapy. **Pharmacotherapy + CBT most effective.**
- Acute panic attacks: **Benzodiazepines** (eg, **Alprazolam,** Clonazepam). Watch for dependence or abuse.

AGORAPHOBIA

- **Intense fear or anxiety about being in places or situations from which escape or obtaining help may be difficult** (eg, open spaces such as bridges, enclosed spaces, crowds, public transportation or being outside of the home alone).
- Although commonly seen with Panic disorder, Agoraphobia is now seen as a separate entity from panic disorders & can occur with other psychiatric disorders.
- The triggering situation causes anxiety or fear out of proportion to the potential danger of the situation.
- **Symptoms last at least 6 months, cause significant social or occupational dysfunction,** & not better explained by another disorder.
- <u>Risk factors:</u> strong genetic factor & may follow a traumatic event

<u>MANAGEMENT</u>

- Similar to Panic disorder: **Cognitive behavioral therapy & SSRIs**

GENERALIZED ANXIETY DISORDER

- More common in females.
- Onset of symptoms usually occurs in early 20s.

<u>DIAGNOSTIC CRITERIA</u>

- **Excessive anxiety or worry a majority of days for at least <u>6 months</u> about <u>various aspects</u> of life.** The **anxiety is usually out of proportion to the event.**
- Associated with at least 3 of the following symptoms: **fatigue,** restlessness, difficulty concentrating, muscle tension, sleep disturbance, irritability, shakiness, & headaches.
- It is not episodic (as in panic disorders), situational (as in phobias) nor focal.
- The symptoms cause significant social or occupational dysfunction.
- Not due to medical illness or substance abuse.

<u>MANAGEMENT</u>

- **Antidepressants – <u>SSRIs first-line</u>** (eg, **Fluoxetine, Paroxetine, Escitalopram),** SNRIs (eg, Venlafaxine).
- **Buspirone can be an adjunct to SSRIs (does not cause sedation).**
- Cognitive behavioral therapy & psychotherapy. Psychotherapy + pharmacotherapy more effective than either alone.
- Benzodiazepines can be used for short-term use only until long-term therapy takes effect (watch for dependence or abuse).
- Beta-blockers or TCAs.

BUSPIRONE

<u>Mechanism of action:</u>

- Partial Serotonin (5HT-1A) receptor agonist & dopamine receptor antagonist.

<u>Indications:</u>

- **Generalized anxiety disorder** (often used in combo with an SSRI). **Does not cause sedation & does not potentiate the CNS depression of alcohol** (almost negligible abuse or addiction potential).
- Takes 1-2 weeks to take full effect.

<u>Adverse effects:</u>

- Headache, nausea, dizziness, restless legs syndrome, & extrapyramidal symptoms.

SOCIAL ANXIETY DISORDER (Formerly Social Phobia)

- Most common type of phobia (public speaking).

DIAGNOSTIC CRITERIA

- Disabling, **persistent (at least 6 months) intense fear of social or performance situation in which the person is exposed to the scrutiny of others** for fear of embarrassment (eg, public speaking, meeting new people, eating or drinking in front of people, using public restrooms).
- Exposure to social situations almost always provokes anxiety & **causes expected panic attacks.**
- May realize feelings are excessive & out of proportion to any actual threat or danger. May avoid those situations.

MANAGEMENT

- **Psychotherapy: initial treatment of choice** - cognitive behavioral therapy (eg, desensitization), relaxation techniques, insight-oriented therapy.

- Pharmacotherapy: **SSRIs** (eg, **Fluoxetine, Sertraline**), SNRIs (eg, Venlafaxine). Adjunctive use of Benzodiazepines can be used until full effect of SSRIs for patients with need of faster relief.

- Most patients with moderate-severe cases benefit from combination pharmacotherapy & psychotherapy.

SITUATIONAL

- **Beta-blockers for performance anxiety & public speaking** (eg, **Propranolol**, Atenolol) 30-60 minutes before the performance.

SPECIFIC PHOBIAS

DIAGNOSTIC CRITERIA

- **Persistent (at least 6 months) intense fear or anxiety of a specific situation** (eg, heights, flying), **object** (eg, pigeons, snakes, blood) or **place** (eg, hospital).
- Exposure to the situation triggers an immediate response
- The fear is out of proportion to any real danger.
- The phobic object or situation is actively avoided or endured with intense fear or anxiety.
- **Everyday activities must be impaired by distress or avoidance** of the situation or object.
- Not due to substance use or medical condition

SUBTYPES

- Animal (eg, spiders, dogs, mice), situational (eg, airplanes, elevators), natural environment (eg, heights, thunder, water) & blood-injection injury (injuries, needle injections, or blood).

MANAGEMENT

- **Exposure & desensitization therapy treatment of choice.**

- Short-term benzodiazepines or beta-blockers can be used in some patients.

MOOD (AFFECTIVE) DISORDERS

MAJOR DEPRESSIVE DISORDER (MDD)/UNIPOLAR DEPRESSION

- Risk factors: family history, **female:** male (2:1). Peak onset of age in the 20s.

PATHOPHYSIOLOGY

- **Alteration in neurotransmitters** - serotonin, epinephrine, norepinephrine, dopamine, acetylcholine, & histamine. Genetic factors.
- Neuroendocrine dysregulation: adrenal, thyroid, or growth hormone dysregulation.
- 15% of patients commit suicide (especially men 25-30y & women 40-50y). Higher suicide rates in patients with a detailed suicide plan, white males >45y, & concurrent substance abuse.
- Patient Health Questionnaire (PHQ)-2 form for initial screen. If positive, may use PHQ-9 form.

DIAGNOSTIC CRITERIA:

- At least 2 distinct episodes of **at least 5 associated symptoms (must include either depressive mood or anhedonia)** almost every day for most of the days for **at least 2 weeks:** depressive mood, anhedonia, fatigue almost all day, insomnia or hypersomnia, feelings of guilt or worthlessness, recurring thoughts of death or suicide, psychomotor agitation or retardation (restlessness or slowness), significant weight change (gain or loss), decreased or increased appetite, & decreased concentration or indecisiveness. Not associated with mania or hypomania.
- **The symptoms must cause significant distress or impairment (social or occupational).**
- The symptoms are not due to substance use, bereavement, or medical conditions.

MANAGEMENT

- Psychotherapy (eg, cognitive behavioral therapy, **interpersonal therapy,** & supportive therapy).
- **SSRIs first-line medical management.** If no effect after 4 weeks, switch to other SSRI.
- Second-line: SNRIs (eg, Duloxetine, Venlafaxine); Bupropion.
- Tricyclic antidepressants. Tetracyclics, MAO inhibitors.
- Electroconvulsive therapy: rapid response in patients unresponsive to medical therapy, unable to tolerate pharmacotherapy (eg, pregnancy), or rapid reduction of symptoms.

SUBTYPES "COURSE SPECIFIERS" OF MDD

1. **SEASONAL AFFECTIVE DISORDER/SEASONAL PATTERN:** the presence of depressive symptoms at the same time each year (ex. most common in the winter – "winter blues" – due to reduction of sunlight & cold weather). Management: SSRIs, light therapy, Bupropion.

2. **ATYPICAL DEPRESSION:** shares many of the typical symptoms of major depression but patients experience **mood reactivity (improved mood in response to positive events).** Symptoms include significant weight gain/appetite increase, hypersomnia, heavy/leaden feelings in arms or legs & oversensitivity to interpersonal rejection. Management: MAO inhibitors.

3. **MELANCHOLIA:** characterized by anhedonia (inability to find pleasure in things), lack of mood reactivity, depression, severe weight loss/loss of appetite, excessive guilt, psychomotor agitation or retardation & sleep disturbance (increased REM time & reduced sleep). Sleep disturbances may lead to early morning awakening or mood that is worse in the morning.

4. **CATATONIC DEPRESSION:** motor immobility, stupor & extreme withdrawal.

SELECTIVE SEROTONIN REUPTAKE INHIBITORS (SSRIs)

Citalopram, Escitalopram, Paroxetine, Fluoxetine, Sertraline, & Fluvoxamine

Mechanism of action:

- Selectively inhibits CNS uptake of serotonin, leading to increased serotonin activity in the CNS.

Indications:

- **SSRIs first-line medical therapy for depression, PTSD, panic disorder, premenstrual dysphoric disorder, & anxiety disorder in most cases –** effective, relatively mild adverse effects and less toxic in overdose compared to other antidepressants (because they don't affect norepinephrine, acetylcholine, histamine, or dopamine).
- **Fluoxetine: only antidepressant approved for treatment of Bulimia.** Fluoxetine has a long-half life (2-4 days) compared to other SSRIs (~1 day). Because of the longer half-life, there is a longer washout period for switching to MAOI (5 weeks) compared to other SSRIs (at least 2 weeks).
- **On average, antidepressants take 4-6 weeks to reach maximum efficacy.** If no response, switch to another SSRI.

Adverse effects:

- **GI** (nausea & diarrhea). Headache, changes in energy level (fatigue, restlessness).
- **Sexual dysfunction** (eg, decreased libido, anorgasmia).
- Anxiety, insomnia, **weight changes**, SIADH, & serotonin syndrome.
- Increased suicidality in children & young adults (black box warning).
- **Avoid Citalopram in patients with long QT syndrome**.

SEROTONIN & NOREPINEPHRINE REUPTAKE INHIBITORS (SNRIs)

Duloxetine, Venlafaxine, Desvenlafaxine

Mechanism of action: inhibits neuronal reuptake of serotonin, norepinephrine, & dopamine.

Indications:

- **Duloxetine** may be used as first line agent, **particularly in patients with significant fatigue or neuropathy pain syndromes in association with depression.**
- Venlafaxine is good for depression & anxiety disorder.

Adverse effects:

- Safety, tolerability & adverse effect profile similar to those of SSRIs including hyponatremia.
- Norepinephrine effects: **hypertension,** sweating, dizziness, dry mouth, & constipation.

Contraindications & cautions:

- MAOI use, renal or hepatic impairment, seizures. Avoid abrupt discontinuation. Use with caution in patients with hypertension. Increased risk of Serotonin syndrome if SNRIs + St John's Wort.

TETRACYCLIC

Mirtazapine

Mechanism of action:

- Increases the release of norepinephrine & serotonin via central presynaptic alpha-2 adrenergic receptor antagonism. High affinity for histamine H1 receptors (leading to its sedative properties).
- Postsynaptic serotonin 5-HT2 and 5-HT3 receptor antagonist, increasing neurotransmission mediated by serotonin 5-HT1 receptors.

Indications:

- **Depression, especially patients with insomnia or significant weight loss** (has appetite stimulating & sedating properties). **Fewer sexual adverse effects** compared to SSRIs.
- **Anxiety disorders** (has anxiolytic properties). May be used with Trazodone.

Adverse effects:

- **Sedation, weight gain (appetite stimulant).**
- Dry mouth, constipation, tremor, dizziness, & agranulocytosis.
- Increased risk of suicidality in children, adolescents, and young adults.

Contraindications:

- Use with MAO inhibitors (may cause Serotonin syndrome).

TRICYCLIC ANTIDEPRESSANTS (TCAs)

Tertiary: Amitriptyline, Clomipramine, Imipramine, & Doxepin
Secondary: Desipramine & Nortriptyline
Mechanism of action: Inhibits reuptake of Serotonin & Norepinephrine.
Indications:

- **Depression,** insomnia, **neuropathies** (eg, Diabetic neuropathic pain, Post-herpetic neuralgia), Migraine, & Urge incontinence.
- **Used less often because of their adverse effect profile & severe toxicity with overdose.**

Adverse effects:

- **Anticholinergic effects most common** (eg, dry mouth, constipation, urinary retention, tachycardia, & orthostatic hypotension - elderly may experience confusion or hallucinations).
- **Weight gain. Prolonged QT interval** (best indicator of overdose).
- Sedation (antihistaminic effect), lowered seizure threshold, & SIADH.

Overdose:

- 3 C's: **Cardiotoxicity:** sinus or **wide complex tachycardia** (due to its Na+ channel blocker effects), **Convulsions (seizures)** or other neurologic symptoms (eg, respiratory depression), & **Coma.**
- Management: **sodium bicarbonate may be used for cardiotoxicity.**

Contraindications/cautions:

- Use of MAO Inhibitors, recent MI, seizure history.

TRICYCLIC ANTIDEPRESSANTS	SPECIFIC FACTS
TERITIARY AMINES	• **Most anticholinergic, antihistaminic (sedating) and antiadrenergic so higher toxicity with overdose**
Amitriptyline	• **Useful in neuropathies & chronic pain** (due to its sodium channel blocking properties) & insomnia.
Clomipramine	• **Useful in Obsessive compulsive disorder (most serotonin specific).**
Doxepin	• Good for chronic pain
Imipramine	• **Useful for enuresis in children** and panic disorder.
SECONDARY AMINES	• **Least anticholinergic, antiadrenergic & antihistaminic (less sedating)**
Desipramine	• **Least sedating (least antihistaminic) and least anticholinergic.**
Nortriptyline	• Good for chronic pain. Best tolerated. • **Least likely to cause orthostatic hypotension.**

- **Exam tip:**
- **In general, SSRIs are first-line medical therapy in most cases** because they are effective, have relatively mild adverse effects and less toxic in overdose compared to other antidepressants.
- **On average, antidepressants take 4-6 weeks to reach maximum efficacy.**
- In patients not responsive to initial SSRI therapy after 4-6 weeks, switch to another SSRI.
- **Duloxetine first-line if depression + neuropathic pain.**
- **Bupropion may be preferred if patient is fearful of sexual dysfunction or weight gain** (also good for **smoking cessation**).

BUPROPION

Mechanism of action:

- Inhibits the neuronal presynaptic uptake of dopamine & norepinephrine.

Indications:

- Major depressive disorder & Seasonal affective disorder (marketed as Wellbutrin).
- **Less GI, weight gain, & sexual adverse effects compared to SSRIs** (useful in depressed patients who are fearful of sexual side effects or weight gain).
- Aid in **smoking cessation** (marketed as Zyban) – useful in depressed smokers trying to quit.

Adverse effects:

- **Seizures** (lowers seizure threshold).
- Dry mouth, nausea, insomnia, agitation, anxiety, weight loss, hypertension, & headache.
- Increased risk of Psychosis at high doses.
- Avoid abrupt withdrawal.

Contraindications:

- **Epilepsy or conditions with increased seizure risk** (eg, **eating disorders, such as Bulimia & Anorexia** or patients undergoing abrupt discontinuation of alcohol, benzodiazepine, barbiturate, or antiepileptic medications).
- Avoid in patients with MAO inhibitor use in the past 2 weeks.

NONSELECTIVE MAO INHIBITORS

Phenelzine, Tranylcypromine, & Isocarboxazid

Mechanism of action:

- Blocks breakdown of neurotransmitters (**increased levels of norepinephrine, serotonin**, dopamine, epinephrine, & tyramine) by inhibiting monoamine oxidase (MAO).

Indications:

- **Refractory depression** or refractory anxiety disorders.

Adverse effects:

- **Orthostatic hypotension most common,** insomnia, anxiety, weight gain, & sexual dysfunction.
- **Hypertensive crisis after ingesting foods high in tyramine (eg, aged or fermented cheese, all aged, smoked, pickled or cured meats/poultry/fish, red wine,** draft beer, & chocolates). MAO inhibition prevents the breakdown of tyramine, leading to hypertension.

Drug interactions:

- **Increased risk of Serotonin syndrome if MAO inhibitors are combined with SSRIs**, SNRIs, St. John's wort, MDMA, cocaine, Meperidine, Tramadol, & Dextromethorphan.
- Wait at least 2 weeks before switching from MAO inhibitors to SSRIs or vice versa (5 weeks for Fluoxetine due to its longer half-life).
- MAOI + TCAs may cause delirium & hypertension.

SEROTONIN RECEPTOR ANTAGONISTS & AGONISTS

Trazodone, Nefazodone

Mechanism of action:

- Trazodone is a serotonin antagonist & agonist - postsynaptic serotonin 5-HT2A and 5-HT2C receptor inhibitor. Weakly inhibits presynaptic serotonin uptake (reuptake inhibition). Its active metabolite is a serotonin receptor agonist.
- Alpha-1 adrenergic receptor antagonist (leads to sedation).

Indications:

- **Antidepressant with anxiolytic & hypnotic effects (useful for insomnia).**
- May be used as a sleep aid (low dose).
- Unlike SSRIs, Trazodone does not affect REM sleep or cause sexual adverse effects.

Adverse effects:

- **Sedation (most common),** dizziness, dry mouth, nausea, orthostatic hypotension, headache.
- **Priapism** rare but classic adverse effect.
- Increased suicidality in children & young adults. Cardiac arrhythmias.
- Nefazodone has a black box warning for rare but serious fulminant hepatitis.

SEROTONIN SYNDROME

- Potentially life-threating syndrome due to **increased serotonergic activity in the CNS.**

ETIOLOGIES

- Most commonly occurs within 24 hours (especially 6 hours) with **initiation or change in serotonergic drugs,** such as SSRIs, SNRIs, TCAs, & MAO inhibitors, Buspirone, Triptans, or combination of those medications with St John's wort, MDMA (ecstasy), cocaine, or amphetamines.

PHYSICAL EXAMINATION

- **Cognitive effects:** altered mental status, confusion, **agitation,** hallucinations, hypomania.
- **Autonomic instability** **hyperthermia,** tachycardia, diaphoresis, blood pressure changes.
- GI serotonin effects: nausea, vomiting, increased bowel sounds, & **diarrhea.**
- Neuromuscular hyperactivity: **spontaneous or inducible clonus, hypertonia (increased DTR), tremor,** akathisia (restlessness).
- **Mydriasis (dilated pupils),** dry mucous membranes, & flushed skin.

DIAGNOSIS

- Clinical diagnosis based on the Hunter criteria.

MANAGEMENT OF MILD

- **Prompt discontinuation of offending drug(s) most important.**
- **Supportive care** mainstay of therapy - supplemental oxygen, IV fluids & **Benzodiazepines** (for agitation, to reduce hyperthermia, and to correct mild increases in heart rate and blood pressure).

MANAGEMENT OF MODERATE

- As above + **Cyproheptadine** (serotonin antagonist).
- Antipyretics should not be used for hyperthermia.

BIPOLAR I DISORDER

- Risk factors: **family history (1st-degree relatives) strongest risk factor** (10 times more likely). Men = women.
- 1% of population. Average age of onset is 20s - 30s. New onset rare after 50y.
- The earlier the onset, the greater likelihood of psychotic features & the poorer the prognosis.

DIAGNOSTIC CRITERIA

- **At least 1 Manic or mixed episode (only requirement).** The manic episodes often cycle with occasional depressive episodes but *major depressive episodes are not required for the diagnosis.*
- **Mania = abnormal & persistently elevated, expansive or irritable mood at least 1 week** (or less if hospitalization is required) with **marked impairment of social/occupational function** At least 3: **Mood:** euphoria, irritable, labile or dysphoric; **Thinking:** racing, flight of ideas, disorganized, easily distracted, expansive or grandiose thoughts (highly inflated self-esteem). Judgment is impaired (eg, spending sprees); **Behavior:** physical hyperactivity, pressured speech, decreased need for sleep (may go days without sleep), increased impulsivity, excessive involvement in pleasurable activities including risk-taking, hypersexuality, disinhibition, & increased goal directed activity.
- Psychotic symptoms (paranoia, delusions, hallucinations) may be seen in these patients.
- Symptoms not due to medical condition or substance use.

MANAGEMENT

- **Mood Stabilizers: Lithium first-line** (acute mania & long-term management). **Lithium also decreases suicide risk.**
- Valproic acid or Carbamazepine useful for rapid cycling or mixed features.
- **2nd-generation (atypical) antipsychotics:** (eg, Risperidone, Quetiapine, Olanzapine & Ziprasidone) are effective as monotherapy or as adjunctive therapy to mood stabilizers (combination of mood stabilizers and antipsychotics is faster & more effective than monotherapy).
- **Psychotherapy:** cognitive, behavioral & interpersonal. Good sleep hygiene recommended.
- Bipolar depression: Lithium, Quetiapine, Lurasidone, or Lamotrigine.
- Antidepressant therapy may be used as adjunct to mood stabilizers for severe depression but **antidepressant monotherapy may precipitate mania or hypomania.**

ACUTE MANIA

- **Antipsychotics (eg, Risperidone or Olanzapine > Haloperidol) or mood stabilizers** (eg, **Lithium,** Valproic acid) are most effective.
- Antipsychotics or benzodiazepines can be used for acute psychosis or agitation.
- Electroconvulsive therapy especially helpful for refractory or life-threatening acute mania or depression (also best treatment for pregnant women with manic episodes).

	MANIA/MIXED	MAJOR DEPRESSION
BIPOLAR I	**Yes**	**Typical but not required.**
BIPOLAR II	**HYPOmania only (no mania)**	**Yes**
CYCLOTHYMIA	No (but may have periods of mood elevation)	No. Associated with relatively mild depressive episodes.
MAJOR DEPRESSIVE DISORDER	No	**Yes**
PERSISTENT DEPRESSIVE DISORDER (DYSTHYMIA)	No	Usually mild but can meet criteria for major in some cases.

"Mixed" symptoms = simultaneous occurrence of ≥3 manic (or hypomanic) symptoms + depression.

LITHIUM

Mechanism of action:

- Exact mechanism of action unknown but thought to alter neuronal sodium transport and influence the reuptake of serotonin and/or norepinephrine.

Indications:

- **Bipolar disorder** (both manic & depressive episodes)
- **Acute mania (mood stabilizer)**
- Schizoaffective disorder

Adverse effects:

- Endocrine: **hypothyroidism, nephrogenic diabetes insipidus, hyperparathyroidism, hypercalcemia, hypermagnesemia,** & sodium depletion. Increased thirst (should drink 8-10 glasses of water daily).
- Neurologic: seizures, tremor, headache, sedation.
- GI – nausea, vomiting, diarrhea, weight gain.
- Arrhythmias. Leukocytosis.
- Narrow therapeutic index: prior to initiating therapy, a basic ECG, chemistries, thyroid function, beta-hCG, and CBC should be performed. Initially levels should be checked after 5 days then every 2-3 days until therapeutic. Once therapeutic, monitor plasma levels every 4- 8 weeks. Levels may be toxic if > 1.5.

Contraindications:

- **Pregnancy** - may be associated with **Ebstein's anomaly** if taken during the first trimester.
- Severe renal disease, cardiac disease.

Cautions:

- **Use with NSAIDs,** thiazide diuretics, ACE inhibitors.
- Impaired renal function associated with increased Lithium levels.

BIPOLAR II DISORDER

- Recurrent major depressive episodes with hypomania.

DIAGNOSTIC CRITERIA FOR BIPOLAR II

- **History of at least 1 major depressive episode + at least 1 hypomanic episode.** Any current or prior Manic episode makes the diagnosis Bipolar I.

- **Hypomania** = abnormal & persistently elevated, expansive or irritable mood **≤ 1 week, does not require hospitalization, not associated with marked impairment of social/occupational function,** & not associated with psychotic features. At least 3 symptoms affecting mood, thinking, or behavior (symptoms otherwise similar to Manic episodes).

MANAGEMENT: same as Bipolar I

- **Mood Stabilizers: Lithium first line (also decreases suicide risk) or second-generation (atypical) antipsychotics** (eg, Risperidone, Quetiapine, Olanzapine, & Ziprasidone).

- Valproic acid or Carbamazepine useful for rapid cycling.

- Psychotherapy: cognitive, behavioral & interpersonal. Good sleep hygiene recommended.

PERSISTENT DEPRESSIVE DISORDER (DYSTHYMIA)

- DSM V combined **Dysthymia** & chronic major depressive disorder into PDD.
- More common in women. Onset often in childhood, adolescence, or early adulthood.

DIAGNOSTIC CRITERIA

- **Chronic depressed mood for at least 2 years in adults** (at least 1 year in children/adolescents) that last most of the day, more days than not. In that 2 year period, the **patient is not symptom free for >2 months at a time.**
- At least 2 of the following conditions must be present - insomnia or hypersomnia, fatigue, low self-esteem, decreased appetite or overeating, hopelessness, poor concentration or indecisiveness.
- May have major depressive episodes or meet the criteria for Major depressive disorder continuously.
- Must never have had a manic episode (rules out Bipolar I) or hypomanic episode (rules out cyclothymic disorder).

MANAGEMENT

- **Combination treatment with psychotherapy & pharmacotherapy more efficacious than either alone.**
- Pharmacotherapy: **SSRIs**, SNRIs, TCAs, & MAO inhibitors.
- Psychotherapy includes interpersonal, cognitive, and insight-oriented psychotherapies.

CYCLOTHYMIC DISORDER

- Similar to Bipolar II but is less severe.
- Approximately 1/3 will eventually develop Bipolar disorder. Men = women.
- May coexist with Borderline personality disorder.

DIAGNOSIS

- Characterized by **at least 2 years** of prolonged, **milder elevations and milder depressions in mood** that **do not meet the criteria for full hypomanic episodes or major depressive episodes** (at least 1 year in children).
- The symptom free periods don't last longer than 2 months at a time for those 2 years.
- Major depressive, manic or mixed episodes do not occur.

MANAGEMENT

- Similar to bipolar I: mood stabilizers (eg, **Lithium,** Valproic acid) or **2nd–generation antipsychotics** (eg, Risperidone, Olanzapine, Quetiapine, Ziprasidone).

PREMENSTRUAL DYSPHORIC DISORDER

- **PMS:** cluster of physical, behavioral and mood changes with cyclical occurrence during the luteal phase of the menstrual cycle.
- **Premenstrual dysphoric disorder: severe PMS with functional impairment** where anger, irritability, & internal tension are prominent (DSM V diagnostic criteria).

CLINICAL MANIFESTATIONS

- **Physical:** abdominal bloating & fatigue most common, breast swelling or pain, weight gain, headache, changes in bowel habits, muscle or joint pain.
- **Emotional: irritability most common,** tension, depression, anxiety, hostility, libido changes, aggressiveness.
- **Behavioral:** food cravings, poor concentration, noise sensitivity, loss of motor senses.

DIAGNOSIS

- **Symptoms occurring 1-2 weeks before menses (luteal phase), relieved within 2-3 days of the onset of menses** plus at least 7 symptom-free days during the follicular phase.
- Patient should record a diary of symptoms for >2 cycles.

MANAGEMENT

- Lifestyle modifications: stress reduction & exercise most beneficial. Caffeine, alcohol, cigarette, & salt reduction. NSAIDs, vitamin B6 & E.
- **SSRIs first-line medical therapy for emotional symptoms with dysfunction** (eg, **Fluoxetine, Sertraline**, Citalopram).
- **Oral contraceptives** (especially **Drospirenone-containing** OCPs) can be used in patients who do not want to take SSRIs.
- Gonadotropin-releasing hormone (GnRH) agonist therapy with estrogen-progestin addback if no response to SSRIs or OCPs.

SUICIDE

RISK FACTORS

- Plan: **previous attempt strongest single predictive factor** (70% of people who committed suicide succeeded on their first try). Organized plan > no organized plans.
- Access to firearms is an increased risk.
- Gender: **females attempt suicide more than men but men are more successful at committing suicide.**
- Age: increases with age. **Elderly white men** have the highest risk in the US.
- Race: whites > blacks.
- Psychiatric disorders: majority who attempt or commit suicide have underlying psychiatric disorders.
- Substance abuse: increased risk.
- Marital status: **alone** > never married > widowed > separated or divorced > married without children > married with children (marriage is protective).
- Others: positive family history of suicide, history of impulsivity, chronic illness. Among highly skilled workers, physicians are at an increased risk of suicide.

MANAGEMENT

- Assuring the patient's safety to prevent the patient from committing suicide.
- Admission and psychiatric evaluation.
- Once safety is established, treatment is aimed at diagnosing and treating any underlying mental disorder, including psychotherapy.

CONDUCT DISORDERS

- Persistent pattern of behaviors that **deviate sharply from the age-appropriate norms and violates the rights of others and animals.**
- These individuals engage in physical and/or sexual violence, lack empathy for their victims, and may lack remorse for committing crimes.
- More common in males. High incidence of ADHD and Oppositional defiance disorder.
- **May progress to Antisocial personality disorder.**

DIAGNOSTIC CRITERIA

- Persistent pattern of **violation of the rights of others or age-appropriate societal norms** with at least 3 behaviors over the last year and at least one incidence within the last 6 months:
- **Aggression to humans or animals** – threatens, intimidates, or bullies others, uses weapons, physically cruel to animals or humans, sexual violence.
- **Destruction of property** – engages in **fire setting, vandalism,** etc.
- **Serious violation of rules** – runs away from home, stays out past curfew, engages in truancy (often before 13 years old).
- **Deceitfulness or theft** – lies to obtain goods and favors, breaks into buildings, cars or homes etc., steals the properties of others. Lacks remorse for actions.
- <18 years of age.

MANAGEMENT

- Multimodal: **behavioral modification,** community and family involvement, parent management training (eg enforcing rules and setting limits).

PROGNOSIS

- Good prognosis: positive relationship with at least 1 parent, adolescent onset of symptoms, female gender, good interpersonal skills, high IQ, good academic performance.
- Poor prognosis: onset of symptoms prior to 10 years, low IQ, poor academic performance.

EXAM TIP

Both ODD and Disruptive mood dysregulation disorder are associated with a disruptive and angry child, blaming others or refusing to follow rules.
ODD is associated with intent behind their behavior.
Children with DMDD do not do it on purpose and may feel remorseful after outbursts.

OPPOSITIONAL DEFIANT DISORDER

- **Disorder in which children are generally defiant towards authority but is <u>not</u> associated with physical aggression, violating others' basic rights or breaking laws** (unlike Conduct disorder).
- Persistent pattern of negative, angry or irritable mood, argumentative, or defiant behavior, & intentional vindictiveness or spitefulness.
- 50% associated with ADHD. May occasionally lead to Conduct disorder.

DIAGNOSTIC CRITERIA

- Characterized by at least 4 symptoms present at least 6 months (with at least one individual that is not a sibling).
- **Angry or irritable mood** (eg, loses temper, anger or resentment, often blames others for their misbehaviors & negative attitude).
- **Argumentative or defiant behavior**: breaks rules, often blames others for their behavior, **argues with authority** & deliberately annoys others.
- **Vindictiveness:** spiteful at least 2 times in the past 6 months.

MANAGEMENT

- **Psychotherapy** – **behavioral modification therapy**, problem-solving skills and conflict management training, & teaching parents child management (parenting skills, parent-child interaction therapy.

DISSOCIATIVE DISORDERS

Dissociation: loss or impaired sense of "self". Temporary alteration in consciousness, memory, personality, behavior, or motor function. Causes impairment of functioning.

DISSOCIATIVE IDENTITY DISORDER

- **Presence of ≥2 DISTINCT IDENTITIES OR STATES OF PERSONALITIES** that take control of behavior (formerly known as multiple personality disorder). The symptoms of the disruption of the identity may be self-reported and/or observed by others.
- Gaps in the recall of events may occur for everyday and not just for traumatic events.
- Most common in women. May be associated with history of **sexual abuse,** PTSD, substance use etc.

DEPERSONALIZATION/DEREALIZATION DISORDER

- **Persistent feelings of detachment or estrangement** from:
  - oneself (depersonalization) eg, "out of body feeling" and/or
  - surrounding environment (derealization)

During these experiences, reality testing is intact & the symptoms cause distress.

DISSOCIATIVE AMNESIA

- **Inability to recall personal/autobiographical information.** Often secondary to sexual abuse, stress, or trauma. It causes significant impairment in functioning.
- **Dissociative fugue**: **abrupt change in geographic location** with loss of identity or inability to recall the past.
- Before determining this diagnosis, neurologic testing must be done to rule out seizures or brain tumor as the cause.

MANAGEMENT OF DISSOCIATIVE DISORDERS

- Psychotherapy.

FEEDING AND EATING DISORDERS

OBESITY

- **Body mass index (BMI) 30 kg/m² or greater or body weight 20% or greater over the ideal weight.**

COMPLICATIONS
- Obesity associated with increased risk for coronary disease, diabetes mellitus II, breast & colon cancers.
- About 50% of patients experience Binge eating episodes

MANAGEMENT
- Behavior modification: exercise & dietary changes, group therapy.
- Medical therapy: antidepressants if there is underlying depression. Treat any complications.
- **Anti-obesity medications: Orlistat** (decreases GI fat digestion); **Lorcaserin** (serotonin agonist).
- Surgical options: include gastric bypass, gastric sleeve, gastric banding, & bariatric surgery.

SCREENING
- USPSTF recommends for screening all adults and children age 6 years and older.

BINGE-EATING DISORDER

DIAGNOSTIC CRITERIA
- **Recurrent episodes of binge eating** - recurrent episodes characterized by eating within a 2-hour period more than people would in a similar period with lack of control during an overeating episode. **Occurs at least weekly for 3 months**.
- Severe distress over binge eating.
- May be triggered by stress or mood changes. Patients are often obese.
- Unlike Bulimia nervosa, Binge-eating episodes are **not associated with compensatory behaviors** (eg, purging or restrictive behaviors) and they are not as fixated on their body shape or weight.

MANAGEMENT
- Psychotherapy (eg, cognitive behavioral therapy, interpersonal, dialectic behavioral).
- Strict diet & exercise plan.
- **Topiramate** (antiepileptic associated with weight loss).
- Stimulants: appetite suppressants (eg, Lisdexamfetamine, Amphetamine).

BULIMIA NERVOSA

- Eating disorder characterized by frequent **binge eating combined with compensatory behaviors** to prevent weight gain.

- Unlike Anorexia, patients with **Bulimia nervosa usually maintain a normal weight (or may be overweight)** & **their compensatory behaviors are ego-dystonic** (troublesome to the patient).

- **More common in females** 10:1.

- Average onset of age in the late teens or early adulthood.

PHYSICAL EXAMINATION

- **Teeth pitting or enamel erosion (from vomiting).**

- **Russell's sign:** calluses on the dorsum of the hand from self-induced vomiting.

- Parotid gland hypertrophy.

LAB FINDINGS

- Hypokalemia, hypomagnesemia (electrolyte imbalance may lead to cardiac arrhythmias).

- **Increased amylase** (salivary gland hypertrophy + vomiting). Metabolic alkalosis from vomiting.

DIAGNOSTIC CRITERIA

- **Recurrent episodes of binge eating** - recurrent episodes characterized by eating within a 2-hour period more than people would in a similar period with lack of control during an overeating episode. **Occurs at least weekly for 3 months**. May be triggered by stress or mood changes.

- **Compensatory behaviors:**
  - **Purging type** - primarily engages in self-induced vomiting, diuretic, laxative or enema abuse.
  - **Non-purging type**: reduced calorie intake, dieting, fasting, excessive exercise, & diet pills.

- Perception of self-worth is excessively influenced by shape and body weight.

MANAGEMENT

- **Psychotherapy:** cognitive behavioral therapy, group therapy, interpersonal therapy. Combination psychotherapy & pharmacotherapy more effective.

- Pharmacotherapy: **Fluoxetine is the only FDA-approved medication for Bulimia nervosa** - has been shown to reduce the binge-purge cycle. Fluoxetine associated with cardiovascular adverse effects especially if electrolyte abnormalities are present.

ANOREXIA NERVOSA

- **Failure to maintain a normal body weight**, fear & preoccupation with body weight, body image, & being thin.
- Most common in teenage girls ages 14-18. 90% are women.
- Frequently seen in athletes, dancers (or other conditions requiring thinness).
- 60% incidence of depression.
- **Anorexia nervosa has the highest mortality rate of all psychiatric conditions** (due to arrhythmias) 5-18%.

CLINICAL MANIFESTATIONS
- **Exhibits behaviors targeted at maintaining a low weight** or certain body image: eg, excess water intake, food-related obsessions (hoarding, collecting). Anorexia nervosa is **ego-syntonic** (their behaviors are acceptable to them and are in harmony with their self-image goals).

- **Restrictive type:** strict, reduced calorie intake, dieting, fasting, excessive exercise, & diet pills.

- **Binge eating/purging type:** primarily engages in self-induced vomiting as well as diuretic, laxative use, or enema abuse.

PHYSICAL EXAMINATION
- Emaciation, hypotension, bradycardia, skin or hair changes (eg, **lanugo**), dry skin, salivary gland hypertrophy, **amenorrhea**, arrhythmias, osteopenia.

- Russel's sign: callouses on the dorsum of the hand from self-induced vomiting.

- Body mass index **(BMI) 17.5 kg/m^2 or less** OR **body weight <85% of ideal weight.**

DIAGNOSTIC CRITERIA
- **Restriction of calorie intake** relative to requirements leading to **significantly low body weight** (less than minimally normal).

- **Intense morbid fear of fatness or gaining weight** or persistent behaviors to prevent weight gain.

- **Distorted body image –** self-perception of being overweight (even though they are underweight).

LABS:
- **Hypokalemia** (GI loss from laxatives or vomiting), increased BUN (dehydration), hypochloremic **metabolic alkalosis** (from vomiting), hypogonadotropic hypogonadism (low estrogen), & hypothyroidism

MANAGEMENT
- Medical stabilization: hospitalization for <75% expected body weight or patients who have medical complications (eg, dehydration). Electrolyte imbalances may lead to cardiac arrhythmias.

- Nutritional rehabilitation: most common complication is refeeding syndrome (increased insulin leads to hypophosphatemia & cardiac complications).

- Psychotherapy: cognitive behavioral therapy, supervised meals, weight monitoring.

- Pharmacotherapy: if depressed eg, **SSRIs (may also help with weight gain);** Atypical antipsychotics (may also help with weight gain).

OBSESSIVE-COMPULSIVE & RELATED DISORDERS

Includes Obsessive-compulsive disorder, Body dysmorphic disorder, Hoarding disorder, Trichotillomania (hair-pulling disorder) & excoriation (skin-picking) disorder.

OBSESSIVE-COMPULSIVE DISORDER (OCD)

- Obsessions: **recurrent or persistent thoughts/images.** These thoughts are inappropriate, intrusive, & unwanted. The patient tries to ignore or suppress the obsessions. They are usually **ego-dystonic** (inconsistent with one's own personal beliefs).

- Compulsions: **repetitive behaviors** (rituals) the person **feels driven to perform** to reduce or prevent stress from the obsession. These **compulsions cause distress, impairment, or are time consuming** (eg, > 1 hour a day).

- Men = women but men often present earlier in their teens. Genetic component.
- Mean age of onset 20y with symptoms often present in adolescence (onset rare after 50y).
- Theorized due to **abnormal communication between the basal ganglia,** orbitofrontal cortex, and the anterior cingulate gyrus.
- Serotonin thought to be primary neurotransmitter involved.
- May be associated with the triad of "uncontrollable urges" – OCD, ADHD, & tic disorders (Tourette).

CLINICAL MANIFESTATIONS

4 major patterns:

- **1. Contamination** - compulsion may include cleaning or hand washing.

- **2. Pathologic doubt** eg, forgetting to unplug iron to avoid potential danger.

- **3. Symmetry/precision** eg, ordering or counting.

- **4. Intrusive obsessive thoughts** without compulsion.

SPECIFIERS

- Good/fair insight: recognizes OCD beliefs are not true or may not be true.
- Poor insight: thinks the OCD beliefs are probably true.
- Absent insight/delusional beliefs: completely convinced that the OCD beliefs are true.

MANAGEMENT

- Combination of cognitive behavioral therapy and pharmacotherapy.

- Cognitive behavioral therapy: **first-line therapy - exposure & response prevention,** psychoeducation.

- Pharmacotherapy **– SSRIs first-line medical therapy** (eg, Fluoxetine, Sertraline, Paroxetine) - higher doses needed compared to depressive disorders; Tricyclic antidepressants (**Clomipramine because it is the most serotonin specific**), SNRIs (eg, Venlafaxine). Augmentation therapy with antipsychotics.

- Severely debilitating or resistant: psychosurgery (cingulotomy) or electroconvulsive therapy.

BODY DYSMORPHIC DISORDER

- Excessive **preoccupation with at least 1 perceived flaw or defect in physical appearance** that is not observable by others or appears slight to others.
- This preoccupation often causes them to be ashamed or feel self-conscious, leading to functional impairment or significant distress.
- **May commit repetitive acts in response to this preoccupation** of physical flaw/defect (mirror checking, skin picking, seeking reassurance) or mental acts (comparison to others).
- Average age of onset 15 years of age. May be associated with anxiety disorder or depression.

MANAGEMENT
- **Antidepressants (eg, SSRIs) &/or Cognitive behavioral therapy.**
- TCAs (eg, Clomipramine) are an alternative to SSRIs.

TRICHOTILLOMANIA

- **Hair-pulling disorder**. 1-2% of the adult population.

RISK FACTORS
- **More common in women** (10:1).
- **Increased incidence with OCD, excoriation (skin picking disorder), & Depressive disorders.**

CLINICAL MANIFESTATIONS
- Hair loss usually involving the scalp, eyebrows, eyelashes but can be hair loss anywhere.
- Physical exam: decreased hair density, coarse hairs in the affected area and hair of different lengths.

DIAGNOSTIC CRITERIA
- Recurrent pulling of hair, resulting in hair loss. Repeated attempts to stop or minimize hair pulling.
- Not due to another medication or psychiatric disorder.

MANAGEMENT
- Cognitive behavior therapy eg, **habit reversal therapy.**
- SSRIs, second generation antipsychotics, N-acetylcysteine, or Lithium

HOARDING DISORDER

- Persistent difficulty discarding possession, regardless of value resulting in accumulation of a large number of possessions that may clutter living spaces to the point they may become unusable.
- The issue is due to the need to save the possessions with distress associated with discarding them.
- Hoarding causes impairment of social, occupational, or other areas of function.

RISK FACTORS
- **Most prevalent in the older population** but behavior often begins in the early teens.
- 20% have associated Obsessive-compulsive disorder.

MANAGEMENT
- **Cognitive behavioral therapy specific for hoarding (very difficult to treat).**

- SSRIs can be used (not as effective unless concurrent OCD).

NEURODEVELOPMENTAL DISORDERS

ATTENTION-DEFICIT DISORDER (ADD) & ATTENTION-DEFICIT HYPERACTIVITY DISORDER (ADHD)

- Neurodevelopmental disorder characterized by **problems paying attention**, **impulsivity** (difficulty controlling behaviors), & **hyperactivity** that is not age-appropriate.
- Many continue to have symptoms as adults (inattentiveness > hyperactivity).
- **67% comorbid with Conduct and Oppositional defiant disorders.**

<u>3 SUBCATEGORIES</u>

- 1. Predominantly inattentive, 2. Predominantly hyperactive/impulsive, & 3. combined type.

<u>DIAGNOSTIC CRITERIA</u>

- The symptoms must be developmentally inappropriate for age, have **symptom onset before 12 years of age** and must be present for **at least 6 months**.
- Symptoms **must occur in at least 2 settings** (eg, school, home, recreational activities).
- **<u>At least 6 inattentive symptoms</u>**:

INATTENTIVENESS
1. Easily distracted: misses details, frequently switches from one activity to another, forget things, easily distracted when multiple things are happening simultaneously.
2. Has difficulty maintaining focus on one task or learning something new.
3. Misses details and may make careless mistakes.
4. Forgets things or loses things (eg, pencils) needed to complete activities and tasks.
5. Difficulty in completing assignments.
6. Becomes bored with a task after a few minutes, unless doing something enjoyable.

and/or

- **<u>At least 6 hyperactivity/impulsivity symptoms</u>**:

HYPERACTIVITY/IMPULSIVITY
1. Fidgets and squirms in their seat.
2. Constantly in motion (may often leave their seat).
3. Talks nonstop or excessively.
4. Impatience.
5. Dashes around, touching or playing with everything in sight.
6. Has trouble sitting for long periods (eg, doing homework, dinner or school).
7. Difficulty doing quiet tasks.
8. Restlessness.
9. Blurts out appropriate or inappropriate comments, shows unrestrained emotions.
10. Interrupts the conversation or the activities of others.

<u>MANAGEMENT</u>

Multimodal approach

- Behavior modification including social skills training, classroom modifications, and parent psychoeducation
- **<u>Stimulants</u>** – **first-line medical treatment of choice** (eg, **Methylphenidate, Amphetamine/Dextroamphetamine,** Dexmethylphenidate).
- <u>Nonstimulants:</u> **Atomoxetine** (norepinephrine reuptake inhibitor).
  <u>Adverse effects:</u> dry mouth decreased appetite, insomnia.
- <u>Adjunctive medications</u>: Alpha agonists (eg, **Guanfacine**, Clonidine); Bupropion, Venlafaxine.

MANAGEMENT OF ADHD & ADD

Multimodal approach

- Behavior modification including social skills training, classroom modifications and parent psychoeducation.

STIMULANTS

Methylphenidate, Amphetamine/Dextroamphetamine, & Dexmethylphenidate.

- Mechanism: stimulant – blocks reuptake and increases the release of norepinephrine and dopamine in the extraneuronal space (sympathomimetic).
- Indications: **first-line medical treatment for ADD & ADHD.** Narcolepsy, excessive daytime sleepiness.
- Adverse effects: **abdominal pain,** insomnia, weight loss, dizziness, vomiting, anxiety, hypertension, tachycardia, growth delays, & addiction.

NONSTIMULANTS

Atomoxetine

- Mechanism of action: selective norepinephrine reuptake inhibitor. Similar efficacy and adverse effect profile as stimulants (but less adverse effects & less addictive ability).
- Adverse effects: dry mouth decreased appetite, insomnia.

OTHER ALTERNATIVES

- Alpha-2 agonists: **Guanfacine**, Clonidine. These drugs also used in Tourette syndrome.
- Bupropion, Venlafaxine.

AUTISM SPECTRUM DISORDER

- Spectrum of developmental disorders characterized by **impairment in social interaction or communication, restricted, repetitive stereotyped behaviors** as well as other signs leading to impaired social functioning.
- Male: female 4:1.
- Should be suspected if there is a rapid deterioration of social or language skills during the first 2 years of life.
- **Symptoms usually recognized between 12 and 24 months old.** M CHAT @ 18 + 24 months

DIAGNOSTIC CRITERIA

- **Social interaction difficulties:** significant emotional discomfort or detachment (eg, avoiding eye contact, no response to cuddling or affection).
- **Impaired communication:** either inability to communicate or has the ability to communicate but chooses not to in social settings. Difficulties in understanding what is not explicitly stated (eg, metaphors, humor in jokes etc.).
- **Restricted, repetitive, stereotyped behaviors** & patterns of activities (eg, peculiar interest in objects, rigid, inflexible thought patterns), repetitive motor patterns.
- Other signs: persistent failure to develop social relationships, failure to show preference to parents over other adults; unusual sensitivity to visual, auditory or olfactory stimuli; unusual attachments to ordinary objects. Savantism (unusual talents).
- These disturbances are not better explained by intellectual disability (intellectual development disorder) or global developmental delay.

MANAGEMENT

- Referral for neuropsychologic testing, behavioral modification strategies, & medications.

PERSONALITY DISORDERS

- 10-15% of population. Pervasive inflexible personality trait causing impaired function or distress.

CLUSTER A DISORDERS

- **Cluster A:** **SOCIAL DETACHMENT** with unusual behaviors: **WEIRD, ODD, ECCENTRIC BEHAVIOR.**

SCHIZOID PERSONALITY DISORDER

- Lifelong pattern of **voluntary social withdrawal & anhedonic introversion** (constricted affect).
- **Most common in males.** Usually early childhood onset.

Think **Schizoids AVOID** people:

- Anhedonic – little pleasure in activities, appears indifferent, lacks response to praise or criticism
- Voluntary social withdrawal – **prefers to be alone** (unlike avoidant PD). No desire for close or sexual relationships, prefers solitary activities.
- Odd-appearing or eccentric.
- Introvert – **loner "hermit-like behavior"**, quiet.
- Detached, flat, cold, constricted affect

MANAGEMENT

- **Psychotherapy:** including individual or group therapy **first-line management.**
- Pharmacologic: ± short-term low dose antipsychotics, antidepressants or psychostimulants.

SCHIZOTYPAL PERSONALITY DISORDER

- Characterized by **odd, eccentric, bizarre behavior and thought patterns** suggestive of Schizophrenia without psychosis (no delusions or hallucinations).
- Usually early adulthood onset. Small percentage may develop Schizophrenia

DIAGNOSTIC CRITERIA:

At least 5 of the following:

- Ideas of reference (excluding delusions of reference), suspiciousness.
- Odd beliefs or **magical thinking** or speech (eg, belief in clairvoyance, telepathy, superstition, bizarre fantasies etc.).
- May talk to self in public.
- Unusual perceptual experiences; distorted cognition and reasoning.
- Inappropriate or restricted affect.
- Pervasive discomfort with close relationships (increased social anxiety, may have few close friends).

MANAGEMENT

- **Psychotherapy first-line treatment** - cognitive behavioral, individual, or group therapy.
- Pharmacologic: short term low-dose antipsychotics for psychotic episodes or suspiciousness occur.

PARANOID PERSONALITY DISORDER

- **Pervasive pattern of distrust & suspiciousness of others.**
- Begins in early adulthood.
- More common in males. More common if family history of Schizophrenia.

DIAGNOSTIC CRITERIA

- Suspicion of others with interpretation of their motives as malevolent without sufficient basis.
- **Preoccupation with unjustified doubts regarding the loyalty & trustworthiness of others**. Reluctance to confide in others. Blames their problems on others.
- Misinterpretation of the benign remarks of others as threatening or demeaning – sees hidden messages, is easily insulted, bears grudges, doesn't forgive.
- Perception of attacks on his or her character that is not apparent to others & may react angrily to counterattack.
- Suspicion regarding the faithfulness of their partner or spouse without justification.

MANAGEMENT

- **Cognitive behavioral therapy first-line treatment** (patients may be suspicious of group therapy).
- Short-term antipsychotics if severe or if psychosis occurs.

CLUSTER B DISORDERS

- Cluster B: "DRAMATIC, WILD, ERRATIC, IMPULSIVE & EMOTIONAL"

ANTISOCIAL PERSONALITY DISORDER

- **Behaviors deviating sharply from the norms, values, & laws of society** (harmful or hostile to society). Their deceitful nature may be masked and may be seemed as charming or nice to those who don't know their history.
- **May commit criminal acts** with disregard to the violation of laws.
- 3 times more common in males.

DIAGNOSTIC CRITERIA

- **Must be at least 18 years old** (must have history by 15 years of age consistent with **Conduct disorder**).

At least 3 of the following:

- **Failure to conform to social norms** with **disregard & violation of the rights of others or committing unlawful acts.**
- Irritability or aggressive towards others (eg, **assaults**).
- Exploiting others for personal gain (eg, lying, manipulating, or deceitful acts).
- Recklessness & disregard for the safety of self or others (eg, **drunk driving common**). Impulsivity.
- Lack of remorse for actions.
- Irresponsibility or failure to maintain work or honor financial obligations.

MANAGEMENT

- Psychotherapy: **establishing limits.** Otherwise, psychotherapy & pharmacotherapy generally ineffective. Avoid medications with abusive potential.

BORDERLINE PERSONALITY DISORDER

- **Unstable, unpredictable mood & affect. UNSTABLE SELF-IMAGE & RELATIONSHIPS.**
- Most commonly seen in women.

DIAGNOSTIC CRITERIA

Think of the B's for Borderline:
- "**B**at" - mood swings
- '**B**lack & white thinking': thinks in extremes "all good" or "bad" - no middle ground (splitting).
- **B**lown up (intense) reaction disproportionate to the event.
- **B**roken: unstable relationships
- **B**reaking up - fear of abandonment
- **B**ad behavior: impulsivity in self-damaging behaviors: suicide, self-mutilation, substance abuse, reckless driving, binge eating, spending. Bad sense of self.

MANAGEMENT
- Behavioral therapy: eg, cognitive, dialectical

HISTRIONIC PERSONALITY DISORDER

Think of the H's for Histrionic:
- **Hey look at me – attention-seeking** with the need to be the center of attention, overly emotional, dramatic, seductive.
- **Hissy fits –** temper tantrums, self-absorbed.
- Come **Hither –** often inappropriate, sexually provocative, seductive.
- **Hype me up** – seeks reassurance & praise often. Can be easily influenced by others.
- **Hyperinflated** - may believe their relationships are more intimate than they really are.

MANAGEMENT
- Behavioral therapy (eg, cognitive, dialectical).

NARCISSISTIC PERSONALITY DISORDER

- **Grandiose often excessive sense of self-importance, superiority, need for admiration, & lack of empathy.**
- Despite this exaggerated self-importance, they may have a fragile self-esteem (eg, difficulty with aging process etc., loss of power, higher incidence of mid-life crises, & may become depressed when they don't get the recognition they feel they deserve).

CLINICAL MANIFESTATIONS
- Inflated self-image – belief he or she is special, entitled, or requires extra special admiration.
- Preoccupation with fantasies of brilliance, wealth, success etc.
- Takes advantage of or exploit others for self-gain (eg recognition or status). Arrogance.
- Envy of others or belief that others are envious of them.
- **Lacks empathy for others**. May reacts to rejection or criticism with rage.

MANAGEMENT
- **Psychotherapy initial treatment of choice** (cognitive behavioral therapy, individual or group therapy).

CLUSTER C DISORDERS

- **Cluster C:** **ANXIOUS, WORRIED & FEARFUL.**

AVOIDANT PERSONALITY DISORDER

- **Characterized by social inhibition due to an intense fear of rejection, affecting their daily lives.**
- **Timid, shy, & lacks confidence.**

DIAGNOSTIC CRITERIA

- Pattern of hypersensitivity, social inhibition, and feelings of inferiority or inadequacy + at least 4 of the following:
- Unwilling to interact with others unless certain of being liked.
- Avoids occupations that require interpersonal contact due to a fear of rejection & criticism.
- Cautious of interpersonal relationships.
- Inferiority or inadequacy complex.
- Averseness to participate in new activities due to fear of embarrassment
- Preoccupation with being rejected in social situations.

MANAGEMENT

- Psychotherapy: eg, social training, cognitive behavioral, or group therapy.

DEPENDENT PERSONALITY DISORDER

- **Characterized by the inability to assume responsibility, dependent or submissive behavior, fear of being alone, & difficulty making day to day decisions.**

DIAGNOSTIC CRITERIA

- Pattern of excessive need to be taken care of, leading to needy or clingy behavior characterized by at least 5 of the following:
- Need for others to assume responsibilities for most things in life
- Difficulty expressing disagreement for fear or decreased approval.
- Difficulty making day to day decision without external help. Often will not initiate things or may volunteer for unpleasant tasks.
- Feeling of helplessness and intense discomfort when they are alone with a quickness to enter a relationship after one ends.
- Preoccupation with fears of being left to take care of self.
- Goes to extreme lengths to obtain approval of others.

MANAGEMENT

- Psychotherapy: cognitive behavioral therapy social skills training and assertiveness skills treatment of choice.

OBSESSIVE-COMPULSIVE PERSONALITY DISORDER

- **Characterized by preoccupation with order, details, & perfectionism without obsessions or compulsions.**
- Their behavior is **ego-syntonic** (they don't see anything wrong with their behaviors).
- 2 times more common in men.

DIAGNOSTIC CRITERIA
- Preoccupation with order, details, & perfectionism, characterized at least 4 of the following:
- Perfectionism that may make completion of a task difficult or in a timely fashion.
- Preoccupation with rules, lists, minute details, & organization that the primary goal of the activity is lost.
- Hesitance to delegate task to others.
- Extreme devotion to work, morals, and ethics.
- Rigid, stubborn, serious, or restricted affect.
- Inability to discard useless objects

MANAGEMENT
- Psychotherapy: eg, social training, cognitive behavioral or group therapy.
- Pharmacologic: ± Beta blockers for anxiety or SSRIs for depression.

PSYCHOSES

DELUSIONAL DISORDER

- Delusion = fixed belief despite evidence to the contrary.
- **Nonbizarre delusion** = false + plausible but highly unlikely (eg, being poisoned).

CRITERIA
- **At least 1 delusion** lasting **at least 1 month WITHOUT other psychotic symptoms + no significant impairment in function.**
- Apart from the delusion, behavior is not obviously odd or bizarre & there is no significant impairment of function.
- Does not meet the criteria for Schizophrenia.
- Not explained by another disorder, substance, or medication.

MANAGEMENT
- **Atypical (2nd-generation) antipsychotics first-line medical management.**
- Psychotherapy may be additive in some patients (with the exception of group therapy).

PSYCHOTIC DISORDERS

- Disorder of abnormal thinking, behavior, & emotion.

Schizophrenia diagnostic criteria:
- **2 or more of the following symptoms** - positive symptoms, negative symptoms, grossly disorganized or catatonic behavior **for at least 6 months**.

Schizophreniform:
- Symptoms of Schizophrenia but **duration between 1- 6 months.**

Brief psychotic disorder:
- At least 1 psychotic symptom with onset & remission **<1 month.**

Schizoaffective disorder:
- **Schizophrenia + mood disorder** (major depressive or manic episode).

SCHIZOPHRENIA

- **Disorder of abnormal thinking, behavior, & emotion.**
- ~1% of population. Men & women are affected equally but men present earlier (early to mid 20s) compare to late 20s as seen in women. Rarely initially presents before 15 or after 55y.
- Men tend to have more negative symptoms & poorer outcome.
- **Strong genetic predisposition** – 50% concordance among monozygotic twins. 40% risk if both parents have schizophrenia. 12% risk if a first-degree relative is affected.
- Substance use is common – nicotine most common (>50%), alcohol, cannabis, and cocaine.

Better prognosis:
- **Later age at onset, acute onset, positive symptoms,** good social support, female gender, few relapses, good premorbid function, mood symptoms, & no family history of mental illness.

Worse prognosis:
- **Early age of onset, gradual onset, negative symptoms**, poor social support, male gender, many relapses, poor premorbid function.
- Pathophysiology: exact cause is unknown but the **positive symptoms are thought to be due to excess dopamine in the mesolimbic pathway** with negative symptoms due to dopamine imbalance in the mesocortical pathway.

DIAGNOSTIC CRITERIA
- **2 or more of the following symptoms -** positive symptoms (eg, hallucination, delusion, disorganized speech), negative symptoms, grossly disorganized or catatonic behavior **for at least 6 months.**
- **At least 1 must be hallucination, delusion, or disorganized speech** & must manifest for a 1 month period.
- **Must impair function.**
- Symptoms not due to the effects of a substance or medical condition.

HALLUCINATIONS	Sensory perception without physical stimuli
Auditory (Most common type)	Sound or a voice. Voice often in "3rd person" or can be command hallucinations.
Visual	Simple (flashing light) or complex (eg, seeing faces).
Olfactory	Stench or foul smells common.
Tactile	Insects on skin or being touched.
Somatic	Sensation arising from within the body.
Gustatory	Can be a part of persecutory delusions (tasting poison in food).

DELUSIONS	A fixed belief held with strong conviction despite evidence to the contrary
Persecutory	Person or force is interfering with them, observing them or wishes harm to the patient
Reference	Random events take on a personal significance (directed at them).
Control	Some agency takes control of the patient's thoughts, feelings & behaviors.
Grandiose	Unrealistic beliefs in one's powers & abilities.
Nihilism	Exaggerated belief in the futility of everything & catastrophic events.
Erotomania	Believes another person is in love with them.
Jealousy	Somebody is suspected of being unfaithful.
Doubles	Believes a family member or close person has been replaced by an identical double.

Positive symptoms: these symptoms are "added to" normal behavior

- **Hallucinations** (sensory perception without physical stimuli) – **auditory most common,** visual, gustatory, tactile, olfactory, or somatic.
- **Delusions** (firmed, fixed beliefs despite evidence to the contrary) – **persecutory, grandiose,** reference, control, nihilism, erotomania, doubles, & jealousy.
- **Disorganized speech** - thoughts are disconnected & tangential rambling.
- Behavioral disturbances.

Negative symptoms: these symptoms "take away" from normal behavior. **6 As** –

- **Absence of normal cognition** - impairment in attention, working memory, & executive function.
- **Affect flattening** – poor eye contact, unchanging facial expression, little change in affect, little spontaneous movement, lack of vocal inflections.
- **Alogia** - poverty of speech, increased latency of response.
- **Avolition** (lack of will) - poor hygiene & grooming, anergy, failure of appropriate role responsibilities.
- **Anhedonia** – lack of interest in stimulating activities, intimacy, or sex.
- **Asociality** - failure to engage with others socially, socially withdrawn.

Not part of diagnostic criteria but findings asked on exams:
Neuroimaging:

- CT scan – **ventricular enlargement** (lateral & third) as well as **decreased cortical volume** & grey matter.
- PET scan – hypoactive frontal lobes, hyperactivity in the basal ganglion.

MANAGEMENT OF SCHIZOPHRENIA

- **Second-generation (atypical) antipsychotics first-line management – Risperidone,** Olanzapine, Quetiapine, Ziprasidone, Aripiprazole, & Lurasidone.
  Mechanism of action: Dopamine antagonists (D4 > D2) & Serotonin 5-HT2 antagonists. Lower risk of extrapyramidal adverse effects but increased risk of metabolic adverse effects. **Clozapine is not used first-line but is the most effective medication for treatment-resistant psychosis** (eg, after 2 medications have been tried). Medications should be tried for at least 4 weeks before efficacy is determined.
- First-generation (typical) antipsychotics: (eg, **Haloperidol,** Droperidol, Fluphenazine, Chlorpromazine, Perphenazine, & Thioridazine). Most effective drugs for positive symptoms. Minimal effect on negative symptoms but **increased risk of extrapyramidal symptoms, tardive dyskinesia, & neuroleptic malignant syndrome**.
- Behavioral therapy & family therapy.
- Long-acting IM versions of Risperidone, Fluphenazine, Paliperidone, Aripiprazole, or Haloperidol can be used in patients who don't take their oral medications regularly.
- Lithium.

ACUTE PSYCHOSIS

- Emergency: (eg, extremely agitated psychotic) - **Haloperidol,** Risperidone, or Paliperidone can be used.
- **Hospitalize patient.**
- Urine toxicology to rule out substance abuse, CBC, chem-7, LFTs, ECG (baseline QTc interval), & fasting glucose.
- Emergency: (eg, extremely agitated psychotic) – intramuscular Ziprasidone, Olanzapine, or Aripiprazole may be used. IM Haloperidol may be used, but has more adverse effects.

ANTIPSYCHOTIC	SPECIFIC FACTS
Risperidone	• One of the most commonly agents prescribed for Schizophrenia. • Long acting injectable form. **Greater incidence of movement disorders**.
Quetiapine	• **Lower incidence of movement disorders (extrapyramidal symptoms).**
Olanzapine	• **Higher incidence of weight gain & Diabetes mellitus.** • Olanzapine & Clozapine have the highest risk of metabolic abnormalities.
Clozapine	• Not first-line due to **increased risk of agranulocytosis & myocarditis.** • **Best drug for medication-refractory Schizophrenia.** • Decreased incidence of suicide.
Ziprasidone	• **Higher risk of prolonged QT interval.** • **Less likely to cause significant weight gain**. Must be taken with food.
Aripiprazole	• Unique mechanism – partial dopamine (D2) agonism. • **Less potential for weight gain**, less sedation but increased akathisia.
Lurasidone	• Safer for use in pregnancy. Must be taken with food. • Can be used in Bipolar depression

ADVERSE EFFECTS OF ANTIPSYCHOTICS

Extrapyramidal symptoms (EPS): due to dopamine blockade in the nigrostriatal pathway.

- **Acute Dystonia** – spasms or sustained contractions of the neck or face (eg, trismus, protrusions of the tongue, facial grimacing, torticollis, & difficulty speaking). Usually occurs hours – days after initiating medication. Acute management: Diphenhydramine or Benztropine.
- Akathisia: feeling of restlessness. Management: reduction of the dose or switch medications. Beta-blockers (eg, Propranolol) first-line medical management, Benztropine, or Benzodiazepines.
- **Parkinsonism**: tremor, rigidity, & bradykinesia.
- **Tardive dyskinesia – repetitive involuntary movements mostly involving the face (eg, lip smacking, teeth grinding, & rolling of the tongue).** Seen with **long-term** use **(especially first-generation).**

Other adverse effects

- **Increased prolactin** (dopamine blockade in the tuberoinfundibular pathway) – more common with first-generation.
- **Metabolic**: hyperlipidemia, weight gain, hyperglycemia, & increased abdominal fat. **More common with second-generation.** Aripiprazole & Ziprasidone least associated with metabolic changes.

- **Neuroleptic malignant syndrome: altered mental status, "lead-pipe" muscle rigidity, autonomic instability** (tachycardia, tachypnea, hyperthermia, fever, blood pressure changes, hypersalivation, & diaphoresis), **incontinence**, **leukocytosis** & rhabdomyolysis (increased CPK, LDH, & LFTs).
    - Management: prompt discontinuation of medication most important. Supportive care (cooling blankets, IV fluids). Dopamine agonists (eg, Bromocriptine or Amantadine). Dantrolene for rigidity & fever may be needed.

- **QT prolongation,** arrhythmias, & seizures. Rash.

- Anti-HAM effects - **antiHistamine, antiadrenergic, & antiMuscarinic (anticholinergic) effects.** More common with first-generation.

- Anticholinergic effects: dry mouth, dry eyes, blurred vision, urinary retention, constipation, & hyperthermia.
- Antihistaminic effects: sedation, weight gain.
- Anti-alpha 1 adrenergic: orthostatic hypotension, sexual dysfunction, & cardiac abnormalities.

TRAUMA & STRESSOR-RELATED DISORDERS

POSTTRAUMATIC STRESS DISORDER (PTSD)

DIAGNOSTIC CRITERIA

- **Exposure** to actual or threatened death, serious injury or sexual violence via 1) direct experience of the traumatic event, 2) witnessing the event in person, 3) learning the event happened to someone close (family member or friend) or 4) experiencing extreme or repeated exposure to aversive details of the traumatic event (eg, first responders collecting human remains during 9/11, war, rape, natural disasters).
- **Traumatic event occurred anytime in the past.**
- **Presence of at least 1 of the following intrusion symptoms** after the event that may lead to significant distress or impairment in function (eg, occupational, social or other areas).
- **Re-experiencing: >1 month** as **repetitive recollections** (eg, distressing dreams) & **dissociative reactions** (eg, flashbacks in which the person feels/acts as if the event is recurring), leading to physiologic distress &/or physiologic reactions.
- **Avoidance** of stimuli associated with the traumatic event (reminders of the events).
- **At least 2 negative alterations in cognition & mood**: inability to remember an important aspect of the event, dissociative amnesia, negative feelings of self, world or others, anhedonia, negative emotions (eg, horror guilt, anger or shame), feelings of detachment or inability to experience positive emotions.
- **At least 2 arousal & reactivity symptoms:** angry outbursts, irritable behavior, reckless or self-destructive behaviors, hypervigilance, sleep disturbances, concentration issues, & exaggerated startle response.

MANAGEMENT

- **SSRIs first-line medical treatment** (eg, Paroxetine, Sertraline, Fluoxetine). Tricyclic antidepressants (eg, Imipramine). MAO inhibitors. May be augmented with atypical antipsychotics.
- **Trazodone may be helpful for insomnia.**
- **Cognitive behavioral therapy:** psychotherapy including individual or group counseling. Relaxation techniques.
- Prazosin may be used for nightmares and hypervigilance.

ACUTE STRESS DISORDER

DIAGNOSTIC CRITERIA

- Symptoms similar to PTSD except the **traumatic event occurred < 1 month ago and the symptoms last < 1 month.**
- The symptoms include intrusive symptoms, avoidance, increased arousal, and negative alterations in thought and mood.

MANAGEMENT:

- **Counseling & psychotherapy first-line** because by definition the symptoms will resolve in 1 month.
- If symptoms > 1 month, treat as PTSD.

- **EXAM TIP**
- Posttraumatic stress disorder (PTSD) and Acute stress disorder (ASD) have the same symptoms. The difference is time of event & duration of symptoms.
- **ASD: trauma occurs < 1 month + symptoms < 1 month in duration**
- **PTSD: trauma occurred at any time in the past + symptoms > 1 month**

ADJUSTMENT DISORDER

- **Maladaptive emotional or behavioral reaction to an identifiable stressor** (eg, job loss, physical illness, leaving home, divorce, etc.) or a non-life threatening event that causes a **disproportionate response** than would normally be expected **within 3 months of the stressor** (does not include bereavement) & **usually resolves within 6 months** of the stressor.

CLINICAL MANIFESTATIONS
- One or both of the following - marked distress out of proportion to the severity of stressor and/or significant impairment in areas of functioning (eg, occupational, social, etc.).
- May manifest as depressed mood, anxiety, or disturbance of conduct.

MANAGEMENT
- **Psychotherapy initial management of choice** (including individual or group therapy).
- Medications may be used in selected cases but they are not the preferred treatment.
- Patients may self-medicate with alcohol or other drugs.

SOMATIC SYMPTOM & RELATED DISORDERS

ILLNESS ANXIETY DISORDER (Formerly HYPOCHONDRIASIS)

- **Preoccupation with having or acquiring a serious illness** despite constant reassurance and medical workups showing no disease.
- Formerly known as *Hypochondriasis.*
- The patient exhibits high level of concern & anxiety about their health.
- Care seeking type: frequently gets tested, "doctor shop".
- Care avoidance may be seen.
- Age of onset usually 20-30 years of age.

DIAGNOSTIC CRITERIA
- **Preoccupation causes the patient to perform excessive health-related behaviors or may develop maladaptive behaviors.**
- **Preoccupation or behaviors must last at least 6 months.**
- Somatic symptoms are usually not present. If they are present, they are mild in intensity.
- Not explained by another disorder (eg, Somatic symptom disorder).

MANAGEMENT
- **Regularly-scheduled appointments with their medical provider** for continued reassurance.
- Psychotherapy: eg, **cognitive behavioral therapy**.
- Comorbid anxiety & depressive disorders should be treated with SSRIs or other antidepressants.

MALINGERING

- **Intentional falsification or exaggeration** of signs & symptoms of a medical or psychiatric illness for **external (secondary) gain** – eg, financial gain (insurance money, lawsuits), food, shelter, avoidance of prison, school, work, military services, to obtain drugs (eg, narcotics).
- Malingering is NOT a mental illness.
- Both factitious disorder and malingering are associated with intentionally faking signs and symptoms. The difference is that in malingering, they feign illness for secondary gain whereas in Factitious disorder the primary motive is to 'assume the sick role' & get sympathy.

FUNCTIONAL NEUROLOGICAL SYMPTOM DISORDER (CONVERSION DISORDER)

- Formerly known as **Conversion disorder** (patients "convert" their psychological distress into neurological symptoms).
- 2-3 times more common in women. Often preceded by a traumatic event.
- May have comorbid depressive, anxiety, or neurological disorder.

DIAGNOSTIC CRITERIA

- **At least 1 symptom of neurologic dysfunction (voluntary motor or sensory)** that **cannot be explained clinically** & not explained by another medical or psychiatric condition.
- Patients are often calm or seem unconcerned about the deficits.
- Symptoms are NOT intentionally produced or feigned.
- **Motor dysfunction:** **paralysis**, aphonia, **mutism**, seizures, gait abnormalities, involuntary movements, tics, weakness, swallowing, globus sensation (lump in throat).
- **Sensory dysfunction:** **blindness,** anesthesia, paresthesias, visual changes, & deafness.
- Causes significant distress and/or impairment in function (social, occupational etc.).

MANAGEMENT

- **Patient education** about the illness first-line treatment.
- Cognitive behavioral therapy with or without physical therapy if education not successful.

FACTITIOUS DISORDER

- **Intentional** falsification or exaggeration of signs & symptoms of medical or psychiatric illness for **"primary gain" (inner need to be seen as ill or injured)** but **NOT for external rewards** (aka secondary gain, as seen in Malingering).
- **Factitious disorder imposed on self –** presents themselves as injured, impaired, or ill.
- **Factitious disorder imposed on another** - presents another as injured, impaired, or ill (eg, child, elder or mentally disabled family member). Considered a form of premeditated child or elder abuse.

CLINICAL MANIFESTATIONS

- **Intentional creation or exaggeration of symptoms of illness** - eg, may hurt themselves to bring on symptoms, alter diagnostic tests, lie, or mimic symptoms. May inject themselves with substances to make themselves sick, etc. Medical history may be dramatic but inconsistent.
- May be **willing or eager to undergo surgery repeatedly or painful tests** in order to **obtain sympathy**. They may "hospital jump", use other aliases, or go to different cities to access care. They often have extensive knowledge about medical terminology, hospitals, or great detail about their "illness" (may even work in healthcare).

DIAGNOSTIC CRITERIA

- **Intentional falsification or exaggeration** of signs & symptoms of a medical or psychiatric illness for **"primary gain"** (motivation of their actions is to **assume the sick role to get sympathy**).
- Induction of an injury or disease with intent to deceive. The deceptive behavior is evident even in the absence of obvious external rewards (as seen in Malingering).
- Presentation of the individual or another individual (imposed on another).
- Behavior is not explained by another psychiatric disorder (eg, Delusional disorder).

MANAGEMENT

- Nonspecific treatment eg, collect information from medical providers & family members to avoid unnecessary procedures. May require confrontation in a non-threatening manner. When confronted, patients often leave against medical advice.
- Child or adult protective services if imposed on another.

SOMATIC SYMPTOM DISORDER (Formerly Somatization Disorder)

- Chronic condition in which the patient has **physical symptoms involving at least 1 body system but no physical cause found on workup.**
- **Excessive thoughts, feelings, or behaviors** related to the somatic symptoms - disproportionate & persistent thoughts about the seriousness of the symptoms, persistently high level of anxiety about symptoms or health, or excessive time & energy devoted to the symptoms & health concerns.
- They frequently seek treatment from many medical providers, resulting in extensive lab work, diagnostic procedures, and/or surgeries.
- May or may not be associated with other medical condition.

RISK FACTORS

- Most common in **young women** (10:1) with onset usually before 30 years age, older age, unemployment, history of sexual abuse, & lower socioeconomic status.

DIAGNOSTIC CRITERIA

- **1 or more vague physical symptoms that are distressing or result in significant disruption of daily life.** These symptoms cannot be explained by a physical or medical cause. At least 2 symptoms increase the likelihood of somatization disorder.

MNEMONIC	SYMPTOM	SYSTEM
Symptoms	Shortness of breath	Respiratory
Described as	Dysmenorrhea	Reproductive
Body	Burning in sexual organ	Psychosexual
Laments &	Lump in throat (dysphagia)	Pseudo neurological
Ailments	Amnesia	Pseudo neurological
Void a	Vomiting	GI
Physical cause	Painful extremities	Skeletal muscle

- Although any one of the somatic symptoms may not be continuously present, the state of being symptomatic is persistent (usually **> 6 months**).
- Specifiers: **with predominant pain** (previously pain disorder in DSM IV) & Persistent.

MANAGEMENT

- **Regularly scheduled visits to a healthcare provider.**
- Psychotherapy (source of the symptoms are psychological). Patients may be reticent to seek mental health counseling (they truly believe there is an organic cause).

- **Exam tip:**
- These 5 disorders seem similar so look for these clues to differentiate them:
- Somatic symptom disorder: physical symptoms (at least 1 body system) with no cause on workup + no intentional falsification (they believe they are ill).
- Functional neurologic disorder: neurologic symptoms or deficits (sensory or motor) with no cause on workup + no intentional falsification (they believe they are ill).
- Illness anxiety: preoccupation one has an undiagnosed serious illness + no intentional falsification (they believe they are ill).
- Factitious disorder: intentional falsification of symptoms for primary gain (assuming the sick role or sympathy).
- Malingering: intentional falsification of symptoms for secondary (external) gain (eg, money, shelter, etc.).

DRUG ABUSE/DEPENDENCE

TOBACCO USE/DEPENDENCE

- Smoking is the most important modifiable risk factor in the US for preventable pulmonary, cardiac, and cancer deaths.
- Smoking cessation should be discussed with all smokers at every clinical contact.

NICOTINE WITHDRAWAL

- Symptoms include restlessness, anxiety, irritability, sleep abnormalities, headaches, depression, increased appetite, weight gain, chest tightness, and nicotine craving.

MANAGEMENT OF DEPENDENCE

- Includes counseling and support therapy, cognitive behavioral therapy.
- Relapse after abstinence is common.
- **Nicotine tapering therapy:** gum, nasal sprays, transdermal patches, inhaler & lozenges.
- **Bupropion:** antidepressant drug often used in combination with nicotine tapering therapy. Mechanism: Dopamine & norepinephrine reuptake inhibitor that reduces nicotine cravings and withdrawal symptoms.
- **Varenicline:** blocks the nicotine receptors, reducing nicotine activity. Partial agonist that mimics the effects of nicotine, reducing the reward effect and preventing withdrawal symptoms. Therapy should begin 1 week prior to quit date and continued 4 months after quit date. Adverse effects: headache, nausea, insomnia, **increased suicidality** or neuropsychiatric conditions.

BUPROPION

Mechanism of action:

- **Antidepressant** drug often used in combination with nicotine tapering therapy. Dopamine & norepinephrine reuptake inhibitor that reduces nicotine cravings and withdrawal symptoms.

Indications:

- Aid in **smoking cessation** (can be combined with nicotine therapy to increase success rates).
- Therapy should begin 1-2 weeks prior to quit date and continued for 4-6 months after quit date.

Adverse effects:

- **Seizures** (lowers seizure threshold), dry mouth, insomnia, weight loss, hypertension, & headache.
- Increased anxiety & agitation.
- Increased risk of Psychosis at high doses.
- Avoid abrupt withdrawal.

Contraindications:

- **Epilepsy or conditions with increased seizure risk (eg, eating disorders such as Bulimia & Anorexia nervosa** or patients undergoing abrupt discontinuation of alcohol, benzodiazepine, barbiturate, or antiepileptic medications).
- **Avoid in patients with recent MAO inhibitor use.**

Caution:

- Hypertension & cardiovascular disease.

OPIOID USE/DEPENDENCE

OPIOID USE & DEPENDENCE

Heroin, Oxycodone, Hydrocodone, Codeine, Morphine, Dextromethorphan, Meperidine, & Methadone

OPIOID INTOXICATION:

- **Euphoria & sedation:** drowsiness, impaired social functioning, impaired memory, slow or slurred speech. May develop nausea, vomiting, seizures, & coma.

- **Physical examination findings:** **pupillary constriction** (narcotics are miotics), **altered mental status & respiratory depression.** May also develop Biot's breathing (groups of quick, shallow inspirations followed by regular or irregular periods of apnea), **bradycardia, hypotension,** nausea, vomiting, flushing. Patients on long-term narcotics may develop constipation (opioid receptors in the GI tract reduce GI motility), hypothermia.

OPIOID WITHDRAWAL

- Lacrimation, hypertension, pruritus, tachycardia, nausea, vomiting, abdominal cramps, diarrhea, sweating, yawning, **piloerections** (goose bumps), **pupil dilation (mydriasis), flu-like symptoms: rhinorrhea,** joint pains, myalgias. Withdrawal is often unpleasant but is not life threatening.

MANAGEMENT

- **Opioid intoxication:** **Naloxone is an opioid antagonist** used in acute intoxication or overdose to acutely reverse the effects of opioids. Onset of action ~2 minutes IV (~5 minutes IM). ~30-60 minutes duration of action. Most commonly used in patients with respiratory depression.

- **Opioid withdrawal:** symptomatic control: Clonidine (decreases sympathetic symptoms), Loperamide for diarrhea, Dicyclomine for abdominal cramps, & NSAIDs for joint pains & muscle cramps. Benzodiazepines may be helpful in some cases of mild withdrawal. Severe symptoms can be treated with detox with Methadone or Buprenorphine + Naloxone.

- Long-term management of dependence: Methadone maintenance program. Suboxone (Buprenorphine + Naloxone), or Naltrexone.

OPIOID DEPENDENCE MANAGEMENT

Methadone

- Mechanism of action: long-acting opioid receptor agonist used in the control withdrawal from opioid in patients with opioid addiction. Can be used in pregnant opioid-dependent women. Given orally.

- Adverse effects: can cause prolonged QT interval.

Buprenorphine

- Mechanism of action: partial opioid receptor agonist. Suboxone is a combination of Buprenorphine + Naloxone (Naloxone prevents intoxication from IV injection).

Naltrexone

- Mechanism of action: competitive opioid antagonist. Precipitates withdrawal if used within 7 days of heroin use. Oral or monthly depot injection.

ALCOHOL WITHDRAWAL

Uncomplicated alcohol withdrawal:
- Onset: 6 – 36 hours after last drink (time may vary).
- Clinical manifestations: **increased CNS activity** - tremors, anxiety, irritability, diaphoresis, palpitations, hypertension, insomnia, & GI (nausea, vomiting, diarrhea).
- Uncomplicated = no seizures, hallucinosis or delirium tremens.

Withdrawal seizures:
- Onset: 6 – 48 hours after last drink. Usually generalized tonic-clonic type.
- Most commonly occurs as a single brief episode.

Alcoholic hallucinosis:
- Onset: 12 – 48 hours after last drink.
- Clinical manifestations: visual auditory and/or tactile **hallucinations.** Patient has a **clear sensorium & normal vital signs.**

Delirium tremens:
- Onset: 2 – 5 days after last drink.
- Clinical manifestations: **delirium (altered sensorium),** hallucinations, agitation. **Abnormal vital signs** (eg, tachycardia, hypertension, fever). Patients often diaphoretic.

MANAGEMENT
- Requires medical treatment & hospitalization. **Alcohol withdrawal can be fatal.**
- **IV Benzodiazepines: Diazepam**, **Lorazepam**, Chlordiazepoxide, & Oxazepam.
  - Mechanism: **potentiates GABA-mediated CNS inhibition.** Alcohol mimics GABA at the receptor sites (GABA is the most abundant inhibitory neurotransmitter in the CNS) so ETOH withdrawal causes increased CNS activity. Benzodiazepines are titrated until the patient is slightly somnolent & then gradually tapered.
- Lorazepam or Oxazepam preferred in patients with advanced cirrhosis or alcoholic hepatitis (Chlordiazepoxide may cause over titration in these patients).
- **IV fluids, IV thiamine (B1), magnesium, multivitamins** (including B12 & folate), & electrolyte repletion.

ALCOHOL DEPENDENCE

- Alcohol abuse becomes dependence when withdrawal symptoms develop or tolerance.

CAGE ALCOHOL SCREENING

≥2 considered a positive screen.

Cutdown	Have you felt the need to cut down on drinking?
Annoyed	Have people told you that they were annoyed at you when you drink?
Guilt	Have you ever felt guilty about your drinking?
Eye opener	Have you ever needed an eye opener to start your day or reduce jitteriness?

MANAGEMENT
- Supportive: psychotherapy: eg, individual, group (eg, Alcoholics Anonymous); Inpatient & residential rehabilitation programs.
- **Disulfiram (Antabuse)** can be a deterrent to alcohol use.
  MOA: inhibits aldehyde dehydrogenase (enzyme needed to metabolize alcohol), leading to increased acetaldehyde when coupled with alcohol intake ⇨ uncomfortable symptoms including: hypotension, palpitations, flushing, hyperventilation, dizziness, nausea, vomiting, & headache.
  CI: cardiovascular disease, diabetes mellitus, hypothyroidism, epilepsy, kidney or liver disease.
- **Naltrexone:** opioid antagonist that reduces alcohol craving & reduces alcohol-induced euphoria.
- Gabapentin, Topiramate.

COCAINE INTOXICATION AND WITHDRAWAL

COCAINE INTOXICATION

- Mechanism: produces a stimulant effect via inhibition of the reuptake of dopamine, norepinephrine, and epinephrine in the synaptic cleft.

- Dopamine plays a role in the "reward" system of the brain.

INTOXICATION

- **Elevated or euphoric mood,** psychomotor agitation, and pressured speech.

- May progress to nausea, vomiting, & seizures.

- Physical examination: findings include sympathetic hyperactivity - increased motor activity, tremor, flushing, hyperthermia, cold sweats, & pupillary dilation. May develop hypertension or hypotension, & tachycardia or bradycardia.

SEVERE INTOXICATION

- Respiratory depression, arrhythmias, hypertension, seizures, repetitive behaviors (eg, picking at skin), agitation, aggression, hallucinations, and paranoia.

- Deadly complications include myocardial infarction, stroke, or intracranial hemorrhage.

MANAGEMENT

- Mild: reassurance and **Benzodiazepines.**

- Severe or psychosis: antipsychotics (eg, Haloperidol), treatment of arrhythmias. Do not place in restraints (may lead to Rhabdomyolysis).

- **Cardiovascular effects: Benzodiazepines are first-line** because most of the cardiovascular effects are centrally mediated via the sympathetic system. Phentolamine can reduce the blood pressure but may cause tachycardia. Nitroglycerin or nitroprusside may be used. If a beta-blocker is used, a mixed alpha-1/beta blocker (eg, Labetalol) is preferred over the other beta blockers.

- Hyperthermia: cooling blankets and possibly ice baths.

COCAINE WITHDRAWAL

- Characterized by craving with resultant dysphoria, **post-intoxication depression,** anhedonia, **hypersomnia,** increased appetite, constricted pupils.
- Patients may develop nightmares, **suicide ideation**, headache, and increased irritability.

MANAGEMENT

- Mainly symptomatic.
- Hospitalization may be required for severe psychiatric symptoms.

PCP INTOXICATION

MECHANISM:

- Phencyclidine (PCP) is a dissociative, anesthetic, hallucinogenic drug that is a NMDA glutamate receptor antagonist "angel dust".
- PCP also activates the dopaminergic neurons.
- It can cause CNS stimulant or depressive effects.
- Short onset of action with a brief duration (1-4 hours).

CLINICAL MANIFESTATIONS:

- Impulsiveness, fear, homicidality, **rage,** psychosis, delirium, psychomotor agitation, **hallucinations, multidirectional nystagmus,** ataxia, tachycardia, erythematous and dry skin.
- In severe cases, it may be associated with hyperthermia, seizures.

MANAGEMENT

- **Supportive care** (eg, airway, breathing and circulation monitoring, placement in a low stimulus environment).
- **Benzodiazepines are the first line agent for chemical sedation if agitated**, hyperthermic, & for PCP-induced hypertension & seizures.
- Antipsychotics (eg, Haloperidol) if psychotic.
- Physical restraints may be required in some cases of severe agitation.

MARIJUANA INTOXICATION & WITHDRAWAL

MECHANISM

- Binds to CB1 & CB2 cannabinoid receptors.

CLINICAL MANIFESTATIONS

- Euphoria, giddiness, anxiety, disinhibition, intensification of sensory experiences, **dry (cotton) mouth, increased appetite,** and motor impairment.
- Some patients may experience fear and depression.
- Psychosis may occur.
- Chronic use can lead to cognitive performance issues.

PHYSICAL EXAMINATION

- Conjunctivitis, tachycardia, and hypotension.

MANAGEMENT

- Treatment is usually not needed. Symptomatic management if needed.

HYPEREMESIS SYNDROME

- Chronic severe emesis in chronic users.
- Managed with cessation of marijuana use and antiemetics (Ondansetron & Metoclopramide).

WITHDRAWAL

- Irritability, insomnia, depression, restlessness, diaphoresis, diarrhea, and twitching.

	INTOXICATION		WITHDRAWAL	
	BEHAVIORAL/MOOD EFFECTS	PSYCHOLOGICAL EFFECTS	ONSET	SYMPTOMS
ETHANOL BENZODIAZEPINES	Disinhibition ***Depression:*** slurred speech, impaired judgment & somnolence. Ataxia. Labile Mood: erratic behavior, aggression ***Flumazenil used to treat benzodiazepine intoxication****	Prolonged reaction time, muscular incoordination, facial flushing **Chronic:** - **Wernicke's encephalopathy**: triad of ataxia, confusion & oculomotor palsy (due to thiamine/B1 deficiency). - **Korsakoff syndrome** amnesia (both retrograde & antegrade) - Hepatomegaly, palmar erythema, cirrhosis, Dupuytrens contractures, gynecomastia, testicular atrophy. - Increased mean corpuscular volume	6-24 hours 6 – 48 hours 2 – 5 days	***Increased CNS activity* tremor,*** insomnia, nausea, vomiting, anxiety, tachycardia, hypertension, increased respirations Seizures, hyperreflexia ***DELIRIUM TREMENS: altered sensorium:*** tactile, visual or auditory hallucinations (ex. ***formication – "something crawling" on them) especially at night,*** altered mental status, seizures, coma, death. ***Often occurs when hospitalized for a nonrelated illness.***
STIMULANTS COCAINE AMPHETAMINES	• **Initial:** elevated/euphoric mood, restlessness, pressured speech • **Psychosis:** mild ⇨ anxiety. Paranoia, ***aggression, agitation,*** hallucinations (Ex. tactile, auditory) • ***Treat cocaine intoxication with benzodiazepines,*** neuroleptics & blood pressure reduction.	• **Neurologic:** ↑motor activity, headache, tremor, flushing, hyperthermia, cold sweats, nausea, vomiting, seizures • ***SYMPATHETIC STIMULATION:*** sweating, tachycardia, ***hypertension, pupillary dilation*,*** peripheral vasoconstriction, myocardial infarction. • Compulsive & stereotyped behavior (ex. picking at skin), rhabdomyolysis.	Varied onset	Craving with resultant dysphoria, agitation, anxiety, diaphoresis, ***hypersomnia, increased appetite.*** **Neurologic:** nightmares, ***suicide ideation*,*** headache, irritability, extreme fatigue, muscle cramps.
OPIOIDS & NARCOTICS	• **Euphoria & sedation:** ***drowsiness,*** impaired social functioning, impaired memory, slow or slurred speech. ***Naloxone (Narcan) used to treat opioid intoxication****	• ***Pupillary constriction**** *(narcotics are miotics).* • ***Respiratory depression,* bradycardia, hypotension,*** coma, nausea, vomiting, hypothermia. • Chronic: pruritus & constipation (opioid receptors in GI tract decreases motility).	6-24 hours (Methadone may take longer)	Neurologic: psychomotor agitation, anxiety, irritability, twitching, yawning dysphoria, insomnia, diaphoresis Vitals: hyperthermia, hypertension, tachycardia Flulike sx: ***rhinorrhea*,*** myalgias, chills, ***piloerections**** (Goosebumps). GI: nausea, vomiting, diarrhea Ocular: ***pupillary dilation*, tearing***
NICOTINE	• Nausea, vomiting, diarrhea, abdominal pain, headache	Tremor, tachycardia, salivation	Usually begin within 24h after last use	Psychomotor: anxiety, restlessness, bradycardia, increased appetite & craving
CANNABIS	• Euphoria, giddiness. • Psychosis in some cases.	Dry mouth (cotton-mouth), conjunctival erythema, tachycardia, hypotension	Usually on seen with heavy usage	Irritability insomnia, restlessness, diaphoresis, diarrhea, twitches.
PCP	• Impulsiveness, homicidality, psychosis, delirium, seizures, ***nystagmus***			Depression, irritability, anxiety, sleep problems
LSD	• Visual hallucinations & synesthesias (seeing sound as color), delusions, pupillary dilation			

GRIEF REACTION

- Altered emotional state as a response to a major loss (eg, death of a loved one).
- Only persistent complex bereavement disorder is considered a mental disorder.
- 5 stages of grief: denial, anger, bargaining, depression, & acceptance.

Normal grief:

- **Usually resolves within 6 months to 1 year.**
- It peaks usually within the first couple of months after the loss. Usually characterized by intense emotions, appetite or sleep disturbances.
- Symptoms may include illusions or hallucinations of the deceased that the patient understands is not real.
- Patients are usually able to function.

Abnormal grief:

- **Severe symptoms, symptoms > 1 year or positive suicidal ideation,** psychosis, illusions or hallucinations that the patient perceives are real.

Persistent complex bereavement disorder:

- Severe grief reactions that persist > 1 year (or 6 months in children) after the death of the bereaved.

MANAGEMENT:

- Psychotherapy.
- Short course of Benzodiazepines may be needed for insomnia in some.

PANCE PREP PEARL OF THE WEEK

NEUROLEPTIC MALIGNANT SYNDROME

•Rare but potentially deadly **complication of Antipsychotics (Dopamine antagonists)** especially 1st generation (typical) antipsychotics

•Most commonly seen in young males early in the treatment.

Fever (most common presenting symptom) + **ALTERED** mental status

Autonomic instability - tachycardia, tachypnea, hyperthermia, fever, blood pressure changes, hypersalivation, diaphoresis & **incontinence**.

Lead-pipe muscle rigidity – almost universal.

Tremor

Elevated WBC (leukocytosis) & CPK (rhabdomyolysis)

Regular-sized pupils (distinguishes it from mydriasis in Serotonin syndrome)

Excessive sweating (diaphoresis)

Delirium (altered mental status changes), **Decreased DTR** (hypOreflexia)

•**Management: Prompt discontinuation of medication most important. Supportive care** (cooling blankets, IV fluids). **Dopamine agonists (eg, Bromocriptine or Amantadine). Dantrolene** for rigidity & fever.

NARCOLEPSY

- Long-term neurological disorder characterized by decreased ability to regulate sleep-wake cycles.
- Elements of sleep interfere with wakefulness and elements of wakefulness interferes with sleep.
- Typically presents initially in the teens and early twenties.

CLINICAL MANIFESTATIONS

- **Chronic daytime sleepiness:** patients are prone to fall asleep throughout the day and develop sleep attacks (rapid dozing off without warning), often at inappropriate times.
- **Cataplexy:** emotionally-triggered transient weakness of the muscles (eg, excitement, laughter, anger). The weakness often begins in the face (eg, slack, ptosis, hypotonic face with an open mouth) and often affects the neck and knees. Patients may develop bilateral weakness or paralysis.
- **Hypnagogic hallucinations:** vivid visual, tactile, or auditory hallucinations occurring as the patient is falling asleep.
- **Sleep paralysis:** complete inability to move for 1-2 minutes immediately after waking or before falling asleep.
- May also develop other sleeping disorders (eg, fragmented sleep, obstructive sleep apnea, restless leg syndrome, sleepwalking, REM sleep behavior disorder).

WORKUP

- Thorough medical history, history and physical examination, sleep history, and neurologic examination. Workup usually includes both polysomnography and multiple sleep latency testing.
- **Polysomnography:** excludes alternative and/or coexisting causes of daytime sleepiness.
  Narcolepsy: spontaneous awakenings, mild reduced sleep efficiency, increased light non-REM sleep, REM sleep within 15 minutes after the onset of sleep (healthy individuals usually experience REM sleep 80-100 minutes after the onset of sleep).

- **Multiple sleep latency test:** identifies the sleep onset rapid eye movements and measure the mean sleep latency. The patient is placed in a sleep-inducing environment and instructed to try to fall asleep.
  - On average, healthy patients fall asleep within 10-15 minutes.
  - Narcolepsy: often fall asleep < 8 minutes. The naps usually include **sleep onset rapid eye movements.**
  - Prior to testing, patients should discontinue antidepressants 3 weeks prior (4 weeks for Fluoxetine) and stimulants or psychoactive medications should be stopped 1 week prior.

MANAGEMENT

- **Modafinil: first-line medical management** (improves control of sleepiness, promotes wakefulness early into the evening).
  - Mechanism: exact mechanism unknown but thought to inhibit dopamine reuptake, increasing dopaminergic signaling.
  - Adverse effects: headache, dry mouth, diarrhea, decreased appetite, nausea, increased blood pressure (used cautiously in patients with arrhythmia history or heart disease).
- Solriamfetol: a reasonable alternative first-line agent.
  - Mechanism: oral selective dopamine and norepinephrine reuptake inhibitor, improving wakefulness. Similar adverse effects to Modafinil.

Cataplexy

- REM-suppressing medications: eg, Fluoxetine, Venlafaxine, Atomoxetine. Sodium oxybate alternative.

CHAPTER 12 – DERMATOLOGIC SYSTEM

ACNEIFORM LESIONS

ACNE VULGARIS

- Inflammatory skin condition associated with papules and pustules involving the pilosebaceous units.
- Pathophysiology: 4 main factors – follicular hyperkeratinization, increased sebum production, *Propionibacterium acne* overgrowth, & and inflammatory response.

CLINICAL MANIFESTATIONS

- Commonly seen in areas with increased sebaceous glands (eg, face, back, chest, upper arms).
- Comedones: small, noninflammatory bumps from clogged pores.
  Open comedones (blackheads) - incomplete blockage.
  Closed comedones (whiteheads) - complete blockage.

- **Inflammatory:** papules or pustules surrounded by inflammation.

- **Nodular or cystic acne:** often heals with scarring.

DIAGNOSIS

- **Mild:** comedones, small amounts of papules &/or pustules.
- **Moderate:** comedones, larger amounts of papules &/or pustules.
- **Severe:** nodular (> 5 mm) or cystic acne.

MANAGEMENT

- Mild: **topical - azelaic acid, salicylic acid, benzoyl peroxide, retinoids. Tretinoin or topical antibiotics** (eg, Clindamycin or Erythromycin).

- Moderate: as above + **oral antibiotics** (eg, **Minocycline or Doxycycline**). Spironolactone.

- Severe (refractory nodular acne): **oral Isotretinoin**

ISOTRETINOIN

Mechanism of action:

- Affects all 4 of the pathophysiologic mechanisms of acne (**most effective medication for Acne vulgaris**).

Indications:

- Usually reserved for severe or refractory acne.

Adverse effects:

- **Dry skin and lips (most common),** dry eyes.
- **Highly teratogenic** - must obtain at least 2 pregnancy tests prior to initiation of treatment & monthly while on treatment, must commit to 2 forms of contraception (used at least 1 month prior to initiation & 1 month after it is discontinued).
- **Increased triglycerides & cholesterol,** arthralgias, myalgias, hepatitis, leukopenia, & premature long bone closure.
- Photosensitivity, worsening of Diabetes mellitus, headache, idiopathic intracranial hypertension, fatigue, & possible psychiatric effects.
- Due to the severe risk of teratogenesis, prescribers and patients in the US must sign up for iPledge.

ROSACEA

- Chronic acneiform skin condition.
- Face most commonly involved. Most common in women age 30-50 years.
- Etiology: unclear etiology: persistent vasomotor instability, capillary vasodilation, and abnormal pilosebaceous activity.

TRIGGERS:
- **Alcohol, hot or cold weather, hot drinks, hot baths, spicy foods, sun exposure,** & medications.

CLINICAL MANIFESTATIONS
- **Acne-like rash (papulopustules) + centrofacial erythema, facial flushing, telangiectasias, skin coarsening with burning, & stinging.** Red eyes.

PHYSICAL EXAMINATION
- **Absence of comedones (blackheads)** in Rosacea distinguishes it from acne.
- **Rhinophyma** (red, enlarged nose). Cutaneous edema.

DIAGNOSIS
- Usually clinical.
- Biopsy definitive (rarely needed).

MANAGEMENT
- Lifestyle modifications: sunscreen, avoid irritants (eg, toners, astringents, menthols, camphor).
- Mild-moderate: **topical Metronidazole first-line for papulopustules,** Azelaic acid, Ivermectin cream. Sulfacetamide, anti-acne topical antibiotics.
- Moderate-severe: oral antibiotics (eg, Tetracyclines), Laser therapy.
- Oral Isotretinoin may be used in refractory cases.
- **Facial erythema: topical Brimonidine**, Laser or intense pulsed light.

FOLLICULITIS

- **Superficial hair follicle infection** or inflammation.
- Risk factors: more common in men, prolonged use of antibiotics, topical corticosteroids

ETIOLOGIES
- ***Staphylococcus aureus* most common.**
- Other gram-positive & gram negatives and fungi.
- *Pseudomonas aeruginosa* is the most common cause of hot tub-related Folliculitis.

CLINICAL MANIFESTATIONS:
- Singular or clusters of **perifollicular papules and/or pustules** with surrounding erythema on hair bearing skin. Often pruritic.

MANAGEMENT (MILD):
- **Topical Mupirocin**, Clindamycin, Erythromycin, or Benzoyl peroxide.

SEVERE OR REFRACTORY:
- Oral antibiotics: Cephalexin or Dicloxacillin.

GRAM-NEGATIVE:
- Daily acetic acid or topical Benzoyl peroxide (usually resolves without treatment).

ERYTHEMA MULTIFORME

- **Type IV hypersensitivity reaction of the skin** often following infections or medication exposure.
- Most common in young adults 20-40 years.

RISK FACTORS

- **Herpes simplex virus most common, *Mycoplasma* spp** (especially in children), *S. pneumoniae.*
- Medications: **sulfa drugs, beta-lactams, Phenytoin, Phenobarbital,** Allopurinol, etc.
- Malignancy, autoimmune, & idiopathic.

CLINICAL MANIFESTATIONS

- Characterized by **target lesions** consisting of three components: **a dusky, central area or blister,** a dark red inflammatory zone **surrounded by a pale ring of edema, and an erythematous halo on the extreme periphery** of the lesion. Most common on the extremities & trunk.
- **Negative Nikolsky sign** (no epidermal detachment). Often febrile.
- **Minor:** target lesions distributed acrally with **no mucosal membrane involvement.**
- **Major:** target lesions acrally progressing centrally + **mucosal membrane involvement** (oral, genital, or ocular). **No epidermal detachment.**

DIAGNOSIS: Usually clinical. Biopsy may be performed if the diagnosis is not clear.

MANAGEMENT

- **Symptomatic:** discontinue offending drug, antihistamines, analgesics, skin care. Corticosteroid + Lidocaine + Diphenhydramine mouthwash for oral lesions.
- Systemic corticosteroids if severe. Antibiotics if Mycoplasma-related; Oral Acyclovir if HSV-related.

STEVENS-JOHNSON SYNDROME (SJS) & TOXIC EPIDERMAL NECROLYSIS (TEN)

- Stevens-Johnson syndrome (SJS) & Toxic epidermal necrolysis (TEN) are **severe mucocutaneous reactions** characterized by **detachment of the epidermis & extensive necrosis.**
- **SJS:** sloughing involving **<10%** of the body surface involvement. **TEN:** **> 30%** body surface area.

RISK FACTORS

- **Medications most common cause,** especially **sulfa drugs & anticonvulsants & Lamotrigine, Allopurinol,** NSAIDs, antipsychotics, & antibiotics.
- Infections less common (eg, *Mycoplasma pneumoniae,* HIV, HSV). Malignancy, idiopathic.

CLINICAL MANIFESTATIONS

- Prodrome of fever & URI symptoms followed by **widespread flaccid bullae** beginning on the trunk & face.
- Pruritic targetoid lesions **(erythematous macules with purpuric centers)** or diffuse erythema with involvement of at least **1 mucous membrane** + involvement **with epidermal detachment (positive Nikolsky sign).**
- The skin is often tender to touch. The lesions start on the face & thorax before spreading to other areas (palms and soles rarely involved).
- Ocular involvement common (corneal ulceration or uveitis). Pulmonary (bronchitis, pneumonitis).

DIAGNOSIS: Clinical. Biopsy: full thickness skin necrosis.

MANAGEMENT

- **Prompt discontinuation of causative agent.**
- **Supportive therapy:** treat like severe burns - burn unit admission, pain control, prompt withdrawal of offending medications, fluid & electrolyte replacement, wound care (eg, gauze, petroleum).

DISORDERS OF THE HAIR AND NAILS

ALOPECIA AREATA

- **Nonscarring immune-mediated hair loss** targeting the anagen hair follicles, (scalp most common).
- Commonly **associated with other autoimmune disorders** (eg, thyroid, Addison's disease, SLE).

CLINICAL MANIFESTATIONS
- **Smooth, discrete, circular patches of complete hair loss** that develop over a period of weeks (painless and not pruritic).

PHYSICAL EXAMINATION
- **Exclamation point hairs** - short hairs broken off a few mm from the scalp with tapering near the proximal hair shaft (exclamation point appearance!) at the margins of the patches. In some cases, hair loss may be diffuse. Hair regrowth may occur (fine white hair regrowth). No erythema, inflammation, or scarring seen.
- **Nail abnormalities**: pitting ~30%, nail fissuring, trachyonychia (roughening of the nail plate), etc.

DIAGNOSIS
- Mainly a clinical diagnosis. Punch biopsy: definitive diagnosis - peribulbar lymphocytic inflammatory infiltrates surrounding the follicles.

MANAGEMENT
- Local: **intralesional corticosteroids**. May be observed in mild cases.
- Extensive: topical corticosteroids.

Prognosis:
- May spontaneously resolve or progress to alopecia totalis (complete scalp hair loss) or alopecia universalis (complete hair loss on the scalp & body – including the eyelashes). Relapse is common.

ANDROGENETIC ALOPECIA

- Genetically predetermined progressive loss of the terminal hairs on the scalp in a characteristic distribution (pattern).
- Most common type of hair loss in men & women. Gradual in onset & usually occurs after puberty.

PATHOPHYSIOLOGY
- **Dihydrotestosterone (DHT) is the key androgen leading to Androgenetic alopecia.** Activation of the androgen receptor shortens the anagen (growth phase) in the normal hair growth cycle.
- Pathologic specimens show decreased anagen to telogen ratio.

CLINICAL MANIFESTATIONS
- Varying degrees of hair thinning & nonscarring hair loss. In males, it begins as bitemporal thinning of the frontal scalp then involves the vertex. In women, it is seen as thinning of the hair between the frontal and vertex of the scalp without affecting the frontal hairline.

DIAGNOSIS: **usually clinical.** Dermoscopy – miniaturized hair and brown perihilar casts.

MEDICAL MANAGEMENT
- **Topical Minoxidil:** best used if recent onset alopecia involving a smaller area. Requires a 4-6 month trial before noticing improvement and must be used indefinitely. Mechanism: widens blood vessels, allowing more blood oxygen and nutrients to promote the anagen (growth) phase. Adverse effects: pruritus & local irritation with flaking.
- **Oral Finasteride**: **5-alpha reductase type 2 inhibitor** - androgen inhibitor (inhibits the conversion of testosterone to dihydrotestosterone). Adverse effects: decreased libido, sexual or ejaculatory dysfunction. Increased risk of high-grade prostate cancer. Category X.
- Hair transplant is effective (if the patient has a sufficient number of donor plugs).

ONYCHOMYCOSIS

- Nail infections caused by fungi.

ETIOLOGIES

- Dermatophytes – Trichophyton & Epidermophyton genera (***T. rubrum*** **most common).** *Candida albicans* (more likely to affect fingernails) & nondermatophyte molds.

RISK FACTORS

- Increasing age, tinea pedis (including close contacts), psoriasis, occlusive shoes, & immunodeficiency.

CLINICAL MANIFESTATIONS

- Nail that is opaque, thickened, discolored and/or cracked. Subungual hyperkeratinization.
- 3 variants: distal lateral, superficial white, and proximal.

- Occurs most common on the great toe.

DIAGNOSIS

- Because only 50% of dystrophic nails are due to fungal infection, **confirmation of fungal infection is essential prior to treatment.** Fungal culture + a rapid test (KOH or PAS).

- KOH wet mount prep: only 60% sensitive. Rapid.

- **Periodic acid-Schiff test most sensitive test** (performed on nail plate clippings). Rapid.

- Fungal cultures: very specific, not sensitive, takes week to get the results but useful to determine the causative organism.

MANAGEMENT

- Management can be initiated if KOH or PAS is positive while waiting for cultures.

- **Systemic antifungals: most effective treatment. Terbinafine first-line for dermatophytes.** Itraconazole for both dermatophytes & Candida.
  - Systemic antifungals associated with **hepatotoxicity & drug-drug interactions.**
  - Contraindications include alcohol use & Hepatitis.

- Topical antifungals: Efinaconazole or Tavaborole. Option in if oral agents are contraindicated or not desired.

PARONYCHIA

- Infection of the lateral & proximal nail folds < 6 weeks.

ETIOLOGIES
- ***Staphylococcus aureus* most common** (especially if rapid), Group A Streptococcus.
- Oral flora if associated with nail biting.
- *Candida* species associated with Chronic paronychia.

PATHOPHYSIOLOGY
- Most commonly occurs after penetrating skin trauma (eg, dishwashing, biting nails, cuticle damage during manicures, ingrown nails).

CLINICAL MANIFESTATIONS
- **Painful, red swollen area around the proximal or lateral nail folds at the cuticle.**
- May have purulent discharge.

MANAGEMENT
Paronychia without abscess:
- Mild: **warm water or antiseptic soaks** 10-15 minutes followed by topical antibiotics (eg, triple antibiotics or Mupirocin).
- Moderate: oral antibiotics – **Cephalexin or Dicloxacillin** are first-line oral therapy.
- Amoxicillin-clavulanic acid or Clindamycin if associated with nail biting.

MRSA:
- Trimethoprim-sulfamethoxazole, Clindamycin, or Doxycycline.

Paronychia with abscess:
- Incision and drainage.

FELON

- **Closed-space infection of the fingertip pulp space** (a Paronychia can progress to a Felon).

ETIOLOGIES
- ***Staphylococcus aureus* most common** (especially if rapid), Group A streptococcus.

PATHOPHYSIOLOGY
- Most commonly occurs after penetrating skin trauma (eg, biting nails, cuticle damage, splinters etc.).
- An abscess develops in the small fingertip pulp compartments.

CLINICAL MANIFESTATIONS
- Severe throbbing **pain, erythema, swelling, and fluctuance to the pad of the fingertip.**

MANAGEMENT
- Fluctuant: **incision and drainage** (single volar longitudinal or high lateral incision).

- Early without fluctuance: elevation, warm water or saline soaks, & oral antibiotics (eg, Cephalexin or anti-staphylococcal Penicillin).

BROWN RECLUSE SPIDER BITE

- Most common in the Southwestern & Midwestern US.
- Brown recluse spiders (*Loxosceles reclusa*) may have a **violin pattern** on its anterior cephalothorax.

PATHOPHYSIOLOGY

- Venom is **cytotoxic & hemolytic** - local symptoms, can be **necrotic**, and associated with lack of severe systemic symptoms.

CLINICAL MANIFESTATIONS

- **Local effects:** local burning & erythema at the bite site for 3-4 hours followed by blanching of the affected area (due to vasoconstriction) followed by an erythematous margin around the ischemic center **"red halo"** for 24-72h followed by a **hemorrhagic bulla that undergoes eschar formation.** 10% may develop skin necrosis.
- Systemic effects: some may develop fever, chills, nausea, vomiting, or a morbilliform rash.

MANAGEMENT

- **Local wound care & pain control the mainstay of management.**
- **Local wound care:** clean the affected area with soap & water, apply cold packs to the bite site (avoid freezing the tissue). If possible, keep the affected body part in elevated or neutral position. **Most wounds heal spontaneously** within days to weeks.
- **Pain control:** NSAIDs (or opioids if more severe). Tetanus prophylaxis if needed.
- Dermal necrosis: debridement (if needed) should be delayed until the lesion is demarcated and clinically stable. In some cases, it may lead to better wound healing. Dapsone has been used in the past.
- Antibiotics only if a secondary infection develops (treat like Cellulitis).

BLACK WIDOW SPIDER BITE

PATHOPHYSIOLOGY

- Black widow spider (*Latrodectus Hesperus*) produces a **neurotoxin.**
- Characteristic **red hourglass shape** on the underside of its belly.

RISK FACTORS

- Outdoor activities, gardening, sleeping outside, etc.

CLINICAL MANIFESTATIONS

- Latrodectism: **local symptoms:** pain at the bite site with the onset of **systemic & neurologic symptoms within 30 minutes to 2 hours - muscle pain (most prominent feature), spasms, & rigidity.** Muscle pain most commonly affects the extremities, back, & abdomen.
- **Usually self-limited** with resolution within 1-3 days.

PHYSICAL EXAM:

- Classic appearance of bite is a **blanched circular patch with a surrounding red perimeter and central punctum (target lesion).**

MANAGEMENT

- Mild: **wound care & pain control** - gently clean the area with mild soap & water. NSAIDs, opioids.
- Moderate to severe: **muscle relaxants** (eg, Benzodiazepines, Methocarbamol).
- Antivenom reserved for patients not responsive to the above medications. Antivenom is not always readily available and if given, usually given after a consult with a toxicologist.

EXANTHEMS

ERYTHEMA INFECTIOSUM

- Also known as **Fifth disease**. Most common in children < 10 years of age.

ETIOLOGY

- Caused by **Parvovirus B19**. Parvovirus B19 infects and destroys reticulocytes, leading to a decrease or transient halt in erythropoiesis (this can lead to Aplastic crisis).
- Transmission: respiratory droplets. 4-14 day incubation period.

CLINICAL MANIFESTATIONS

- Nonspecific viral symptoms (eg, coryza, fever, malaise) followed by **erythematous malar rash with a "slapped cheek"** appearance & **circumoral pallor** for 2-4 days. The malar rash is followed by **lacy, reticular maculopapular rash on the extremities** (especially upper) that usually spares the palms and soles, resolving in 2-3 weeks.
- **Arthropathy or arthralgias in older children & adults.**
- Associated with **increased fetal loss during pregnancy** (hydrops fetalis, CHF, spontaneous abortion).
- **Parvovirus may cause Aplastic crisis in patients with Sickle cell disease** or G6PD deficiency.

DIAGNOSIS: usually clinical. Serologies (eg, Parvovirus-specific IgM).

MANAGEMENT

- Supportive: anti-inflammatories (Acetaminophen or NSAIDs). Self-limited disease.

RUBEOLA (MEASLES)

- Caused by the **Measles virus, part of the Paramyxovirus family.**
- Transmission: respiratory droplets, person to person, airborne. ~6-21 day incubation period.

CLINICAL MANIFESTATIONS

- URI prodrome malaise, anorexia **high fever + 3 Cs (cough, coryza, conjunctivitis)** followed by Koplik spots.
- **Koplik spots: small 1-3 mm pale white or blue papules with an erythematous base on the buccal mucosa** opposite the second molars (pathognomonic). Koplik spots precede the rash by 48 hours.
- Exanthem: **morbilliform (maculopapular), brick-red rash beginning at the hairline,** spreading cephalocaudally and centrifugally that darkens and coalesces. **Rash usually lasts 7 days.**
- Lymphadenopathy, pharyngitis.

DIAGNOSIS

- Primarily a clinical diagnosis. IgM antimeasles antibodies.
- PCR of viral ribonucleic acid from throat, nasopharyngeal, or urine samples

MANAGEMENT

- **Supportive mainstay of treatment** (eg, Acetaminophen, Ibuprofen), oral hydration.
- Vitamin A reduces morbidity & mortality in children with Rubeola.
- Measles immune globulin (for individuals at high risk for complications).

COMPLICATIONS

- **Diarrhea most common.** Otitis media, Conjunctivitis, & Encephalitis.
- **Pneumonia most common cause of Measles-related deaths.**

HAND, FOOT, AND MOUTH DISEASE

- Primarily caused by **Coxsackie virus (especially type A).** Coxsackie virus is an Enterovirus that is part of the Picornavirus family.
- Most common in children < 5 years of age.
- Transmission: primarily fecal-oral and oral-oral.
- **Most common in summer & early fall.**

CLINICAL MANIFESTATIONS
- Mild fever, URI symptoms, & decreased appetite starting 3-5 days after exposure.
- **Oral enanthem:** erythematous macules that become **painful oral vesicles surrounded by a thin halo of erythema** that undergo ulceration (especially seen on the buccal mucosa & the tongue). Followed by exanthem.

- **Exanthem:** greyish-yellow vesicular, macular or maculopapular lesions on the distal extremities (often including the palms and soles). Less commonly, vesicles may be seen on the torso and face. The exanthem is not usually painful nor pruritic.

DIAGNOSIS
- Mainly a clinical diagnosis
- Coxsackievirus-specific immunoglobulin A. Viral culture.

MANAGEMENT
- Supportive: antipyretics (eg, Acetaminophen, Ibuprofen), hydration, topical Lidocaine.
- Complications include Aseptic meningitis & Guillain-Barré syndrome.

HERPANGINA

- Primarily caused by **Coxsackie virus, especially type A** (A1-A6, A8, A10). Coxsackie virus is an Enterovirus that is part of the Picornavirus family.
- Most common in children 3-10 years of age.
- Most common in summer & early fall.

CLINICAL MANIFESTATIONS
- Sudden onset of high fever, **stomatitis – small yellow-white papulovesicular lesions on the posterior pharynx (soft palate, uvula, & tonsillar pillars) that ulcerate** before healing (small, yellow or white ulcers with red rims). Anorexia due to pain common. Pharyngitis, odynophagia.

- In older children, may be accompanied with malaise, headache, vomiting, neck stiffness, or back stiffness.

DIAGNOSIS
- Mainly a clinical diagnosis
- Coxsackievirus-specific immunoglobulin A. Viral culture.

MANAGEMENT
- **Supportive: self-limited** - antipyretics (eg, Acetaminophen, Ibuprofen), oral hydration.

- Complications include Aseptic meningitis & Guillain-Barré syndrome.

INFECTIOUS DISEASES

CELLULITIS

- Acute spreading infection of the deeper dermis & subcutaneous tissues.
- Bacterial entry usually occurs after a break in the skin, such as underlying skin problems (eg, Impetigo, Tinea), trauma (eg, bites, wounds, pressure ulcers), and surgical wounds.

ETIOLOGIES
- **Most commonly caused by Group A *Streptococci.***
- ***Staphylococcus aureus*** is an important but less common cause.

CLINICAL MANIFESTATIONS
- **Localized macular erythema** (flat margins **not sharply demarcated**), swelling, warmth, and tenderness.
- Systemic symptoms not common – fever, chills, regional lymphadenopathy, myalgias, vesicles, bullae hemorrhage. May develop lymphangitis (streaking).

DIAGNOSIS: primarily a clinical diagnosis.

MANAGEMENT
- Oral antibiotics: **Cephalexin, Dicloxacillin.** Clindamycin or Erythromycin if penicillin-allergic.
- IV antibiotics: **Cefazolin**, Ampicillin-sulbactam, Ceftriaxone, & Clindamycin.
- **Cat bite (*Pasteurella multocida*): Amoxicillin-clavulanate;** Doxycycline if PCN allergic.
- Dog or human bite: Amoxicillin-clavulanate. Clindamycin + either Ciprofloxacin or Trimethoprim-sulfamethoxazole.

MRSA:
- Oral: **Clindamycin, Doxycycline. Trimethoprim-sulfamethoxazole** (good for Staph but doesn't cover Streptococcus).
- IV: **Vancomycin** or Linezolid.

ERYSIPELAS

- Variant of Cellulitis involving the upper dermis and cutaneous lymphatics.

ETIOLOGIES
- **Group A *Streptococcus* (*S. pyogenes*) most common.** *S. aureus.*

CLINICAL MANIFESTATIONS
- **Intensely erythematous, raised area with sharply demarcated borders**, tenderness, & warmth.
- **Most commonly involves the lower extremities, face** or skin with impaired lymphatic drainage. Ear involvement (Milian sign).
- Unlike Cellulitis, often associated with systemic manifestations (eg, fever, chills, & leukocytosis).

DIAGNOSIS
- Clinical. Ultrasound with Gram stain and culture of expressed fluid if underlying abscess.

MANAGEMENT
- Oral: **Penicillin, Amoxicillin, Cephalexin.** In patients with Penicillin allergy Clindamycin, Trimethoprim-sulfamethoxazole, or Linezolid can be used.
- IV: **IV Cefazolin, Ceftriaxone**, or Flucloxacillin may be required if systemic symptoms are present.
- MRSA: Vancomycin (if PCN-allergic or MRSA is suspected).

LYMPHANGITIS

- Inflammation of the lymphatic channels due to infectious or noninfectious causes.
- It can be a complication of a distal infection that gains access to the lymphatic vessels, spreading towards regional lymph nodes.

CLINICAL MANIFESTATIONS

- **Red, tender streaks extending proximally** from the site of Cellulitis.
- **May involve regional lymph nodes** (lymphadenitis) or systemic symptoms (eg, fever & chills).

MANAGEMENT

- Based on the underlying cause. If it is a complication of Cellulitis, it can be treated like Cellulitis.

MANAGEMENT ASSOCIATED WITH CELLULITIS

- Oral: **Cephalexin, Dicloxacillin.** Clindamycin or Erythromycin if penicillin-allergic.
- IV: **Cefazolin**, Ampicillin-sulbactam, Ceftriaxone + Clindamycin.
- MRSA: oral – **Clindamycin, Doxycycline. Trimethoprim-sulfamethoxazole** (good for Staphylococcus but doesn't cover Streptococcus). **IV – Vancomycin** or Linezolid.

FURUNCLE & CARBUNCLE

- **Furuncle (abscess): deep infection of the hair follicle** (in contrast to folliculitis which is superficial).
- Carbuncle is a coalescence or interconnection of several furuncles into a single mass with purulent drainage from multiple follicles.

ETIOLOGIES:

- ***Staphylococcus aureus* most common.** Streptococcus 2nd most common.

CLINICAL MANIFESTATIONS:

- Erythematous, tender, **indurated nodule with fluctuance** (abscess) may have a central plug.
- May be associated with or without surrounding cellulitis.
- Systemic symptoms (eg, fever or chills not common).

MANAGEMENT

- **Incision and drainage mainstay of treatment.**
- Warm moist compresses with a dry covering if not fluctuant or as adjunctive treatment for open and draining abscesses.
- **Antibiotics typically reserved for associated Cellulitis**, severe (eg, associated with fever or chills, rapid progression), recurrent or persistent Furunculosis.

IMPETIGO

- Highly contagious superficial vesiculopustular skin infection.
- Most common bacterial skin infection in children (highest incidence 2-6 years).
- Risk factors: poor personal hygiene, poverty, crowding, warm & humid weather, and skin trauma.

TYPES

- **Nonbullous: most common type.** Impetigo contagiosa: **papules, vesicles, & pustules** with weeping and later **development of "honey-colored, golden crusts."** Occurs typically at sites of superficial skin trauma (eg, insect bite), primarily on exposed surfaces of the **face** & arms. Associated with regional lymphadenopathy. ***Staphylococcus aureus* most common cause.** Group A *Streptococcus* 2nd most common.

- Bullous: vesicles form large bullae (rapidly) with rupture and development of thin "varnish-like crusts." Fever, diarrhea. *Staphylococcal aureus* most common cause. Rare (usually seen in newborns or young children).

- Ecthyma: ulcerative pyoderma caused by Group A *Streptococcus* (heals with scarring). Not common.

DIAGNOSIS

- Usually clinical. Gram stain and wound culture.

MANAGEMENT

- **Mild: Mupirocin topically initial drug of choice** (tid x 10 days). Bacitracin. Retapamulin. Wash the area gently with soap & water. Good skin hygiene.

- Extensive disease or systemic symptoms: **systemic antibiotics - Cephalexin** or Dicloxacillin. Macrolides.

- If community-acquired MRSA: Doxycycline, Clindamycin, or Trimethoprim-Sulfamethoxazole.

COMPLICATIONS

- Cellulitis most common (10%). Acute glomerulonephritis (1-5%).

- Impetigo does not lead to Rheumatic fever.

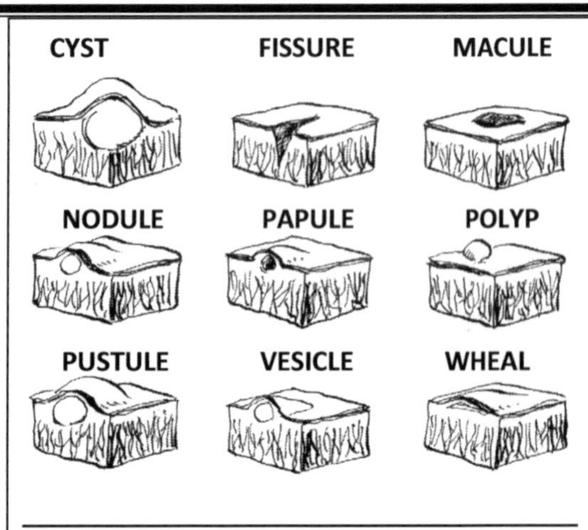

MACULE: flat nonpalpable lesion <10mm.
PATCH: flat nonpalpable lesion >10 mm.

PAPULE: solid, raised lesions <5mm in diameter.
NODULE: solid, raised lesions >5mm in diameter.

PLAQUE: raised, flat-topped lesion >10mm.

VESICLE: circumscribed, elevated fluid-filled lesion <5mm.
BULLA: circumscribed, elevated fluid-filled lesion >5mm.

PUSTULE: pus-filled vesicle or bulla.

WHEAL: transient, elevated lesion (local edema).

PETECHIAE: small punctate hemorrhages that don't blanch.

DERMATOPHYTOSIS

- **Fungal skin infections: Trichophyton,** Microsporum, Epidermophyton.
- Infects keratinized tissues in the stratum corneum of the skin, hair & nails by ingesting keratin.
- Risk Factors: increased skin moisture (eg, occlusive gear), Immunodeficiency (HIV, DM), peripheral vascular disease.

TINEA CAPITIS

- Superficial fungal infection of the scalp. "Ring worm" is a common term.

ETIOLOGIES
- 90% caused by the fungus **Trichophyton** tonsurans in the US. Microsporum.

RISK FACTORS
- Poor hygiene, direct contact, **preadolescents**, more common in African-Americans.

CLINICAL MANIFESTATIONS

The 4 ways Tinea capitis can present are:
- **Patches of alopecia with black dots:** multiple black dots are due to broken hair shafts due to endothrix infection.

- **Scaly patches with alopecia:** single or multiple patches with hair loss. Erythema & pruritus may be present.

- **Kerion:** severe manifestation characterized by an inflammatory plaque with pustules and thick crusting. Often painful.

- Favus: a less common form of tinea capitis characterized by cup-like shaped yellow crusts composed of dried scalp secretions, fungi, skin cells and dead inflammatory cells.

DIAGNOSIS
- Clinical diagnosis

- KOH prep: most common initial test - fungal element inside or surrounding the hair.

- Wood's lamp: no fluorescence with Trichophyton spp. Fluorescence with Microsporum.

- Culture: definitive diagnosis.

MANAGEMENT
- **Oral Griseofulvin: first-line treatment.** Used for 6-12 weeks. **Can cause hepatitis**, GI, headache, & Disulfiram reaction. Griseofulvin better absorbed with fatty food (eg, peanut butter).

- 2nd line: **Oral Terbinafine**. Less common - Itraconazole or Fluconazole.

- Lifestyle: use of antifungal by all house members, avoid sharing hats, clippers, and combs.

TINEA BARBAE: papules, pustules & hair follicles.

TINEA PEDIS

- "Athlete's foot" – most common dermatophyte infection - *Trichophyton rubrum, Trichophyton interdigitale* (formerly *Trichophyton mentagrophytes*), and *Epidermophyton floccosum.*
- Transmission: direct contact (eg, walking barefoot in gyms or swimming pool areas).
- Most common in adolescents and young men.

CLINICAL MANIFESTATIONS

- **Interdigital: most common – pruritic, erythematous erosions or scales between the toes** (may be associated with interdigital fissures). Most common in the third and fourth digital interspaces.
- Hyperkeratotic: diffuse hyperkeratotic rash involving the soles, lateral and medial surfaces of the feet with a "moccasin" distributive pattern.
- Vesiculobullous: pruritic vesicular or bullous eruption with underlying erythema, especially involving the medial surfaces of the foot (may be painful).

DIAGNOSIS

- Clinical diagnosis
- KOH prep: of skin scraping most common initial test - segmented hyphae.
- Wood's lamp: no fluorescence with Trichophyton spp. Fluorescence with Microsporum.
- Culture: definitive diagnosis.

MANAGEMENT

- **Topical antifungals first-line** (eg, Butenafine, Tolnaftate, Ciclopirox, azoles) – 4 week duration. Terbinafine 1% cream x 1 week. Burrow's solution added for Hyperkeratotic lesions.
- PO Terbinafine, Fluconazole or Itraconazole if topical medications are ineffective. Griseofulvin.
- Clean shoes with antifungal spray, keep cool/dry.

TINEA CRURIS

- Superficial **fungal infection** of the groin or inner thighs. AKA "Jock itch".

ETIOLOGIES

- Fungi of the **Trichophyton** genera (***T. rubrum* most common)** or *Epidermophyton floccosum.*

RISK FACTORS

- Males, copious sweating (eg, close contact sports, wearing tight clothing), immunocompromised.
- Tinea pedis may be the source of infection.

CLINICAL MANIFESTATIONS

- **Pruritus hallmark.**
- **Annular patches or plaques, diffuse erythema** to the inner thighs or groin with **sharply demarcated raised border** that may have tiny vesicles. Often spares the scrotum and the mucosa.

DIAGNOSIS

- Clinical diagnosis based on history and physical.
- **KOH prep: best initial diagnostic test** – scrapings from lesion reveals segmented hyphae.
- Fungal cultures definitive diagnosis.

MANAGEMENT

- **Topical antifungals first-line** - **Clotrimazole, Butenafine, Terbinafine**, & Ketoconazole. In addition, use of desiccant powders in the inguinal area with the avoidance of tight-fitting clothing and noncotton underwear. Putting on socks before underwear.
- Oral antifungals: if topical ineffective or extensive – Terbinafine or Griseofulvin.

TINEA CORPORIS:

- Superficial **fungal infection of the body** (trunk, legs, arms, or neck). Does not include the feet, hands, groin, nails, or the scalp.

ETIOLOGIES
- Fungi of the **Trichophyton and Microsporum** genera. ***T. rubrum*** **most common.**

TRANSMISSION
- **Direct contact - common in preadolescents** (eg, wrestlers).
- Infection from other animals (eg, kittens and puppies)
- Infection from another part of the body.

CLINICAL MANIFESTATIONS
- Single or multiple **pruritic**, erythematous, scaly, **circular or oval plaques or patches with central clearing and well-defined raised borders** that spread outwardly. May have pustules.

DIAGNOSIS
- **KOH prep: best initial test** – scrapings from lesion reveals segmented hyphae.
- Culture: definitive diagnosis (slower method).

MANAGEMENT:
- **Topical antifungals first-line:** "azoles" (eg, Clotrimazole, Ketoconazole), Butenafine, Terbinafine, Naftifine, Ciclopirox, and Tolnaftate. Duration is usually 1-3 weeks.
- Oral antifungals: if topical ineffective or extensive – Itraconazole or Terbinafine. Griseofulvin or Fluconazole second-line systemic therapies.

INTERTRIGO

- Inflammatory condition of the **intertriginous areas** (two skin surfaces in close proximity) such as inguinal folds, axilla, intergluteal folds, & inframammary folds.
- ***Candida spp.*** **most common.**

RISK FACTORS
- **Warm moist environment** (eg, **skin folds,** hyperhidrosis, incontinence, **obesity**), **immunocompromised** (eg, **Diabetes mellitus,** HIV), & constrictive clothing.
- Can be a complication of irritant diaper dermatitis.

CLINICAL MANIFESTATIONS: **pruritus.** Pain if maceration occurs.
Physical examination
- **Erythematous "beefy red" macerated plaques** & erosions with peripheral scaling and **erythematous satellite lesions** (papules and pustules).

DIAGNOSIS
- **Usually clinical**. Fungal cultures definitive.
- KOH preparation of skin scrapings – **budding yeast with or without pseudohyphae**.

MANAGEMENT
- **Topical antifungals first-line** (eg Nystatin, Clotrimazole or Ketoconazole). Topical corticosteroids may be adjunctive. Oral antifungals in severe cases.

PREVENTION
- Proper hygiene, keeping intertriginous areas cool and dry. Weight loss.

SCABIES

- A highly contagious skin infection due to the mite ***Sarcoptes scabiei.***

PATHOPHYSIOLOGY

- Female mites **burrow into the skin to lay eggs, feed & defecate** (scybala are the fecal particles that precipitate a hypersensitivity reaction in the skin).

CLINICAL MANIFESTATIONS

- **Intense pruritus especially at night**.
- Infected patients may remain without symptoms for up to 4-6 weeks.

PHYSICAL EXAMINATION

- Multiple, **small erythematous papules, excoriations**.
- **Linear burrows (pathognomonic)** – commonly found in the **intertriginous zones,** including the scalp & **web spaces** between the fingers & toes. Usually spares the neck & face.
- **Red itchy pruritic papules or nodules on the scrotum, glans or penile shaft, or body folds are pathognomonic.**

DIAGNOSIS

- Clinical. Skin scrapings: mites, eggs, and feces seen with magnification.

MANAGEMENT

- **Permethrin topical drug of choice.** Applied topically from the neck down for 8-14 hours before showering. A repeat application after 1 week is recommended. Safe in pregnancy and lactation.
- **Lindane:** cheaper. **DO NOT use after bath/shower (causes seizures** due to increased absorption through open pores). Contraindications: **Teratogenic, not usually used in breastfeeding women & children <2y.**
- 6-10% sulfur in petroleum jelly for pregnant women/infants.
- Ivermectin if extensive.
- **All clothing, bedding etc. should be placed in a plastic bag at least 72 hours then washed & dried using heat.**
- All close contacts should be treated simultaneously as well.

PEDICULOSIS (LICE)

PUBIC LICE

- Pediculosis pubis (also known as phthiriasis pubis).

TRANSMISSION: usually sexually transmitted (especially in teenagers and young adults).

CLINICAL MANIFESTATIONS: **pruritus of the involved area is the chief complaint. Nits may be seen.**

DIAGNOSIS

- Clinical diagnosis (visual of lice or nits). Microscopic examination of hair shafts.

MANAGEMENT

- **Topical Permethrin or Pyrethrins first-line**.
- Treatment repeated after 9-10 days if lice remain.
- Sexual partners should be treated simultaneously.
- Clothing and bedding should be laundered in hot water.

HEAD LICE (*Pediculus humanus capitis*)

- Transmission: person to person. Fomites (hats, headsets, clothing, bedding etc.).
- **Head lice: girls** > boys. Less common in African-Americans.
- Outbreaks commonly affect children 3-12 years old, warmer and & humid weather.

CLINICAL MANIFESTATIONS: **intense itching** (especially occipital area), **papular urticaria near lice bites.**
Physical examination:

- Visualization of crawling nymphs or adult lice. The presence of nits alone does not confirm infestation.
- **Nits:** white, oval-shaped egg capsules at the base of the hair shafts.

MANAGEMENT

- **Permethrin topical drug of choice.** Capitis: Permethrin shampoo left on x10 minutes. **A fine tooth comb should be used to remove the nits.** Pubis/Corporis: Permethrin lotion x at least 8-10 hours. Safe in children at least 2 months of age. Reapplication in 7-10 days recommended to destroy any newly hatched lice. Petroleum jelly can be used in addition to suffocate the lice.
- Malathion is a first-line alternative to Permethrin. It causes paralysis in arthropods (organophosphate cholinesterase inhibitor). Requires 8-12 hour treatment period.
- Benzyl alcohol, Spinosad and topical Ivermectin. Spinosad has ovicidal activity so combing to remove the nits are not necessary.
- **Lindane** adverse effect - **neurotoxic** (headaches, seizures – do not use after shower or a bath). Usually avoided in children.
- Oral Ivermectin can be used in cases that are refractory to topical therapies.

AFTERCARE:

- **Contact items (eg, bedding & clothing) should be laundered in hot water with detergent & dried in hot drier for 20 minutes.** Toys that cannot be washed are placed in air-tight plastic bags x 14 days.
- Avoid sharing contact items. Prophylactic treatment for individuals who share bedding.

BODY LICE (*Pediculus humanus corporis*)

TRANSMISSION

- Usually sexually transmitted.
- Strongly related to poor body hygiene (eg, homeless population, prisons, and crowded unsanitary conditions, natural disasters or refugees from war).

PATHOPHYSIOLOGY

- Unlike head & pubic lice, body lice do not live on the skin.
- Body lice live and lay their eggs in seams of clothing or bedding and move to the skin only to feed.

DISEASE TRANSMISSION

- **Body lice can be a vector for diseases** to humans, such as relapsing fever, epidemic typhus, and trench fever.

CLINICAL MANIFESTATIONS

- **Pruritus** is usually the chief complaint (reaction to the louse saliva) & excoriations.

DIAGNOSIS: clinical - identification of the louse or its nits in clothing, especially in the seams.

MANAGEMENT

- **Hygiene improvement first-line treatment** - bathe thoroughly.
- Infested clothing and bedding should be heat washed, dry cleaned, or discarded.
- Ironing especially in the seams will also destroy lice.
- Permethrin 5% cream (8-10 hour application).

MOLLUSCUM CONTAGIOSUM

- Benign infection with Molluscum contagiosum virus (***poxviridae*** family).

TRANSMISSION
- Highly contagious - direct contact (skin to skin) most common. Fomites.
- Most common in children, sexually active adults, & patients with HIV.

CLINICAL MANIFESTATIONS
- **Single or multiple firm dome-shaped, flesh-colored to pearly-white, waxy papules** 2-5 mm in diameter **with central umbilication.**
- Curd-like material may be expressed from the center if lesion is squeezed.

DIAGNOSIS
- Usually a clinical diagnosis.
- Histology: Henderson-Paterson bodies (keratinocytes containing eosinophilic cytoplasmic inclusion bodies).

MANAGEMENT
- **No treatment needed in most cases** (spontaneous resolution in 3-6 months usually).
- Curettage (rapid resolution) – first-line when therapy is indicated.
- Cryotherapy, Podophyllotoxin. electrodesiccation. Imiquimod.
- Topical retinoids may be needed in severe cases.

COMMON, FLAT, & PLANTAR WARTS

- Caused by **Human papillomavirus infection.**

PATHOPHYSIOLOGY
- HPV infects keratinized skin, causing excessive proliferation & retention of the stratum corneum.
- Types: common (vulgaris), plantar (plantaris), flat (plana).

CLINICAL MANIFESTATIONS
- Common & plantar warts: firm, hyperkeratotic papules between 1-10 mm with red-brown punctations (**thrombosed capillaries are pathognomonic).** Borders may be rounded or irregular. Common on the hands.
- Flat warts: numerous, small, discrete, flesh-colored papules measuring 1-5 mm in diameter & 1-2mm in height. Typically seen on the face, hands & shins.

DIAGNOSIS
- Clinical diagnosis, serologies. Immunofluorescence.
- Histology: koilocytotic squamous cells with hyperplastic hyperkeratosis.

MANAGEMENT
- **Most warts resolve spontaneously within 2 years** if immunocompetent.
- Topical: over the counter salicylic acid & plasters. Podophyllin, 5-fluorouracil.
- Cryotherapy (liquid nitrogen) or electrocautery or Imiquimod.
- Intralesional interferon or bleomycin if other treatments fail.
- Excision is associated with recurrence.

CONDYLOMA ACUMINATA

- Also known as **Condyloma acuminata.** Caused by **Human papillomavirus infection.**

- Complications include squamous cell carcinoma (eg, cervix, anal, penile, vaginal, and vulvar cancers).

CLINICAL MANIFESTATIONS
- Tiny, **painless** papules evolve into **soft, fleshy, cauliflower-like lesions** ranging from skin-colored to pink or red, occurring in clusters in the genital regions & oropharynx.

- Lesions persist for months & may spontaneously resolve, remain unchanged, or grow if not treated.

DIAGNOSIS
- Clinical diagnosis, serologies.
- Acetic acid application: **whitening of the lesion with acetic acid.**

- Histology: koilocytotic squamous cells with hyperplastic hyperkeratosis.

MANAGEMENT
- Treatment depends on location, size & number of warts. ~80% will experience spontaneous resolution of lesions.

- Cryotherapy (liquid nitrogen), trichloroacetic acid. Electrocauterization or surgical excision are effective but can lead to scarring.

- Second-line: topical Podophyllotoxin or Podofilox. Topical Imiquimod or Sinecatechins can be used on external warts. Podophyllotoxin not used for anogenital warts. Laser CO2 vaporization is less effective than other techniques.

VACCINES:
- **Gardasil 9 (preferred):** targets the same as Gardasil (**6, 11, 16, 18**) as well as HPV types 31, 33, 45, 52, & 58.

- Gardasil: quadrivalent HPV vaccine that targets **HPV 6, 11, 16, 18.**

DOSING:
- <15y: 2 doses of HPV vaccine at least 6 months apart.

- 15y or older or immunocompromised: should receive *3 doses over a minimum of 6 months.* Classically administered at day 0, at 2 month & at 6 months. Minimum interval between first 2 doses is 4 weeks, minimum interval between the second & 3rd is 12 weeks.

- HPV vaccine is contraindicated if pregnant or lactating.

KERATOTIC DISORDERS

SEBORRHEIC KERATOSIS

- **Most common benign epidermal skin tumor.**
- Pathophysiology: benign proliferation of immature keratinocytes.
- Most common in fair-skinned elderly with prolonged sun exposure.

CLINICAL MANIFESTATIONS

- Well-demarcated round or oval **velvety warty lesions** with a **greasy or "stuck on" appearance.** Varied possible colors (eg, flesh-colored, grey, brown, & black).

DIAGNOSIS

- Usually clinical.
- Biopsy can be performed if the diagnosis is uncertain. Biopsy reveals well-demarcated proliferation of keratinocytes with characteristic small keratin-filled cysts.

MANAGEMENT

- **No treatment needed – benign (no premalignant potential).**
- Cosmetic or symptomatic management includes cryotherapy (most common treatment used), curettage, electrodesiccation, or laser therapy.

ACTINIC KERATOSIS

- **Most common premalignant skin condition (may progress to Squamous cell carcinoma).**
- Pathophysiology: proliferation of atypical epidermal keratinocytes.
- Risk factors: prolonged sun exposure, lighter skin, increasing age, & males.

CLINICAL MANIFESTATIONS

- **Dry, rough, macules or papules that feel like "sandpaper", often with transparent or yellow scaling.**
- Can range from skin-colored to **erythematous or hyperkeratotic (hyperpigmented) plaques.**
- May have a projection on the skin (cutaneous horn).

DIAGNOSIS

- Clinical: based on inspection & palpation.
- Punch or shave biopsy may be performed to distinguish AK from SCC. Classic findings include **atypical epidermal keratinocytes** & cells with large hyperchromatic pleomorphic nuclei from the basal layer upwards (no invasion into the dermis).
- Lesions that are greater than 1 cm in diameter, indurated, ulcerated, rapidly growing, and lesions that fail to respond to appropriate therapy should be considered for biopsy.

MANAGEMENT

- Avoid sun exposure. Use of sunscreen.
- Localized AK: surgical - **liquid nitrogen cryotherapy most commonly used treatment,** dermabrasion, electrodesiccation & curettage.
- Multiple AK: medical (eg, topical 5-fluorouracil & Imiquimod) – most commonly used in areas with multiple lesions.

NEOPLASMS

SQUAMOUS CELL CARCINOMA

- Malignancy of keratinocytes that invades the dermis or beyond characterized by hyperkeratosis & ulceration.
- **<u>Bowen's disease</u> = squamous cell carcinoma in situ** (has not invaded the dermis).
- 2nd most common skin cancer. **Slow growing** (rarely metastasizes)

<u>RISK FACTORS</u>

- **Sun exposure major risk factor (often preceded by Actinic keratosis). HPV infection**.
- Lighter-skin, Xeroderma pigmentosum, chronic wounds, old scars or burns, & chronic immunosuppression (eg, post-transplant).

<u>CLINICAL MANIFESTATIONS</u>

- **Erythematous, elevated thickened nodule** with adherent **white scaly or crusted, bloody margins**.
- May present as a **nonhealing ulceration or erosion** slowly evolving.
- Most commonly involve the lips, hands, neck, & head.

<u>DIAGNOSIS</u>

- <u>Biopsy</u>: atypical keratinocytes & malignant cells with large, pleomorphic, hyperchromatic nuclei in the epidermis, extending into the dermis. May form nodules with laminated centers ("epithelial/keratinous pearls").

<u>MANAGEMENT</u>

- **Surgical excision with clear margins is the most frequently used treatment.**
- <u>Electrodesiccation & curettage:</u> may be used for small, well-defined superficial lesions in low risk noncritical sites.
- <u>Mohs micrographic surgery</u>: recurrent/aggressive tumors and cosmetically sensitive areas.
- <u>Cryotherapy</u> can be used for small, well-defined, low risk lesions & Bowen's disease.
- <u>Radiation therapy</u> may be a nonsurgical choice in selected patients or as adjuvant therapy.

KAPOSI SARCOMA

- Vascular cancer associated with **Human herpesvirus 8 infection.**
- **Most commonly seen in immunosuppressed patients (eg, HIV** with CD4 count $<100/mm^3$ or post-transplant). Sporadic: older men of Mediterranean origin. Endemic: eastern & southern Africa.
- May affect the skin, lungs, lymph nodes and GI tract. Cutaneous KS most commonly is seen on the lower extremities, face oral mucosa & genitalia.

<u>CLINICAL MANIFESTATIONS</u>

- Painless nonpruritic **macular, papular, nodule(s), plaque-like brown, pink, red or violaceous lesions.**

<u>DIAGNOSIS</u>

- Biopsy – angiogenesis, inflammation and proliferation (whorls of spindle-shaped cells with leukocytic infiltration & neovascularization) & immunohistologic staining.

<u>MANAGEMENT</u>

- **HAART therapy if associated with HIV.**
- Chemotherapy. Radiation therapy for local disease.

MALIGNANT MELANOMA

- A type of cancer developing from the melanocytes most commonly affecting the skin.
- **Most common cause of skin cancer-related death. Aggressive with high malignant potential.** 3% of all skin cancer but 65% of all skin cancer-related deaths.
- Most commonly METS to the regional lymph nodes, skin, liver, lungs, & brain.

RISK FACTORS
- **UV radiation** associated with 80% of cases, blistering sunburns, family history, > 3 burns before the age 20, tanning booth use, large number of nevi.
- Caucasians, light hair/eye color, & Xeroderma pigmentosum.

- Although it is most common on sun exposed areas, it can occur anywhere on the body.

MAJOR SUBTYPES:
- **Superficial spreading: most common type** (70%). May arise de novo or from a pre-existing nevus. Most common on the **trunk in men and legs in women.**

- Nodular: 2nd most common type. May be associated with rapid vertical growth phase.

- Lentigo maligna: most common on face.

- **Acral lentiginous: most common type found in darker-skinned individuals**. May be seen on the palms, soles, & nail beds.

- Desmoplastic: most aggressive type.

CLINICAL MANIFESTATIONS
- **"ABCDE" Asymmetry; Borders: irregular; Color:** variation; **Diameter: usually 6mm or greater, Evolution** (suspect in a lesion with recent or rapid change in appearance).

- Lesions on the upper back, upper arm, neck, & scalp decrease the likelihood of survival.

DIAGNOSIS
- **Full-thickness wide excisional biopsy** + lymph node biopsy.

- *Shave biopsy discouraged.*

MANAGEMENT
- **Complete wide surgical excision** with sentinel lymph node biopsy.
  - > 1 – 2 mm thick, 2 cm of marginal tissue recommended.
  - 2-4 mm thick (T3) – 2cm marginal tissue.

- Adjuvant therapy in some high risk: interferon-alfa, immune therapy (eg, Nivolumab, Ipilimumab), or radiotherapy. Talimogene (modified HSV).

BASAL CELL CARCINOMA

- **Most common type of skin cancer in the US.** Most common cancer in humans.
- **Slow growing: locally invasive but very low incidence of metastasis.**

RISK FACTORS

- Lighter-skinned individuals, prolonged sun exposure, Xeroderma pigmentosum (genetic disorder with inability to repair damage caused by UV light exposure).

CLINICAL MANIFESTATIONS

- Flat firm area with **small, raised, translucent, pearly, or waxy papule with raised, rolled borders & central ulceration** with overlying **telangiectatic vessels.** Often friable **(bleeds easily).**
- Most commonly seen on the **face, nose,** neck, or trunk.

DIAGNOSIS

- **Punch or shave biopsy** - clusters of basaloid cells with a palisade arrangement of the nuclei at the periphery of the clusters.
- Excisional biopsy may also be performed.

SURGICAL MANAGEMENT

- **Mohs micrographic surgery for facial involvement**, difficult cases, high-risk cases, or recurrent cases (best long-term cure rates & tissue sparing benefit).
- Electrodesiccation & curettage used most commonly on non-facial tumors with low risk of recurrence.
- Surgical excision used for tumors with either low or high risk of tumor recurrence. Cryosurgery.

PAPULOSQUAMOUS DISORDERS

PERIORAL DERMATITIS

- Most commonly seen in **young adult women** (20 – 45).

RISK FACTORS

- History of **topical corticosteroid use.**
- Fluorinated toothpaste.

CLINICAL MANIFESTATIONS

- Erythematous grouped papulopustules, which may become confluent into plaques with scales. May have satellite lesions.
- Classically spares the vermillion border.
- Uncommonly, it may affect the periorbital or paranasal skin.

MANAGEMENT

- **Elimination of topical corticosteroids and irritants** (eg, cosmetics and irritating skin care products). Self-limited.
- **Topical Pimecrolimus, Metronidazole, or Erythromycin first line medical therapy.** Topical Azelaic acid.
- Oral: Tetracyclines may be needed if extensive or refractory.

CONTACT DERMATITIS

- Inflammation of the dermis & epidermis from direct contact between a substance & the surface of the skin. Either **irritant or allergic.**
- **Irritant: most common type.** Causes include chemicals (eg, solvents, cleaners, & detergents), alcohols, or creams. Irritant contact diaper dermatitis – prolonged exposure to urine, feces (or harsh detergents from washable diapers). May develop superimposed Candida infection.
- **Allergen: nickel most common worldwide, poison ivy,** oak or sumac; other metals, chemicals (eg, fragrances, glue, hair dyes), detergents, cleaners, acids, prolonged water exposure.

PATHOPHYSIOLOGY
- **Allergic: type IV hypersensitivity reaction** (T cell lymphocyte-mediated – **delayed by days**).
- **Irritant: non-immunologic reaction (immediate)**.

CLINICAL MANIFESTATIONS
- Acute: erythematous papules or vesicles **(may be linear or geometric)**. Often associated with **localized pruritus, stinging, or burning**. May ooze, develop edema, & progress to blisters or bullae.
- Chronic: lichenification fissuring and scales.

DIAGNOSIS
- Mainly a clinical diagnosis.
- **Patch testing** may identify potential allergens to prevent future exposures.
- Histology not usually needed but will show spongiosis (intercellular edema in the epidermis).

MANAGEMENT
- **Identification & avoidance of irritants is the most important aspect of management.**
- **Topical corticosteroids first-line medical treatment** (eg, **ointments**). Oral corticosteroids in severe or extensive reactions.
- Topical calcineurin inhibitors (eg, Tacrolimus or Pimecrolimus) are alternatives.

GENERAL MEASURES:
- Cool saline or astringent compresses, cool baths, skin emollients.
- If oozing or weeping, drying agents (eg, aluminum acetate) can be used.
- Burrow's solution. Itching can be relieved with antihistamines or calamine lotion.

DIAPER RASH

- A type of **irritant contact dermatitis**.
- Most commonly involves areas in contact with the diaper (eg, buttocks, genitalia, upper thighs, and lower abdomen) with sparing of the skin folds. If superimposed *Candida infection* occurs, it involves the skin folds.

ETIOLOGIES: **prolonged exposure to urine & feces** (or harsh detergents from washable diapers).

CLINICAL MANIFESTATIONS
- Acute: erythematous papules. May develop maceration, superficial erosions.
- If severe, may be associated with extensive erythema, painful erosions and nodules.

MANAGEMENT
- **General skin care: first-line treatment.** Frequent diaper changes, barrier of petroleum or zinc oxide, use of disposable diapers, periods of rest without a diaper, and keeping the affected area clean and dry.
- Low-potency corticosteroids & antifungals may be used in severe cases or in *Candida* superinfections.

TOXICODENDRON DERMATITIS

- **Caused by poison ivy** (most common in the east), **poison oak** (west of the Rocky Mountains), and **poison sumac** (in the southeast).

- Urushiol, composed of oleoresins, initiate a type IV hypersensitivity reaction with direct contact with the leaves.

CLINICAL MANIFESTATIONS
- Well-demarcated erythematous papules or vesicles (**may be linear or geometric**). Often associated with **localized pruritus, stinging, or burning** of skin that mat have come in contact with plant parts.

MANAGEMENT
- Symptomatic treatment: cool compresses, oatmeal baths. High-potency topical steroids may decrease itching. Systemic glucocorticoids if extensive.
- Avoided by the use of protective clothing and washing the exposed area with detergent soap as soon as possible.

ACUTE PALMOPLANTAR (DYSHIDROTIC) ECZEMA

- Recurrent pruritic vesicular rash affecting the palms and/or soles.

- Most common onset is < 40 years of age.

TRIGGERS
- Sweating, emotional stress, warm & humid weather, metals (eg, nickel).

CLINICAL MANIFESTATIONS
- **Pruritic "tapioca-like" small tense vesicles on the soles, palms & fingers** (eg, lateral digits).

- Later **desquamation**, papules, scaling, lichenification, and erosions may occur.

- Bullae may occur if severe.

MANAGEMENT
- **Topical corticosteroid ointments preferred** (medium-high potency). Usually spontaneously resolves over several weeks.

- Oral corticosteroids for severe cases.

- Topical psoralen + ultraviolet A therapy for frequent episodes not controlled with corticosteroids.

GENERAL MEASURES
- Cold compresses, aluminum subacetate (Burrow's solution) or with hazel for weeping wet skin.

- Avoidance of triggers or irritants.

- Use of lukewarm water & soap-free cleansers to wash hands, drying hands after washing, applying emollients immediately after hand drying, & using cotton gloves under nonlatex gloves when performing wet work (eg washing dishes).

LICHEN PLANUS

- Acute or chronic inflammatory dermatitis (cell-mediated immune response).

INCREASED INCIDENCE
- **Hepatitis C,** drug reactions, graft vs host, & malignant lymphoma.
- Most commonly in adults.

CLINICAL MANIFESTATIONS
- Pruritic rash most common on the extremities, especially the volar surfaces of the wrist and the ankles.
- May involve the mouth, scalp, genitals, nails, & mucous membranes.

PHYSICAL EXAMINATION
- **6 Ps: purple, polygonal, planar, pruritic, papules or plaques with fine scales** & irregular borders that may have **Wickham striae** (fine white lines on the skin lesions or on the oral mucosa).
- May also develop **Koebner's phenomenon** - new lesions at sites of trauma (also seen in Psoriasis).
- Nail dystrophy. May cause scarring Alopecia.

DIAGNOSIS
- Primarily a clinical diagnosis.
- Biopsy & immunofluorescence is confirmatory - saw-tooth lymphocyte infiltrate at the dermal epidermal junction.

MANAGEMENT
- **Topical corticosteroids first line** with occlusive dressings. Antihistamines for pruritus.
- Second-line: PO or intralesional corticosteroids, topical Tretinoin or photosensitizing Psoralen + ultraviolet light therapy (generalized eruptions).
- The rash usually resolves spontaneously in 8-12 months.

LICHEN SIMPLEX CHRONICUS (NEURODERMATITIS)

- **Skin thickening in patients with Atopic dermatitis** secondary to **repetitive rubbing & scratching** - "itch-scratch" cycle.

CLINICAL MANIFESTATIONS
- Scaly, well-demarcated, rough hyperkeratotic plaques **with exaggerated skin lines.**

MANAGEMENT
- **Avoid scratching the lesions, topical corticosteroids** (high-strength), antihistamines, & occlusive dressings.

ATOPIC DERMATITIS (ECZEMA)

- Rash due to **defective skin barrier susceptible to drying, leading to pruritus & inflammation.**
- **Atopic triad: eczema + allergic rhinitis + asthma**.
- Pathophysiology: disruption of the skin barrier (filaggrin gene mutation) and disordered immune response. Most manifest in infancy and almost always by age 5.
- Triggers: heat, perspiration, allergens, & contact irritants (eg, wool, nickel, food, synthetic fabrics).

CLINICAL MANIFESTATIONS
- **Pruritus hallmark – required for diagnosis.**
- Erythematous, ill-defined blisters, papules or plaques. Later the lesions dry, crust over, & scale. **Most common in flexor creases** (eg, antecubital & popliteal folds) in older children & adults.
- Infantile atopic dermatitis usually affects the face and extensor part of the extremities (from crawling and rubbing the skin).
- **Nummular eczema:** sharply defined discoid or **coin-shaped lesions**, especially on the dorsum of the hands, feet, & extensor surfaces (knees, elbows).

DIAGNOSIS: clinical. Increased IgE supports the diagnosis.

ACUTE MANAGEMENT
- **Topical corticosteroids first-line. Antihistamines for itching**. Wet dressings (eg, Burrow's solution). Antibiotics if secondary infection develops (eg, *Staphylococcus aureus*).
- Topical calcineurin inhibitors (eg, Tacrolimus, Pimecrolimus) are alternatives to steroids (do not cause skin atrophy).
- Systemic: phototherapy (UVA, UVB & narrow-band UVB), Cyclosporine, Azathioprine, Mycophenolate mofetil, Methotrexate. Dupilumab.

CHRONIC MANAGEMENT
- **Maintain skin hydration**: hydration & skin emollients twice daily & within 3 minutes of exiting a lukewarm shower or tepid bath.
- Oral antihistamines for pruritus (cetirizine, fexofenadine, loratadine). Hydroxyzine, Diphenhydramine.
- **Trigger avoidance (heat, low humidity),** or irritants (eg, soaps, detergents, washcloths, frequent baths).

PITYRIASIS ROSEA

- Etiology: uncertain etiology. May be associated with **viral infections** (eg, Human herpesvirus 6 or 7).
- Primarily seen in older **children & young adults** (rare > 35y). Increased incidence in spring & fall.

CLINICAL MANIFESTATIONS
- **Herald patch (solitary salmon-colored macule)** on the trunk, 2-6 cm in diameter followed by general exanthem 1-2 weeks later: **smaller, very pruritic** 1 cm **round or oval salmon-colored papules** with white circular **(collarette) scaling** in a **Christmas tree pattern** (oriented along skin cleavage lines).
- Confined to the **trunk & proximal extremities** (*face, palms, and soles usually spared*).

DIAGNOSIS: primarily clinical. In young adults, RPR should be ordered to rule out secondary Syphilis.

MANAGEMENT
- **No management needed for most - education, reassurance, & treatment of pruritus (if present) is the management of choice** (resolves spontaneously in 6-12 weeks).
- Treatment for pruritus includes PO antihistamines, topical corticosteroids, & oatmeal baths.
- Lotions or emollients for scaling.
- UVB phototherapy may be helpful if severe & started in the first week of eruption.
- Oral Acyclovir or Erythromycin may speed up healing but are not routinely used.

PSORIASIS

- Immune-mediated multisystemic disease with a genetic predisposition.

PATHOPHYSIOLOGY

- Keratin hyperplasia & proliferating cells in the **stratum basale + stratum spinosum** due to **T cell activation** & cytokine release.

- This causes greater epidermal thickness & **accelerated epidermis turnover.**

CLINICAL MANIFESTATIONS

- **Plaque: most common type. Raised, well-demarcated, pink-red plaques or papules with thick silvery white scales. Most common on the extensor surfaces** of the elbows & knees, scalp (most common initial spot), & nape of the neck. Usually pruritic.

- **Auspitz sign: punctate bleeding with removal of plaque or scale**. Auspitz sign is not specific to Psoriasis (may be seen in Actinic keratosis as well).

- **Koebner's phenomenon:** new isomorphic (similar) lesions at the sites of trauma (also seen in Eczema and Vitiligo).

- **Nail involvement: pitting** (25%). Yellow-brown discoloration under the nail (**oil spot**) pathognomonic. Separation of nail from nail bed (onycholysis).

OTHER VARIANTS

- **Guttate:** small, erythematous "tear drop" papules with fine scales, discrete lesions & confluent plaques. Spares the palms & soles. **Often appears after Streptococcal pharyngitis.**
- Inverse: erythematous (lacks scale). Most commonly seen in body folds (eg, groin, gluteal fold, axilla).
- Pustular: deep, yellow pustules that coalesce to form large areas of pus. Fever, leukocytosis may be seen.
- Erythroderma: generalized erythematous rash involving most of the skin (worst type).

DIAGNOSIS

- Usually clinical.

MANAGEMENT

Mild-Moderate:

- **Topical corticosteroids first-line** (high-potency).
- Vitamin D analogs (**Calcipotriene**), topical coal tar, topical Retinoids/Vitamin A analogs (eg, Tazarotene).
- Calcineurin inhibitors (eg, Pimecrolimus & Tacrolimus can be used on delicate areas, such as face and penis).

Moderate-severe:

- **Phototherapy: UVB,** PUVA (oral Psoralen followed by ultraviolet A).

Severe:

- Systemic treatment eg, Cyclosporine, Retinoids (Acitretin), biologic agents (eg, TNF inhibitors Etanercept, Adalimumab, & Infliximab).

- Methotrexate is usually the last resort (due to liver lung and marrow effects) except in Psoriatic arthritis, where it is the first-line management of severe disease.

PITYRIASIS (TINEA) VERSICOLOR

- Fungal skin infection due to overgrowth of the yeast ***Malassezia furfur*** (part of the normal skin flora).
- Most common in adolescents & young adults.

RISK FACTORS
- Hot & humid weather (tropical climates), excessive sweating, & oily skin.

CLINICAL MANIFESTATIONS
- **Hyper or hypopigmented, well-demarcated round or oval macules with fine scaling**. The lesions often coalesce into patches most common on the upper trunk & proximal extremities (less often the face & intertriginous areas).

- The involved skin **fails to tan** with sun exposure.

DIAGNOSIS
- **KOH prep** from skin scraping: **hyphae & spores ("spaghetti & meatballs"** appearance).

- **Wood's lamp: yellow-green fluorescence** (enhanced color variation seen with versicolor).

MANAGEMENT
- **Topical: first-line - Selenium sulfide, Sodium sulfacetamide, Zinc pyrithione, & "azoles".**

- Systemic therapy: Itraconazole or Fluconazole in adults if widespread or if failed topical treatment. Ketoconazole and Fluconazole can be used but associated with hepatotoxicity. Because Fluconazole is delivered to the skin via the sweat, patients must not shower a few hours after oral administration.

INFANTILE SEBORRHEIC DERMATITIS

- Also known as **Cradle cap**

PATHOPHYSIOLOGY
- Not fully understood but circulating maternal hormones in infancy may lead to increased sebaceous gland overactivity + **hypersensitivity reaction** to ***Malassezia furfur*** may play a role.

CLINICAL MANIFESTATIONS
- **Erythematous plaques with fine yellow or white greasy scales on the scalp.**

DIAGNOSIS
- Usually clinical.

MANAGEMENT
- **Observation** – cradle cap is **benign, self-limited**, and usually resolves by one year of age.

- **Application of an emollient to the scalp** (eg, mineral oil, vegetable oil, baby oil, or white petrolatum) overnight or 15 minutes prior to shampooing with **baby shampoo or removal of scales with a soft brush.**

- Ketoconazole (cream or shampoo) or low-potency topical corticosteroids may be used in more extensive or persistent cases.

SEBORRHEIC DERMATITIS

PATHOPHYSIOLOGY
- Not fully understood but **increased sebaceous gland activity** + **hypersensitivity reaction** to ***Malassezia furfur*** (a yeast that is part of the normal skin flora) may play a role.
- More severe in patients with neurologic disease (eg, **Parkinson disease**) and patients with **HIV.**
- More common in men.
- Tends to worsen during fall & winter months (UV light helpful) & during times of stress.

CLINICAL MANIFESTATIONS
- **Erythematous plaques with fine white scales & greasy appearance.**
- Common in **areas with high sebaceous gland secretion** – scalp **(dandruff)**, eyelids, beard mustache, nasolabial folds, chest, & groin.
- May be associated with burning & pruritus.

DIAGNOSIS:
- Usually clinical.

MANAGEMENT
- Mild: **topical treatment first-line - Selenium sulfide, Sodium sulfacetamide, Zinc pyrithione. Ketoconazole** (shampoo or cream), or Ciclopirox. Low-potency **Corticosteroids.**
- Calcineurin inhibitors (Pimecrolimus, Tacrolimus) do not cause facial atrophy.
- Severe or resistant: oral antifungals (eg, Itraconazole, Fluconazole, Ketoconazole, Terbinafine).

CUTANEOUS DRUG REACTIONS

- Medication-induced changes in the skin & mucous membranes. Most are hypersensitivity reactions.
- **Most cutaneous drug reactions are self-limited** if the offending drug is discontinued.
- Triggers: antigen from foods, insect bites, drugs, environmental, exercise-induced, & infections.

PATHOPHYSIOLOGY:
1. **Type I: Ig-E mediated:** eg, **urticaria & angioedema**. Immediate.
2. **Type II: cytotoxic, antibody-mediated** (drugs in combo with cytotoxic antibodies cause cell lysis).
3. **Type III: immune antibody-antigen complex.** eg, drug-mediated vasculitis & serum sickness.
4. **Type IV: delayed (cell mediated)** - morbilliform reaction eg, **Erythema Multiforme.**
5. Non-immunologic: cutaneous drug reactions due to genetic incapability to detoxify certain medications (ex. anticonvulsants & sulfonamides).

EXANTHEMATOUS DRUG ERUPTION

- **Morbilliform or maculopapular drug eruption** characterized by macules or small papules after the initiation of drug treatment.
- Most commonly occurs 5-14 days after initiation of the offending medication or within 1-2 days in previously sensitized individuals.

PATHOPHYSIOLOGY

- **Type IV (delayed) hypersensitivity reaction.**
- Any drug can cause it but Penicillin, sulfa-containing medications, NSAIDs, & Allopurinol are common causes.

CLINICAL MANIFESTATIONS

- Generalized distribution of **bright red macules & papules** that coalesce to form plaques, primarily involving the trunk & proximal extremities.
- Systemic symptoms include low-grade fever and pruritus.

MANAGEMENT

- **Prompt withdrawal of the offending medication is the mainstay of treatment.** Most cutaneous drug reactions are self-limited once the offending drug is discontinued.
- **Symptomatic treatment: oral Antihistamines (H1 blockers).** Second-generation (eg, Cetirizine, Loratadine & Fexofenadine) or first-generation (eg, Diphenhydramine, Hydroxyzine, Chlorpheniramine).
- Oral corticosteroids (short course) usually reserved for severe cutaneous reactions.

ANGIOEDEMA

- Self-limited, localized subcutaneous (or submucosal) swelling resulting from extravasation of fluid into the interstitium.
- **Affects the mucosal tissues of the face, lips, tongue, larynx, hands, feet, & genitalia.**
- Onset in minutes to hours with spontaneous resolution in hours to a few days.

TYPES:

- **Mast-cell (histamine) mediated** eg, allergic reactions.
- **Bradykinin-mediated** eg, **Angiotensin converting enzyme inhibitor-induced** or hereditary (due to C1 esterase inhibitor deficiency).

CLINICAL MANIFESTATIONS

- Mast-cell mediated: angioedema that may be accompanied with other allergic reaction symptoms (eg, urticaria, flushing, generalized pruritus, bronchospasm, stridor, throat tightness, & hypotension).
- Bradykinin-induced: angioedema without allergic reaction symptoms.

WORKUP

- If there is no information to suggest an external cause and the patient has isolated Angioedema (without pruritus or urticaria), then C4 levels and a C1 inhibitor antigenic level should be obtained.

IMMEDIATE MANAGEMENT

- Immediate assessment & **ongoing airway protection is paramount. Epinephrine if severe.**

Mast-cell mediated:

- **Epinephrine** (if severe), **glucocorticoids, and antihistamines.**

Bradykinin-mediated:

- C1 inhibitor concentrate, Ecallantide (kallikrein inhibitor), Icatibant (bradykinin—beta2 receptor antagonist). Fresh frozen plasma if other therapies are not available.
- Danazol at lowest dose may be needed for long-term management in hereditary causes.

URTICARIA (HIVES)

- Edema of the superficial layers of the skin due to histamine-related increased vascular permeability.
- **Type I (IgE) immediate hypersensitivity reaction** leading to **superficial localized edema and erythema of the dermis**, mucous membranes, & subcutaneous tissues.
- Pathophysiology: release of vasodilators (eg, **histamine,** bradykinin, kallikrein, & prostaglandins) from mast cells & basophils in the skin.

TRIGGERS: food, medications, heat or cold, stress, insect bites, environmental, & infection. Chronic (> 6 weeks) is usually idiopathic.

CLINICAL MANIFESTATIONS

- Sudden onset of **circumscribed hives or wheals (blanchable, raised, erythematous areas on the skin or mucous membranes)** that may coalesce. Often associated with **intense pruritus.**
- **Hives are usually transient** (often disappearing within 24 hours and new crops often occur).

MANAGEMENT

- **Antihistamines (H1 blockers) initial management of choice.** Second-generation (eg, Cetirizine, Loratadine, & Fexofenadine) often preferred over first-generation (eg, Diphenhydramine, Hydroxyzine, Chlorpheniramine) because 2nd-generation associated with less anticholinergic effects, minimally sedating, and less drug-drug interactions.
- H2 blockers (eg, Ranitidine) may be added if no response to H1 antagonists.
- Glucocorticoids may be needed in severe, recurrent, or persistent cases.
- Epinephrine if severe or concern for airway compromise. Eliminate known precipitants.

VENOUS STASIS DERMATITIS

- Inflammatory skin changes associated with **chronic venous insufficiency** (due to DVT, varicose veins, or superficial thrombophlebitis).

CLINICAL MANIFESTATIONS

- **Leg pain classically worse with prolonged standing**, prolonged sitting with the feet dependent and **improved with ambulation and leg elevation.**
- Pain classically described as a burning, aching, throbbing, cramping, or "heavy leg".

PHYSICAL EXAM FINDINGS

- Stasis dermatitis: **eczematous rash** (pruritic, inflammatory papules, crusts or scales), excoriations, weeping erosions & **brownish or dark purple hyperpigmentation of the skin** (hemosiderin deposition).
- **Venous stasis ulcers** (especially at the **medial malleolus**) may be seen.
- Leg edema, increased leg circumference, varicosities, & erythema with normal pulse and temperature.
- Atrophie blanche: atrophic, hypopigmented areas with telangiectasias & punctate red dots.

MANAGEMENT

- **Best initial steps are leg elevation, compression stockings, & exercise.**
- Treatment of the underlying venous insufficiency is the mainstay of treatment.
- Gentle skin cleansing. Petroleum-based emollients for dry skin and pruritus.
- Topical corticosteroids for acute lesions (erythema, vesicles, oozing, and pruritus).

PIGMENT DISORDERS

VITILIGO

- Acquired skin disorder characterized by skin depigmentation.

PATHOPHYSIOLOGY
- Not fully understood but **autoimmune destruction of melanocytes leading to skin depigmentation** thought to be play a major role.
- May be associated with other autoimmune diseases.

CLINICAL MANIFESTATIONS
- **Irregular discrete white macules & patches** (total depigmentation).
- Commonly involves the dorsum of the hands, axilla, face, fingers, body folds, & genitalia.

DIAGNOSIS
- Clinical. Wood's lamp: fluorescence.
- Biopsy rarely needed – loss of epidermal melanocytes.

MANAGEMENT
- **Localized: topical corticosteroids**. Topical calcineurin inhibitors great for facial involvement. Cosmetic camouflage. Sunscreen.
- Disseminated: systemic phototherapy (eg, narrow band UVB) plus topical or oral corticosteroids.
- Laser therapy, grafts, & cultured epidermal suspensions may be effective on limited areas.

MELASMA (CHLOASMA)

- **Hypermelanosis (hyperpigmentation) of sun exposed areas** of the skin.

RISK FACTORS
- **Increased estrogen exposure (OCPs, pregnancy)**
- **Sun exposure**, exposure to phototoxic drugs
- Family history, women with darker complexions

CLINICAL MANIFESTATIONS
- **Mask-like hypermelanotic** (brown-pigment) **symmetrical macules**, especially on the face & neck.
- Dermal melasma has a bluish-grey appearance.

DIAGNOSIS
- Clinical diagnosis.
- Woods lamp may be helpful to determine the pattern of pigment deposition. Appearance is unchanged under black light in dermal Melasma. May be enhanced in epidermal Melasma.
- Histology: increased melanin deposition in all layers of the epidermis.

MANAGEMENT
- **Sun protection** (sunscreen, avoidance of the sun, wearing a wide-brimmed hat) during & after treatment + **Triple therapy often used** = Fluocinolone acetonide 0.01% + Hydroquinone 4% + Tretinoin 0.05%.
- Topical bleachers: (eg, **Hydroquinone** or Azelaic acid). Topical retinoids. Chemical peels.
- Laser therapy may be needed for dermal Melasma.

SKIN INTEGRITY

BURN SIZE Rule of Nines Not used for 1st degree burns.

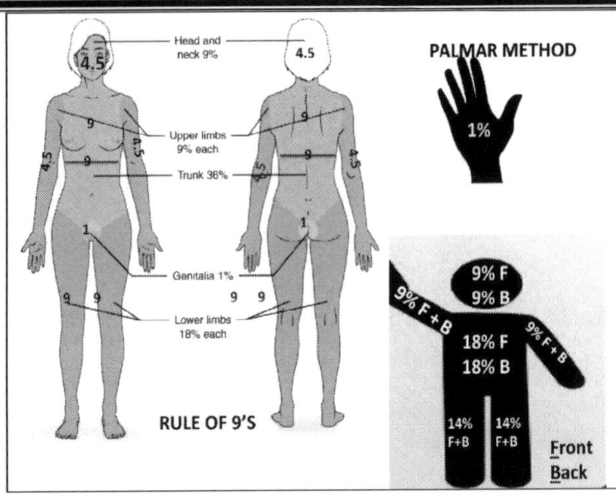

Palm size classically has been considered to represent 1% of TBSA (it accurately represents 0.4% with entire hand representing 0.8%)

Minor Burns: <10% TBSA burn* in adults*
<5%TBSA burn in young /old*
<2% full thickness burn
- Must be isolated injury
- Must not involve face, hands, perineum, feet
- Must not cross major joints. Must not be circumferential

MAJOR BURNS: >25% TBSA burn* in adults*
>20%TBSA burn in young/old*
>10% full thickness burn
- Burns involving the face, hands, perineum, feet
- Burns crossing major joints, circumferential burns

Lund-Browder chart is the most accurate method for estimating TBSA in both children & adults.

THERMAL BURNS

First degree:
- Involves minor damage to the **epidermis.** Manifests as **erythema, pain, tenderness to palpation, & dry appearance without blistering.**
- Capillary refill intact (blanches with pressure). Usually heals within 7 days without scarring.

Second degree: affects the epidermis and the dermis. Characterized by **blistering.**
- **Superficial partial thickness:** affects the epidermis and superficial portion of the dermis (papillary).
  - Characterized by **blistering, erythematous, pink, moist skin.**
  - **Very tender to touch with intact capillary refill.**
  - Heals within 7-21 days. They typically heal without scarring but may leave pigment changes.

- **Deep partial thickness:** affects the epidermis and deeper portion of the dermis (reticular).
  - Characterized by red yellow or pale skin, **blistering, not painful** (except with pressure), **absent capillary refill,** decreased 2 point discrimination.
  - Heals within 3 weeks – 2 months with scarring.

Third degree
- **Full thickness.**
  - Characterized by waxy, white, leathery, & dry skin.
  - Painless, absent capillary refill, lack of blistering, & lack of sensation.
  - Usually does not spontaneously heal well (may need skin grafting).

Fourth degree
- Skin into the underlying fat, muscle, and bone.
  - Skin is black, charred and dry.
  - Painless, loss of capillary refill.
  - Usually requires tissue reconstruction & debridement.

INITIAL BURN CARE

- **Cooling: room temperature tap water or cooled, saline-soaked gauze; not with ice directly to the skin,** soap and water to cleanse and dressing.
- Pain and Tetanus status addressed.
- With all burns, 24 hour follow up is needed if the patient is not admitted to assess burn status, assure dressing change competence, and any adjustment of analgesia as needed.

First-degree burns:

- **Superficial burns generally do not require dressings or topical antibiotics.**
- They do require follow up to monitor for progression.

Partial and full thickness burns:

- **Usually requires dressings and topical antibiotics.**
- Application of topical antibiotic, followed by a layer of nonadherent gauze over the burn, a layer of fluffed dry gauze and an outer layer of elastic gauze.
- **Topical antibiotics:** antimicrobial ointments, silver-containing agents, bismuth-impregnated petroleum gauze, Chlorhexidine, and Mafenide.

TOPICAL ANTIBIOTICS IN BURNS

- Antimicrobial ointments, silver-containing agents, bismuth-impregnated petroleum gauze, Chlorhexidine, and Mafenide.

ANTIMICROBIAL OINTMENTS:

- **Bacitracin zinc-Polymyxin B sulfate, Neomycin**: single or combination agents that can be used for superficial burn wound or partial thickness burns. Compared to Silver sulfadiazine, they are easier to apply and remove and can be used on sensitive areas (eg, face, perineum, ears). Mupirocin effective against MRSA.

  Adverse effects: systemic absorption of Polymyxin B can cause nephrotoxicity or neurotoxicity (rarely systemically absorbed). Neomycin is associated with allergic reactions.

- **Silver-containing agents: Silver sulfadiazine (SSD) & Silver nitrate**. Activated silver has antimicrobial and anti-inflammatory properties. **Silver sulfadiazine is the most commonly used burn dressing.**

  Adverse effects: **SSD cannot be used on the face** (can cause yellowing of the skin), **not used in women who are pregnant, breastfeeding or infants < 2 months old. Sulfa allergies, oculotoxic** (not used near the eyes), does not penetrate the eschar, may cause pseudoeschar formation, & impedes reepithelialization (should be discontinued when epithelialization is seen).

- **Bismuth-impregnated petroleum gauze:** often the preferred dressing for skin graft donor sites and for covering fresh skin drafts. May be useful in children as it is only applied once.

- **Mafenide acetate:** carbonic anhydrase inhibitor that is an alternative to SSD.

  Adverse effects: pain when first applied, metabolic acidosis, allergic reactions (eg, rash, pruritis, hives, erythema, eosinophilia), and respiratory complications (tachypnea).

- **Chlorhexidine:** long-lasting antimicrobial cleanser that does not interfere with reepithelialization (compared to SSD).

MODERATE TO SEVERE BURNS

Diagnostic studies for major burns:

- CBC (hematocrit may be increased initially), electrolytes (hyperkalemia is the most common abnormality seen early on), creatinine kinase along with UA and myoglobin to evaluate for rhabdomyolysis; carboxyhemoglobin and serum lactate for carbon monoxide and cyanide poisoning in smoke inhalation patients.

Fluid resuscitation:

- **Parkland (Modified): 4** mL/kg **per percent total burn surface area** (TBSA) - counting moderate (partial thickness) and severe (full thickness) burn area only **plus** normal 24 hour maintenance fluid requirements. Add maintenance fluid with glucose for children <5 years of age.
    - **Half of the fluid is given over the first 8 hours.**
    - **The remaining half is given over the next 16 hours.**
- Isotonic crystalloid fluids – **Ringer's lactate is the resuscitation & maintenance fluid of choice for the first 24 hours.** Some experts add 5% dextrose to children < 20 kg to prevent hypoglycemia.
- Monitoring fluid status: urine output should be maintained at 1 to 2 mL/kg/hr in children < 30 kg and 0.5 – 1 ml/kg/hr if 30 kg or greater. Heart rate is a better monitor of circulatory status than blood pressure. Output of at least 0.5 mL/kg/hr in adults.

PRESSURE INJURY (DECUBITUS ULCER)

- Ulcers resulting from vertical pressure.
- Commonly seen on bony prominences (eg, sacrum, calcaneus, & ischium).

RISK FACTORS

- Elderly, immobilization & incontinence.

PATHOPHYSIOLOGY:

- Pressure impairs delivery of oxygen and nutrients and waste removal from the affected area. Moisture causes skin maceration, leading to skin breakdown.

ULCER STAGES:

Stage I	superficial, **nonblanchable redness** that does not dissipate after pressure is relieved.
Stage II	epidermal damage extending into the **dermis**. Resembles a **blister or abrasion**.
Stage III	full thickness of the skin and may extend into the **subcutaneous layer.**
Stage IV	Deepest. Extends beyond the fascia, extending into the **muscle, tendon, or bone**.

- If slough or eschar obscures the extent of tissue loss, this is an unstageable ulcer (slough or eschar must be removed to determine if it is stage 3 or 4).

MANAGEMENT

- Wound care with a moist wound environment. Pain control (non-opioid oral medication if mild) & opioid analgesics for moderate to severe pain.
- Debridement if necrotic tissue is present. Negative pressure wound therapy. Optimize nutrition (protein and caloric intake, especially stage 3 and 4).
- **Pressure redistribution:** position and re-position and using support surfaces (eg, air-fluidized beds, powered mattresses).
- Stage 1: transparent film for protection.
- Stage 2: dressing that maintain a moist wound environment - transparent films or occlusive dressings (hydrocolloids or hydrogels) if there is no infection is present.
- Stages 3 & 4: debridement of necrotic tissue (mechanical, surgical or enzymatic). Surgical debridement for thick eschars or extensive tissue necrosis.

	1ST DEGREE	2ND DEGREE		3RD DEGREE	4TH DEGREE
	SUPERFICIAL	**SUPERFICIAL PARTIAL THICKNESS**	**DEEP PARTIAL THICKNESS**	**FULL THICKNESS**	
DEPTH	• Epidermis (Intact epidermal barrier)	• Epidermis + Superficial portion of dermis (papillary)	• Epidermis into deep portion of dermis (reticular)	• Extends through entire skin	• Entire skin into underlying fat, muscle, bone.
APPEARANCE	• Erythematous (red) • Dry	• Erythematous, pink • Moist, weeping • ⊕ ***BLISTERING***	• Red, yellow, pale white • Dry • ⊕ ***BLISTERING***	• Waxy, white • Leathery, Dry	• Black, charred, eschar • Dry
SENSATION	• PAINFUL • Tender to touch	• ***Most PAINFUL of all burns*** • ***Very tender to touch***	• ***Not usually painful*** • ±pain with pressure. • May have decreased 2 point discrimination	• PAINLESS	• PAINLESS
CAPILLARY REFILL	• ⊕ ***refill intact:*** *blanches with pressure*	• ⊕ ***refill intact:*** *blanches with pressure*	• ***Absent capillary refill***	• Absent	• Absent
PROGNOSIS	• Heals within 7 days • No scarring	• Heals within 14-21 days • No scarring (but ± leave pigment changes)	• ***3 weeks – 2 months*** • ***Scarring common*** (may need skin graft or excision to prevent contractures)	• Months • Does not spontaneously heal well	• Does not heal well. • Usually needs debridement of tissues & tissue reconstruction.
	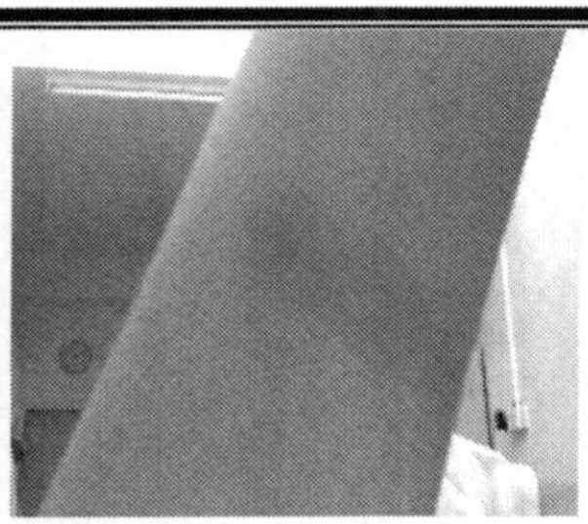	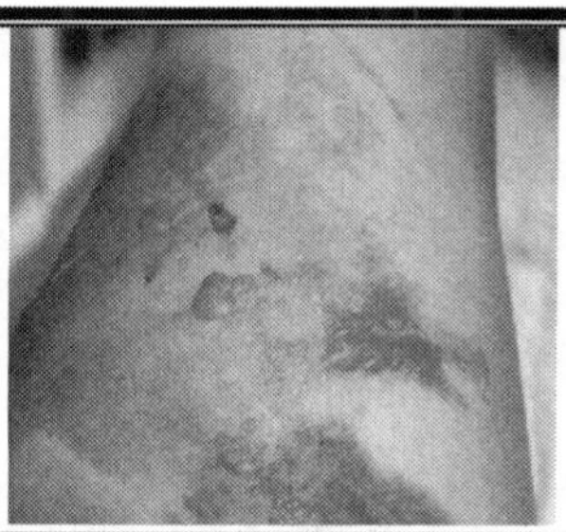	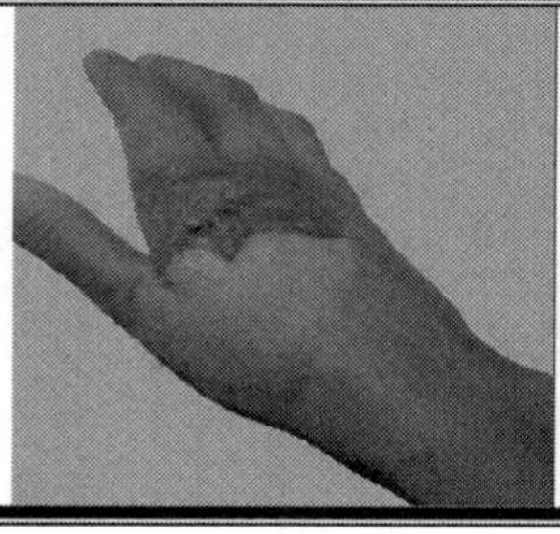	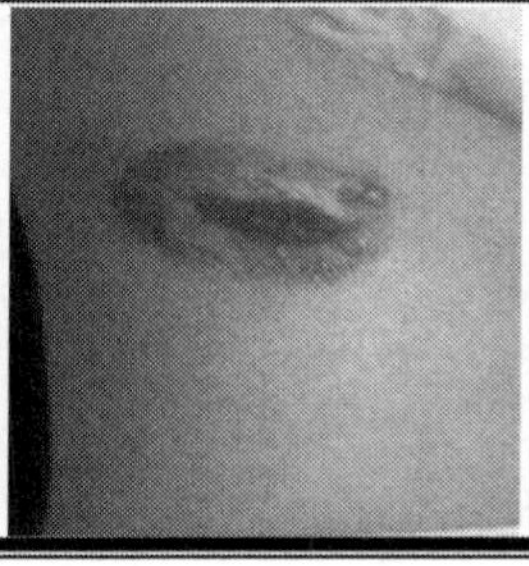	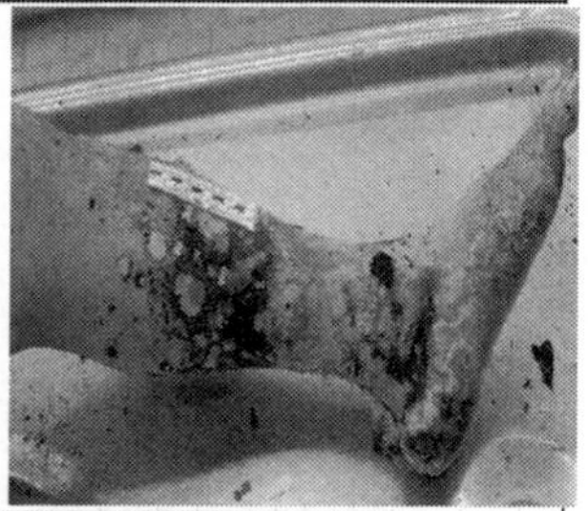

SMOKE INHALATION INJURIES

Upper airway obstruction:

- Smoke inhalation injuries are usually limited to the upper airways (steam can travel to the lower airways).

PHYSICAL EXAM FINDINGS

- Burns of the face & neck, hoarseness, stridor, dysphagia, singed nasal hairs, soot in the mouth (or nose), & black sputum.
- Respiratory distress may not be present until hours after.

LABS

- ABG or VBG (carboxyhemoglobin level), CBC, electrolytes, UA, Chest radiographs (include soft tissue neck radiographs in children), and ECG.

MANAGEMENT

- Early airway protection: maintain and secure the airway (low threshold for intubation) with tracheostomy if necessary.
- Supportive: bronchodilators (B2 agonists, anticholinergics).
- Carbon monoxide poisoning: high oxygen therapy – 100% Nonrebreather 10-12 L/min (goal is usually Carboxyhemoglobin levels < 10%).
- Hydrogen cyanide poisoning: hydroxocobalamin, cyanide kit (Amyl nitrite for inhalation, IV sodium nitrite or thiosulfate) in select patients.

CARBON MONOXIDE POISONING

- Carbon monoxide is an odorless, tasteless, colorless, nonirritating gas that has over 200 times the affinity for hemoglobin than oxygen.

ETIOLOGIES

- **Fire-related smoke inhalation most common.** Other causes include poorly functioning or improperly vented heating systems, motor vehicles operating in poorly ventilated areas (eg, garages).

CLINICAL MANIFESTATIONS

- **Neurologic: headache most common symptom**, nausea, malaise, altered mental status, seizures, brain hypoxia, coma; **Cardiac:** cardiac dysrhythmias, dyspnea, angina.
- Physical examination:
- **Bright-red retinal vessels on funduscopy.**
- **Cherry-red skin is a classic, but not common finding** (it is usually seen postmortem).

DIAGNOSIS

- Most pulse oximeters can't differentiate between HbO_2 and carboxyhemoglobin.
- Workup for inhalation injuries: **ABG or VBG - increased carboxyhemoglobin level** (level doesn't correlate with severity), methemoglobin CBC, CK, troponin, electrolytes, UA, chest radiograph (usually normal initially) and ECG. May need to include soft tissue neck radiographs in children.

MANAGEMENT

- Mild: **high-flow oxygen therapy mainstay – 100% Nonrebreather** 10-12 L/min **(goal is usually Carboxyhemoglobin levels < 10%).**
- Severe: **Hyperbaric oxygen in severe cases** (eg, increased carboxyhemoglobin > 25% + acidosis with pH < 7.1 + severe neurologic symptoms).

CYANIDE POISONING

CLINICAL MANIFESTATIONS

- Rapidly-developing coma, apnea (with severe lactic acidemia), cardiac derangements.

DIAGNOSIS

- Via history and physical examination. Cyanide levels

MANAGEMENT

- Hydrogen cyanide poisoning: hydroxocobalamin, cyanide kit (Amyl nitrite for inhalation, IV sodium nitrite or thiosulfate) in select patients.

HIGH VOLTAGE ELECTRIC INJURIES

- Determine current intensity (household usually ~110V), type of current – alternating current (AC) or direct current (DC), tissue resistance, duration & type of contact, area, "vertical" more dangerous than "horizontal", water immersion.
- **Electricity favors the path of least resistance** (eg, **nerves, muscle and blood**). Skin has the most resistance as well as fat & bone. Tissues with the highest resistance (eg, skin, fat, and bone) tend to suffer the greatest level of damage.
- **AC currents are 3-5 times more damaging than a direct current of equal voltage and current.** AC currents can cause muscle contraction (causing patient to hold on tight to the source). DC current can often violently propel the victim from the current source (due to single, large muscle spasm) & trauma (eg, posterior shoulder dislocation).
- In general, **morbidity is often greater with low voltage** injuries than with high voltage because high-voltage injuries tend to propel the individual away from the source, reducing overall contact time. Low voltage injuries, cause muscle contracting, prolonging contact time.

CLINICAL MANIFESTATIONS

- **Cardiac: arrhythmias** - low-voltage AC may produce ventricular fibrillation. High-voltage AC/DC may produce asystole. **ECG is recommended to look for cardiac changes.**
- **Musculoskeletal: rhabdomyolysis** (urinalysis is performed to look for myoglobinuria). Neurological.

WORKUP

- ECG, cardiac enzymes if chest pain, UA (for rhabdomyolysis).

MANAGEMENT

- Thermal burn management as needed. Patients may need to be placed on telemetry.
- Outpatient: asymptomatic patients with household burns may be discharged if normal ECG on presentation and normal physical examination.
- Admission: if >600V, admit even if asymptomatic. Keep urine output at 100ml/hr & alkalinize the urine to protect the kidney.

PEMPHIGUS VULGARIS

- **Life-threatening,** chronic autoimmune **blistering disorder** of the mucous membranes and skin.
- **Type II hypersensitivity reaction** where **autoantibodies (IgG) against desmoglein,** a component of the desmosome, lead to acantholysis (separation of the dermis). Normally, desmosomes connect keratinocytes in the skin.

RISK FACTORS
- Most common in patients in their 30s-40s. Middle Eastern
- Medications, especially **Penicillamine, Captopril**, Cephalosporins, and Phenobarbital.

CLINICAL MANIFESTATIONS
- **Mucosal membrane (painful erosion or ulceration) initially (intraoral most common)** followed by **painful, flaccid skin bullae** (blisters) that **rupture easily,** leaving painful denuded skin erosions that bleed easily. Palms and soles usually spared.
- Physical examination: **Positive Nikolsky sign** – superficial **detachment of skin under pressure/trauma** (pulls off in sheets).

DIAGNOSIS
- Skin biopsy (eg, punch): intraepithelial splitting with acantholysis (separation of epidermal cells). Direct immunofluorescence: **IgG throughout the epidermis**, basal keratinocytes in a pattern that resembles a "row of tombstones".
- ELISA: anti-desmoglein or anti-epithelial autoantibodies.

MANAGEMENT
- **Systemic: high-dose corticosteroids 1st line + local wound care** (treat like burns). Treat secondary infections with antibiotics.
- Steroid-sparing immunosuppressants: Methotrexate, Azathioprine, Mycophenolate, or Cyclophosphamide can be used in addition to or in refractory cases. IVIG or Rituximab.

BULLOUS PEMPHIGOID

- Autoimmune disorder leading to blister formation & severe pruritus. **Primarily seen in the elderly**.
- Type II hypersensitivity reaction - IgG autoantibodies against hemidesmosomes & basement membrane zone causing **subepidermal blistering**. Drug-induced (eg, loop diuretics, Metformin).

CLINICAL MANIFESTATIONS
- Prodrome of **pruritus** with eczematous or **urticarial plaques** followed by **tense large bullae that don't rupture as easily** most commonly involving the groin, axilla, trunk, & flexural areas. Blister roof contains epidermis.

PHYSICAL EXAMINATION: **negative Nikolsky sign** (no epidermal detachment).

DIAGNOSIS
- Skin biopsy: with **direct immunofluorescence gold standard** - linear C3 and IgG along the dermal-epidermal junction, **subepidermal blisters, & eosinophilia.**
- ELISA: autoantibodies against BP antigen 230 & 180.

MANAGEMENT
- **Topical corticosteroids** (high-potency) **first-line for mild disease** (< 20% of BSA) or applied to early lesions to prevent blisters. Antihistamines for pruritus.
- **Systemic corticosteroids if severe** or nonresponsive to topical.
- Immunosuppressants (Azathioprine).

ACANTHOSIS NIGRICANS

- Common benign disorder of the skin characterized by velvety hyperpigmented plaques on the skin.

ETIOLOGIES
- Metabolic: **obesity is the most common cause**, endocrine (eg, **disorders with insulin resistance**, such as Diabetes mellitus and Cushing syndrome).
- Hypothyroidism, acromegaly, polycystic ovary disease, genetic, medications (eg, Nicotinic acid) and rarely malignancies (GI, uterus, lung, breast, and ovarian).

PHYSICAL EXAM
- **Poorly-defined, velvety, hyperpigmented thickened plaques on the skin.**
- Most common on skin folds (eg, neck, forehead, groin, navel, and axillae).

MANAGEMENT
- Not treatable other than treating the underlying cause.
- Lifestyle: controlling blood glucose levels via diet and exercise.
- Keratolytics: topical Tretinoin or topical vitamin D analog (eg, Calcipotriene)

HIDRADENITIS SUPPURATIVA

- AKA Acne inversa - chronic inflammatory skin condition.
- Most commonly affects the **axillae** (**most common**), perianal, groin, inframammary regions, & apocrine gland-rich areas.

PATHOPHYSIOLOGY
- Not fully understood but now thought to be due to by **chronic follicular hair follicle obstruction** followed by follicular rupture and an associated inflammatory reaction.

RISK FACTORS
- **Obesity, females, smoking,** history of Acne, family history, mechanical friction, & medications

CLINICAL MANIFESTATIONS
- Characterized by **deep-seated inflammatory nodules and abscesses, draining tracts, & fibrotic hypertrophic scars.**

MANAGEMENT
- Lifestyle: dietary changes (avoid high glycemic foods), smoking cessation, local skin care, eliminate irritants (eg, synthetic & tight-fitting clothing, harsh cleaning products), reduction of skin friction.
- **Mild disease: topical Clindamycin first-line**. Intralesional injections of Triamcinolone for small cysts.
- Systemic Antibiotics: Tetracyclines, Clindamycin + Rifampin.
- Deep, recurrent infections: punch debridement if small, unroofing of larger ones with washout.
- Painful abscess: incision & drainage.

LIPOMA

- Benign subcutaneous tumors composed of mature adipocytes enclosed by a thin fibrous capsule.
- **Most common benign soft-tissue neoplasm.**

CLINICAL MANIFESTATIONS

- **Soft, painless subcutaneous nodules** ranging in size from 1 to >10 cm that are **easily mobile.**
- Most common on the trunk, neck, forearm, and proximal extremities.

DIAGNOSIS

- **Usually a clinical diagnosis** that may be confirmed after complete surgical excision.
- Biopsy indicated if pain, rapidly enlarging, firm, or restricts movement.
- Radiologic imaging prior to surgical excision may be need if large (> 10cm), painful, fixated, or deep.

MANAGEMENT

- **No treatment needed**.
- May perform compete surgical excision for cosmetic reasons or if rapidly enlarging.

EPIDERMAL (PILAR, SEBACEOUS) CYST

- **Epidermoid or pilar cysts** are benign encapsulated subepidermal nodules filled with fibrous tissue and keratinous (cottage cheese like) material.
- Sebaceous cyst, the name commonly used to describe **epidermoid or pilar cysts**, is a misnomer because both secrete keratin (not sebum) and do not originate from the sebaceous glands.

PATHOPHYSIOLOGY

- Cysts result from plugging of the follicular orifices.
- Most commonly seen in third and fourth decades of life (rare before puberty). Male: female 2:1.

CLINICAL MANIFESTATIONS

- Skin-colored dermal **freely mobile, compressible cyst or nodule**, often with a **clinically visible central punctum** (dark comedone).
- **Ruptured, infected cysts become fluctuant, painful, larger and erythematous** – may lead to **foul-smelling yellowish cheese-like discharge**.

DIAGNOSIS

- **Usually a clinical diagnosis.**
- Histology: cyst wall composed of stratified squamous epithelium.

MANAGEMENT IF NOT INFECTED

- **Inflamed or not inflamed: no treatment needed** – may spontaneously resolve without therapy. Intralesional injection of Kenalog in inflamed lesions can hasten resolution.
- **Complete surgical excision with the cyst wall intact is the most effective treatment** if cosmetically desired by the patient or if recurrent (ideally performed once the inflammation or infection has subsided).

INFECTED

- Incision & drainage.

PYODERMA GANGRENOSUM

- Ulcerative skin lesion secondary to immune dysregulation.
- Misnomer as it is not infectious nor gangrenous as the name implies.

RISK FACTORS
- **Associated with inflammatory diseases - Inflammatory Bowel disease (Crohn, UC)**, Rheumatoid arthritis, spondyloarthropathies etc.
- May be preceded by trauma.
- May be associated with solid tumors or hematologic malignancies.

CLINICAL MANIFESTATIONS
- Inflammatory, erythematous blue-red papules or pustules progressing to a **painful, necrotic ulcer with irregular purple/violet raised or undermined borders & purulent base.**

DIAGNOSIS
- Clinical diagnosis in a majority of cases. Clinical or histological diagnosis of exclusion.
- Biopsy: neutrophilic infiltration (usually not needed).

MANAGEMENT
- **Superficial or localized: topical Corticosteroids (high potency)** or Tacrolimus (calcineurin inhibitor). Local wound care.

- **Rapid growth, deep or refractory: systemic Corticosteroids or Cyclosporine.**

- 3rd line: Intravenous immunoglobulin (IVIG), Cyclophosphamide, Chlorambucil.

KELOIDS

- Hypertrophic benign raised scarring.

PATHOPHYSIOLOGY:
- **Excess production of Type I & III collagen** during wound healing.
- **Most common darker-skinned** individuals.

CLINICAL MANIFESTATIONS:
- Grossly exaggerated scar that often grows pedunculated (especially on the earlobes, face & upper extremities).

MANAGEMENT
Difficult to treat - no single treatment proven effective. Treatment is often combined.
- **Corticosteroid injections first-line management** (intralesional Triamcinolone). Associated with a high recurrence rate. Often combined with silicone gel sheets.
  Adverse effects: hypopigmentation, skin atrophy, injection pain, and telangiectasias.

- Second-line: laser therapy or cryotherapy.

- Intralesional 5-fluorouracil, pressure therapy, radiotherapy or surgical excision.

DERMATITIS HERPETIFORMIS

- Pruritic autoimmune skin disorder **strongly <u>associated with Celiac disease</u> (gluten sensitive enteropathy).**

PATHOPHYSIOLOGY

- **IgA immune complex deposition** in the dermal papillae.

CLINICAL MANIFESTATIONS

- **Intensely pruritic, papulovesicular rash most common on the extensor surfaces** (eg, forearms, elbows, knees), buttocks, back, & scalp.

DIAGNOSIS

- Both clinical findings and IgA antibodies for celiac disease (eg, transglutaminase or endomysial antibodies).
- Definitive diagnosis: direct immunofluorescence – Ig deposition within the papillary dermis.

MANAGEMENT

- **Gluten free diet – mainstay of long-term management.**
- **Dapsone first-line short-term management.** Adverse effects of Dapsone include hematologic (eg, hemolysis, methemoglobinemia, and agranulocytosis), drug sensitivity reaction, peripheral neuropathy, hemolysis in patients with G6PD deficiency. Administration with Cimetidine has been shown to decrease the toxic effects of Dapsone.
- Short-term potent topical corticosteroids may be useful for pruritus.
- Other sulfonamide drugs: Sulfapyridine & Sulfasalazine can be used in patients intolerant of Dapsone.

PYOGENIC GRANULOMA

- AKA lobular capillary hemangioma - benign vascular tumor of the skin or mucous membranes.
- Pyogenic granuloma is a misnomer - it is neither pyogenic nor a granuloma.

RISK FACTORS

- Most common in children & young adults especially **after skin trauma**, hormonal changes - **increased incidence in pregnancy** (higher incidence of **oral mucosal or gingival involvement).**
- Medications (eg, Indinavir & chemotherapy).

CLINICAL MANIFESTATIONS

- **Solitary glistening, <u>friable</u> red (raspberry-like) nodule or papule (may bleed or ulcerate).**
- **Rapid growth** - usually evolves over a period of weeks. Most common on arms, hands, fingers, & legs.

DIAGNOSIS

- Histology – proliferation of capillary vessels with stromal edema and inflammation.

MANAGEMENT

- Pedunculated: shave excision or curettage followed by cautery of the base.
- Nonpedunculated (sessile): surgical excision followed by wound closure with sutures. Results in less postoperative bleeding & lower recurrence rate.
- Topical Imiquimod or Alitretinoin gel. Injectable sclerosing agents.

ERYTHEMA NODOSUM

- Form of panniculitis (inflammation of the fat layer below the skin).

ETIOLOGIES

- **Infections: most common identified etiology, especially Streptococcal infection**, Tuberculosis, sarcoidosis, fungal (eg, **Coccidioidomycosis**).
- Inflammatory disorders: **Sarcoidosis,** inflammatory bowel disease, Leukemia, Behçet disease.
- **Estrogen exposure** (eg, OCPs, pregnancy).

CLINICAL MANIFESTATIONS

- **Painful, erythematous inflammatory nodules seen on the anterior shins** (range in colors from pink, red to purple). Usually bilateral.
- May also occur on other parts of the body.

DIAGNOSIS

- Usually clinical.

MANAGEMENT

- The lesions are generally self-limited & usually resolve spontaneously within a few weeks (excellent prognosis). Treat the underlying cause.
- NSAIDs for pain.
- Persistent: corticosteroids (if underlying cause is not infectious in nature).

CHERRY ANGIOMA

- Cherry-red papules on the skin due to abnormal mature capillary proliferation.
- Most commonly seen in middle-aged and older adults.
- The somatic oncogenic mutations in *GNAQ* and *GNA11*, similar to those found in port wine stains and Sturge-Weber syndrome, have been seen with increased frequency.

CLINICAL MANIFESTATIONS

- Cluster of cherry-red top purple papules that may be flat-topped or domed-shaped (0.1 – 0.4 cm in diameter). They blanch with pressure.
- Most commonly seen on the trunk and may bleed profusely if they are injured.

DIAGNOSIS

- Clinical. Examination with a dermatoscope will reveal purple, red, or blue-black lagoons

MANAGEMENT

- They do not generally require treatment.
- If cosmetically unappealing or subject to bleeding, options include:
  - **Electrocautery:** after local anesthesia with 1% lidocaine.
  - Shave excision and electrocauterization of the base can be employed for larger lesions.
  - Cryotherapy
  - Laser therapy for superficial lesions

PORPHYRIA CUTANEA TARDA

- Hypersensitivity of the skin to abnormal porphyrins when they are exposed to light, leading to blistering skin disease of sun-exposed areas.
- Occurs due to decreased activity of the enzyme uroporphyrinogen decarboxylase.
- May be sporadic (80%) or inherited (20%).

RISK FACTORS

- **Liver disease** (eg, **Hepatitis C**, **alcoholism,** Hemochromatosis), estrogen use, smoking.

CLINICAL MANIFESTATIONS

- Chronic blistering photosensitivity of sun-exposed areas and the hands, which can lead to hyper- or hypopigmentation or scarring.

DIAGNOSIS

- Increased plasma total porphyrins or uroporphyrins in a 24-hour urine collection.

MANAGEMENT

- Phlebotomy (especially if iron-overloaded) or low-dose Hydroxychloroquine.
- Sun avoidance until plasma porphyrin levels have normalized. Treat underlying cause.

PHOTO CREDITS

First degree burn
By Bejinhan (Own work) [CC-BY-SA-3.0 (http://creativecommons.org/licenses/by-sa/3.0) or GFDL (http://www.gnu.org/copyleft/fdl.html)], via Wikimedia Commons
Child silhouette
By Ezra Katz (File:ParentChildIcon.svg) [CC-BY-SA-3.0 (http://creativecommons.org/licenses/by-sa/3.0)], via Wikimedia Commons
Second degree burn
By Cjr80 (Own work) [CC-BY-SA-3.0 (http://creativecommons.org/licenses/by-sa/3.0)], via Wikimedia Commons
Fourth degree burn
By Goga312 (Own work) [CC-BY-SA-3.0 (http://creativecommons.org/licenses/by-sa/3.0) or GFDL (http://www.gnu.org/copyleft/fdl.html)], via Wikimedia Commons
Rule of 9's
By OpenStax College [CC-BY-3.0 (http://creativecommons.org/licenses/by/3.0)], via Wikimedia Commons

Third degree
By Craig0927 (Own work) [Public domain], via Wikimedia Commons

Palm silhouette
By SimonWaldherr (Own work) [CC-BY-SA-3.0 (http://creativecommons.org/licenses/by-sa/3.0)], via Wikimedia Commons

CHAPTER 13 – INFECTIOUS DISEASES

ANTIBIOTICS

PENICILLINS

- Mechanism of action: bactericidal via **inhibition of cell wall synthesis** (via **beta-lactam** ring).

NATURAL PENICILLINS

- **Penicillin G** benzathine-procaine (IM), Penicillin G (IM or IV), **Penicillin VK** (PO).
- Spectrum of activity: most potent gram positive coverage of all Penicillins. Also covers *N. meningitidis* and *Treponema pallidum*.
- Indications: **Strep pharyngitis, oral or dental infections, & Syphilis.**

PENICILLINASE-RESISTANT

- **Nafcillin** (IV), **Oxacillin** (IV, IM), **Dicloxacillin** (PO).
- Spectrum of activity: gram-**positive coverage**, especially **beta-lactamase producing *Staphylococcus aureus*.** Not active against Enterococcus, MRSA, or gram-negatives.

AMINOPENICILLINS

- **Amoxicillin, Ampicillin**.
- Spectrum of activity: great **gram-positive & negative coverage** (including *H. influenzae, E.coli, Listeria, Proteus, & Salmonella*).
- Indications: **UTIs in pregnancy, Listeria monocytogenes, acute Otitis media, Lyme disease,** dental infections & Enterococcal infections.

AMINOPENICILLINS WITH BETA-LACTAMASE INHIBITORS

- **Amoxicillin-clavulanate, Ampicillin-sulbactam.**
- Spectrum of activity: gram-positive, gram-negative and anaerobic coverage.
- Indications: **Acute otitis media, Acute sinusitis, animal and human bites, dental infections, skin & soft tissue infections.**

ANTI-PSEUDOMONAL PENICILLINS (EXTENDED SPECTRUM)

- **Piperacillin-tazobactam**, Ticarcillin-clavulanate, Carbenicillin.
- Reserved for Pseudomonal infections.

ADVERSE REACTIONS

- **Hypersensitivity** – drug class most commonly associated with hypersensitivity reactions
- **GI:** nausea, vomiting or diarrhea
- **Neurotoxicity –** may cause seizures at higher doses
- Acute interstitial nephritis
- **Hematologic:** thrombocytopenia, neutropenia, methemoglobinemia
- IV administration of Penicillin G benzathine or Penicillin procaine is associated with cardiopulmonary arrest and death. It should be given IM in the buttocks (upper outer quadrant) or thigh (anterolateral)

CEPHALOSPORINS

MECHANISM OF ACTION

- Structurally and functionally similar to the penicillin family with a **beta-lactam** ring but are intrinsically **effective against beta-lactamase producing bacteria**.

SPECTRUM OF ACTIVITY

- Categorized by generations based on their spectrum of activity.
- **Increasing level of gram-negative activity & loss of gram-positive activity as you go from first to fourth generation.**
- In general, Cephalosporins are not effective against *Enterococci*, MRSA, *L. monocytogenes*, or *Clostridioides difficile*.

FIRST GENERATION

- **Cephalexin** (PO), **Cefazolin** (IV), Cefadroxil (PO).
- Spectrum of activity: great for **gram-positive cocci,** anaerobes, & gram-negatives rods (eg, *E. coli, Haemophilus influenzae, Proteus mirabilus, Klebsiella pneumoniae*).
- Indications: **skin & soft tissue infections (staph, strep)**, Surgical prophylaxis.

SECOND GENERATION

- **Cefaclor** (PO), **Cefuroxime** (IV, IM, PO), **Cefoxitin** (IV), Cefotetan (IM, IV).
- Spectrum: broader gram-negative coverage (*Neisseria spp, M. catarrhalis*) with weaker gram-positive coverage. Cefoxitin has excellent coverage against *Bacteroides fragilis*.
- Indications: **skin, respiratory/ENT & urinary tract infections.** Cefotetan & Cefoxitin used for **anaerobic infections** (abdominal infections). Inpatient PID treated with IV Doxycycline + either Cefoxitin or Cefotetan.

THIRD GENERATION

- **Ceftriaxone** (IM/IV), **Ceftazidime** (IM, IV)**,** Ceftibuten, Cefotaxime, Cefixime.
- Spectrum: **broader gram-negative coverage** (including Serratia & enteric organisms). **Good CNS penetration (especially Ceftriaxone).**
- Indications: **bacterial meningitis, Gonorrhea, community acquired pneumonia (hospitalized)** combined with Macrolides, Lyme disease involving the heart or brain. **Ceftazidime has coverage vs. *Pseudomonas*.**

FOURTH GENERATION: **Cefepime** (IV).

- Spectrum of activity: gram-negative coverage including ***Pseudomonas aeruginosa***. Gram positive: only methicillin-susceptible organisms.

FIFTH GENERATION: Ceftaroline (IV).

- Spectrum: gram-positives **(including MRSA)** & gram-negatives.
- Does not cover Pseudomonas or anaerobes.

ADVERSE REACTIONS

- Allergic reaction: **5-15% cross reactivity with Penicillins** (therefore should not be used in any patient with an anaphylactic reaction to Penicillins). 1-2% hypersensitivity reaction in patients without a Penicillin allergy.
- Cefotetan & Cefoxitin can increase the risk of bleeding (hypoprothrombinemia due to effect on vitamin K-dependent clotting factors).
- Cefotetan causes a Disulfiram-like reaction (due to blockage of the second step in alcohol oxidation).
- Ceftriaxone has inadequate biliary metabolism especially in neonates so **Cefotaxime preferred over Ceftriaxone in neonates** (eg, **neonatal meningitis).**

CARBAPENEMS

- **Imipenem-Cilastatin** (IV), **Meropenem** (IV), **Ertapenem** (IM, IV)

MECHANISM OF ACTION
- Synthetic beta-lactam antibiotic. Addition of **Cilastatin reduces deactivation of Carbapenems** by the proximal renal tubule. Good CSF penetration.
- Indications: restricted use. **Neutropenic fever**, severe infections.

SPECTRUM OF ACTIVITY
- **Imipenem has the broadest spectrum of all antibiotic classes.** They are not effective against MRSA, bacteria without peptidoglycan cell walls (eg, Mycoplasma) and some Pseudomonas species.
- Ertapenem does not cover any Pseudomonas species.

ADVERSE REACTIONS
- **CNS toxicity (especially with Imipenem)** - includes **seizures,** myoclonus, and altered mental status. The risk of CNS toxicity is **greater in patients with impaired renal function or underlying CNS disease**.
- GI: nausea, vomiting, diarrhea. Eosinophilia & neutropenia (less likely than other beta-lactams).
- Hypersensitivity: 5-10% of patients with Penicillin allergy are also allergic to Carbapenems.

MONOBACTAM

- **Aztreonam** (IV)

Mechanism of action:
- Beta-lactam antibiotic that inhibits and disrupts cell wall synthesis, however, it is a **beta-lactam with no cross reactivity with other beta-lactam antibiotics**.

Spectrum of activity:
- **Primarily gram-negative aerobes only** (including *Pseudomonas & Enterobacteriaceae*). Lacks reliable activity against gram positive organisms & anaerobes.

Indications:
- Used most often clinically in patients with Penicillin allergies, renal insufficiency, those who cannot tolerate Aminoglycosides, or for synergism with Aminoglycosides.

Adverse reactions:
- Generally nontoxic but adverse reactions include: hepatitis, GI symptoms, phlebitis, & skin rashes.

POLYMYXIN

- Routes: topical, ophthalmic & otic. IM/IV.
- Mechanism of action: **alters permeability of the outer membrane** of gram-negative organisms.
- Spectrum of activity: narrow spectrum – primarily **gram-negative organisms (including *Pseudomonas aeruginosa*).**

Indications:
- **Topically for infections of the eye, ear, & skin.** May be part of triple therapy ointment, with Neomycin and Bacitracin. May be used as part of bowel prep for surgery.

Adverse reactions:
- Topical: allergic contract dermatitis.
- **IM/IV forms: nephrotoxicity & neurotoxicity so primarily used in topical forms.**

VANCOMYCIN

- Mechanism of action: cell wall inhibition (by inhibition of phospholipids & **peptidoglycans).**

SPECTRUM OF ACTIVITY:

- Narrow: **gram-positive only** - *S. aureus* (including Methicillin-Resistant *Staphylococcus Aureus* - **MRSA)**, Methicillin-Resistant *Staphylococcus epidermis* (MRSE), *S. pneumoniae* & *Enterococcal* infections. **Synergy with aminoglycosides.**

INDICATIONS:

- Oral: ***Clostridioides difficile* colitis.** Otherwise, oral Vancomycin has **poor tissue penetration.**
- **IV: MRSA & MRSE** infections. Restricted use by the CDC.

ADVERSE REACTIONS

- **Red man syndrome: flushing & pruritus due to histamine release** during rapid IV infusion. **Prevented by giving the infusion slowly** over 1-2 hours and **antihistamine administration**. Severe histamine release may lead to anaphylaxis in some patients.
- Fever and/or chills; Thrombophlebitis at the IV site
- **Ototoxicity:** tinnitus or hearing loss. May be reversible in some cases.
- **Nephrotoxicity:** especially if given with other antibiotics with similar adverse reactions (such as Aminoglycosides).
- Monitoring: trough levels may be needed in patients with renal impairment for renal dosing, patients on other nephrotoxic medications or in severe infections.

TETRACYCLINES

Doxycycline, Tetracycline, Minocycline

MECHANISM OF ACTION:

- **Protein synthesis inhibitor** (binds to **30S ribosomal** subunit). Bacteriostatic.

SPECTRUM OF ACTIVITY:

- **Broad spectrum of activity** - good against gram positive, gram negative, atypical organisms, and organisms other than bacteria.

INDICATIONS:

- **Doxycycline drug of choice: *Chlamydia spp*** - including *C. trachomatis* STIs, pelvic inflammatory disease, lymphogranuloma venereum; *Chlamydia pneumophila* pneumonia, *Chlamydia psittaci*), ***Mycoplasma pneumoniae*, Lyme disease, Rocky Mountain spotted fever, *Vibrio cholerae*,** Q fever, Bubonic plague, Cat scratch fever. Acne.
- **Tetracycline** & Minocycline used for **Acne.**

ADVERSE REACTIONS

- **Poor GI tolerance:** may cause diarrhea and gastritis.
- Deposition in calcified tissue: **deposition in teeth causes teeth discoloration** & may affect growth (**Not usually given in children < 8 years of age for more than 21 days**).
- Hepatotoxic (especially in pregnancy) - **contraindicated in pregnancy**.
- Photosensitivity; Pseudotumor cerebri.
- **Impaired absorption if given simultaneously with dairy products, Ca, Al, Mg, Fe.**
- Contraindicated in patients with renal impairment (except Doxycycline).
- Tetracycline can cause vestibular adverse reactions (hearing loss, tinnitus).

MACROLIDES

Azithromycin, Clarithromycin, Erythromycin

MECHANISM OF ACTION:

- **Binds to the 50S ribosomal subunit, inhibiting protein synthesis.**
- Bacteriostatic at low doses, bactericidal at high doses.

SPECTRUM OF ACTIVITY:

- **Broad spectrum of activity:** good against gram-positive, gram-negative, atypical organisms, and organisms other than bacteria (eg, *Babesia microti*).

INDICATIONS:

- **Erythromycin:** Strep pharyngitis (PCN allergic patients), pneumonia, *C. diphtheriae*, topical use in Acne. **Safe in pregnancy.** Less gram-negative activity compared with others in the class.
- **Azithromycin:** Pneumonia - **best macrolide for atypical coverage (*Mycoplasma, Chlamydia, & Legionella*), *Chlamydia trachomatis.*** Acute bacterial exacerbations of Chronic bronchitis (ABECB). **Anti-inflammatory in the lung.** Compared to Erythromycin, increased activity vs. *H. influenzae & M. catarrhalis* but less activity vs. *Staphylococcus* spp. & *Streptococcus* spp. Clarithromycin & Azithromycin are drugs of choice for Mycobacterium avium complex.
- **Clarithromycin:** Community-acquired pneumonia, legionella, *H. pylori*, sinusitis, bronchitis ABECB.

Adverse reactions

- **GI upset: increased peristalsis** - diarrhea and abdominal cramps, especially Erythromycin.
- **Ototoxicity:** may cause deafness (usually reversible).
- **Prolonged QT interval.**
- Cytochrome P-450 inhibition - **many drug-drug interactions (especially Erythromycin)** - may **increase levels of Warfarin, Digoxin,** Theophylline, Carbamazepine & statins.
- Contraindications: **patients on Niacin or statins (increased muscle toxicity).**
- **Acute cholestatic hepatitis (especially Erythromycin estolate).**
- With the exception of Erythromycin, avoid the other Macrolides in pregnancy (Clarithromycin is embryotoxic).

BACITRACIN

- Routes: **topical, ophthalmic,** IM injection

MECHANISM OF ACTION:

- **Cell wall synthesis inhibitor** and inhibitor of proteases and other bacterial enzymes. Mixture of cyclic peptides that are bactericidal and bacteriostatic.
- Spectrum of activity: **gram-positive only.** Little effect against anaerobes and gram-negatives.

INDICATIONS:

- **Topical preparation for minor skin injuries, scrapes, cuts, and burns.**
- May be part of triple therapy ointment, with Neomycin and Polymyxin B.
- Superficial ocular infections of the cornea and conjunctiva.

ADVERSE REACTIONS:

- Topical associated with allergic contract dermatitis. Patients with allergic reaction to neomycin may also be sensitive to Bacitracin.
- **IM form is nephrotoxic so primarily used in topical form.**

CLINDAMYCIN

- Oral, IV, topical

MECHANISM OF ACTION:
- **Lincosamide (binds to 50S** ribosomal subunit), inhibiting protein synthesis.
- Bacteriostatic or bactericidal depending on drug concentration and susceptibility of the bacteria.

SPECTRUM OF ACTIVITY:
- Narrow spectrum - primarily for **gram-positive & most anaerobes especially above the diaphragm** (little gram-negative coverage). Has **some MRSA coverage** (however there is increasing resistance). Resistance activity in general is similar to that of Erythromycin.

INDICATIONS:
- Anaerobic infections (aspiration pneumonia, intra-abdominal infections), gynecologic infections (eg, bacterial vaginosis, severe PID), skin, soft tissue, bone and joint infections, streptococcal pharyngitis, acne vulgaris. Prophylaxis against infective endocarditis, babesiosis, anthrax, malaria, Toxic shock syndrome & infections due to *Bacteroides fragilis* & *Clostridium perfringens.*

ADVERSE REACTIONS
- GI: **diarrhea, abdominal cramps, nausea, vomiting. GI symptoms most common adverse reaction.**
- ***C. difficile* colitis:** due to altered flora & the fact that *Clostridioides difficile* is inherently resistant to Clindamycin leads to *C. difficile* overgrowth & **Pseudomembranous colitis.**
- May be toxic in patients with renal & hepatic impairment.
- IV administration - thrombophlebitis, metallic taste.
- Topical administration can cause dermatitis, pruritus, and burning.
- Vaginal administration – vaginal candidiasis, pruritus, & vulvovaginitis.

CHLORAMPHENICOL

- Oral and IV

Mechanism of action:
- Binds to 50S ribosomal subunit, inhibiting bacterial protein synthesis.

Spectrum of activity:
- **Broad spectrum of activity** - good against gram-positive, gram-negative, anaerobes, & other organisms (eg, *Rickettsia rickettsii*, the causative agent of Rocky Mountain spotted fever).

Indications:
- **Drug of choice for Rocky Mountain spotted fever during pregnancy.**
- Because of **high incidence of toxicity**, it is **usually reserved for severe infections** (eg, severe anaerobic infections or other life threatening infections not responsive to other antibacterials).

Adverse reactions
- **Bone marrow suppression: Aplastic anemia**, reversible anemia, hemolytic anemia (especially if GPD deficient).
- Overgrowth of *Candida albicans* common.
- **Gray baby syndrome** due to abnormal mitochondrial activity in neonates due to drug, leading to gray skin, cyanosis, abdominal distention, & hemodynamic collapse.
- Drug interactions: may increase levels of Phenytoin, Warfarin, and Chlorpropamide

AMINOGLYCOSIDES

- **Gentamicin, Amikacin, Tobramycin, Neomycin, Streptomycin**

MECHANISM OF ACTION:

- **Binds irreversibly to the 30S ribosomal subunit**, inhibiting bacterial protein synthesis (bactericidal).

SPECTRUM OF ACTIVITY:

- **Gram-negative aerobic bacilli only (including *Pseudomonas*).** There is a **synergistic effect when combined with a beta-lactam or Vancomycin.** Not good for gram-positive or anaerobic coverage (aminoglycoside entry into bacterial cells is via an oxygen-transport system).

INDICATIONS:

- Gentamicin: hospital-acquired pneumonia, gram-negative bacteremia, GU infections, septic shock, neonatal meningitis (used with Ampicillin), Yersinia, Tularemia, Septic shock.
- Tobramycin: slightly increased activity against Pseudomonas. Topical use for Keratitis.
- Neomycin: similar use as Tobramycin. Used as bowel prep. Topically (component of Neosporin & Corticosporin). Topical for Otitis externa (must be able to visualize the tympanic membrane).
- Amikacin: reserved for serious infections.
- Streptomycin: Tuberculosis, Tularemia, & Yersinia infections.

ADVERSE REACTIONS

- **Nephrotoxicity: acute tubular necrosis.**
- **Ototoxicity**: (vestibular & cochlear). Cautious use of Gentamicin with other ototoxic drugs, such as Cisplatin, Furosemide, Bumetanide, Ethacrynic acid & high-dose NSAIDs.
- **Neuromuscular paralysis. increased muscular weakness in patients with Myasthenia gravis.**
- Needs to be renally dosed in patients with renal impairment. **Monitor serum drug levels** - **peak** levels are typically evaluated **30 minutes after completion of the infusion. Trough** levels should be drawn immediately before next dose is administered.
- Reduced activity in sites with acidic pH. Contact dermatitis with topical Neomycin.

LINEZOLID

- Oral & IV

MECHANISM OF ACTION:

- Inhibits protein synthesis (50S ribosomal unit). Bacteriostatic vs. *Staphylococcus* & *Enterococci*. Bactericidal vs. *Streptococcus* & *Clostridium perfringens*.

SPECTRUM OF ACTIVITY:

- **Mainly used for resistant gram-positive organisms, including MRSA, Vancomycin-resistant *Enterococcus faecalis & faecium (VREF)*.** Also covers atypical organisms - Mycoplasma, Chlamydia, Legionella. Not good vs. gram negatives.

ADVERSE REACTIONS

- Nausea, vomiting, diarrhea, headache. Lactic acidosis.
- Hematologic: anemia, thrombocytopenia (especially with treatment duration >2 weeks).
- Neurologic: irreversible nerve damage (peripheral neuropathy), ocular toxicity.
- MAO inhibition: avoid large amounts of foods with tyramine and sympathomimetics. Increased risk of serotonin syndrome when administered with serotonergic medications (eg, selective serotonin reuptake inhibitors).

METRONIDAZOLE

- Oral, IV and topical

MECHANISM OF ACTION:

- Forms metabolites that inhibit bacterial DNA synthesis. In anaerobic bacteria, it is activated by ferredoxin (present in anaerobic parasites) to form reactive cytotoxic products.

SPECTRUM OF ACTIVITY:

- **Effective against protozoa & anaerobes – drug of choice for "anaerobes below the diaphragm".** Anaerobes include *B. fragilis, C. difficile, & Gardnerella vaginalis.* Protozoa include *Entamoeba histolytica, Giardia lamblia, Trichomonas spp.* Also covers *H. pylori.*

INDICATIONS:

- Intra-abdominal infections, vaginitis, vaginosis, Pseudomembranous colitis, & Amoebic liver abscess.

ADVERSE REACTIONS

- **Disulfiram-like reaction** if used with alcohol (**acetaldehyde** accumulation)
- **Neurotoxicity –** peripheral neuropathy
- Metallic taste, headache, nausea, dizziness

DAPTOMYCIN

IV form

MECHANISM OF ACTION:

- Binds & depolarizes bacterial cell membranes, causing inhibition of protein, DNA & RN synthesis (cyclic lipopeptide)

SPECTRUM OF ACTIVITY:

- **Gram-positive only (including MRSA, VRE, *Enterococcus faecium* and *faecalis*).**
- Indications: **complicated skin infections** (multi-drug resistant gram-positives)

ADVERSE REACTIONS

- **Muscle toxicity** (increased CPK and rhabdomyolysis). Monitor creatine phosphokinase (CPK) levels at least weekly during therapy. Concomitant use with statins increase muscle toxicity risk.
- GI symptoms, arthralgias.
- Eosinophilic pneumonia, hypersensitivity
- Inactivated by surfactant, so not used in the treatment of Pneumonia

TRIMETHOPRIM-SULFAMETHOXAZOLE

- Oral and IV

MECHANISM OF ACTION:
- **Folic acid antagonist & inhibitor of folic acid synthesis.** Bactericidal.

SPECTRUM OF ACTIVITY:
- **Broad spectrum** - excellent **gram-negative & gram-positive coverage. Second best PO coverage vs. MRSA** (Linezolid is first but is not used as commonly as TMP/SMX).
- **Not active vs. Group A strep** (so Cephalexin often added for Streptococcal coverage during empiric oral treatment for suspected MRSA cellulitis).

INDICATIONS:
- **Soft tissue infections with MRSA, UTIs, PCP treatment & prophylaxis,** Acute bacterial exacerbation of chronic bronchitis, Toxoplasmosis, Shigellosis, Otitis media (children), & Traveler's diarrhea.

ADVERSE REACTIONS
- **Rash, photosensitivity, & folate deficiency are the primary adverse reactions.**
- GI: loss of appetite, nausea, vomiting. Dizziness, tinnitus, fatigue & hyperkalemia.
- Hematologic abnormalities (due to folic acid inhibition). May cause hemolytic anemia in patients with G6PD deficiency.
- May increase levels of Warfarin & Digoxin
- **Contraindications:** people with increased folic acid requirements - **pregnancy, nursing mothers, & neonates < 6 weeks** (causes kernicterus). **Sulfa allergies**

NITROFURANTOIN

Oral
- MECHANISM OF ACTION: inhibits DNA, RNA, protein, and cell wall synthesis. It is excreted in the urine where the active metabolites attack multiple bacterial sites.
- SPECTRUM OF ACTIVITY: gram-positive & gram-negative coverage, including Enterococcus spp. **Not effective against Proteus or *Pseudomonas* spp.**
- Administration: **should be taken with meals to decrease adverse reactions & increase absorption.**

INDICATIONS:
- **Uncomplicated acute Cystitis treatment and prophylaxis only** (not used for acute Pyelonephritis or other GU infections).
- **Safe in pregnancy** (except at term between 38-42 weeks' gestation or during labor).

ADVERSE REACTIONS
- GI: nausea, vomiting, diarrhea and anorexia. Hepatotoxicity.
- **Pulmonary toxicity:** hypersensitivity pneumonitis & chronic pulmonary fibrosis, **especially if > 65 years of age.**

CONTRAINDICATIONS:
- Acute or chronic renal failure.
- Not used in the treatment of Acute cystitis in men.
- Because of the possibility of hemolytic anemia secondary to immature erythrocyte enzyme systems, it is **contraindicated in pregnant patients at term (38-42 weeks' gestation), during labor and delivery, or in neonates < 1 month of age.**

FLUOROQUINOLONES

MECHANISM OF ACTION:

- **DNA gyrase inhibition** – removes excess positive supercoiling in the DNA helix (primary target for gram-negative bacteria).
- **Topoisomerase IV inhibition** – affects separation of interlinked daughter DNA molecules (primary target for many gram-positive bacteria).

SECOND GENERATION: increased activity vs. aerobic gram-negative bacteria.

- **Ciprofloxacin: best gram-negative coverage of all FQ,** including ***Pseudomonas,*** **enteric organisms,** *H. influenzae, Neisseria.* Indications: **UTI, pyelonephritis, gastroenteritis,** PID, malignant Otitis externa, Sinusitis, Gonococcal arthritis, Anthrax.
- Ofloxacin & Lomefloxacin: enhanced coverage of *Staphylococcus* and *Streptococcus* spp. Indications: same as above + acute bacterial exacerbation of chronic bronchitis & community acquired pneumonia.

THIRD GENERATION: increased activity vs. gram-positive & atypical organisms

- **Levofloxacin:** better activity vs. *S. pneumoniae.* Indications: **Community acquired Pneumonia,** Pyelonephritis, Prostatitis, acute Cystitis, Gastroenteritis.
- **Moxifloxacin: best gram-positive, anaerobic & atypical coverage** of the 3 generations. Poor Pseudomonas coverage. Indications: **intra-abdominal infections** (can be used as monotherapy), respiratory infections, Sinusitis, ophthalmic infections, & skin infections.
- Gatifloxacin ophthalmic.

ADVERSE REACTIONS

- GI: (most common) - nausea, vomiting, diarrhea
- CNS dysfunction: headache, memory impairment, agitation, delirium, seizures, peripheral neuropathy, **may exacerbate Myasthenia gravis.**
- **Arthropathy:** may be associated with **tendinitis or tendon rupture** in adults. **Contraindicated in pregnancy & in children <18y (articular cartilage derangements).**
- Photosensitivity. **May cause QT prolongation**
- Increased risk of hyperglycemia or hypoglycemia, aortic aneurysm
- Renal or hepatic dysfunction
- **Fluoroquinolone use should be avoided for the treatment of uncomplicated infections** (eg, acute sinusitis, simple cystitis) **when the risks outweigh the benefits.**

QUINUPRISTIN/DALFOPRISTIN

MECHANISM OF ACTION

- **Streptogramin class.** Binds to 50S subunit to inhibit protein synthesis. Bacteriostatic (cidal to some bacteria).

SPECTRUM

- **Mainly gram-positive, including MRSA & VRSA** (Vancomycin-resistant *Staphylococcus aureus*).
- Covers ***Vancomycin-resistant Enterococcus faecium*** only (*not Enterococcus faecalis*).
- Positive atypical coverage against Mycoplasma & Legionella.
- Has limited gram-negative activity.

ADVERSE EFFECTS:

- **Thrombophlebitis** (so only given via a central line).

ADVERSE EFFECTS, ADVERSE REACTIONS AND COMMENTS

PENICILLINS	**Hypersensitivity reaction.** Anaphylaxis in 0.05% (skin test does not predict it). Neurotoxicity. Hematologic side effects. **PCN & Cephalosporins associated** with nephrotoxicity **(Interstitial nephritis).**
AMPICILLIN	**Maculopapular rash in patients with Infectious mononucleosis** >90%, diarrhea.
CEPHALOSPORINS	**10% cross reactivity in patients allergic to PCN. Disulfiram reaction** (2nd/3rd), diarrhea. Uncommon S/E: increased LFTs, neutropenia, thrombocytopenia.
AZTREONAM	Beta-lactam that has no cross reactivity with PCN or cephalosporins.
VANCOMYCIN	**"Red Man syndrome"** (Histamine release-occurs when infused too rapidly). Avoided with slow infusion over 1-2 hours. Ototoxic (reversible), nephrotoxic.
MACROLIDES	**GI upset** (less with newer ones). Cytochrome P450 inhibition, **PROLONGED QT INTERVAL.** **Caution if patient is on niacin or statins** (increased muscle toxicity).
FLUOROQUINOLONES	**Tendon rupture**, growth plate arrest, damage to articular cartilage **(not given if <18y or in pregnant women). May exacerbate Myasthenia Gravis.** Photosensitivity, **QT prolongation.** Ciprofloxacin inhibits the CP450 system.
CLINDAMYCIN	**May cause *C. difficile* colitis.** Does not have good CSF penetration.
TETRACYCLINES	GI upset, **deposition in teeth** causing **teeth discoloration**; hepatotoxic. **(not given to children <8 years of age for > 21 days or in pregnancy). Photosensitivity.** Not given simultaneously with dairy products, Ca, Al, Mg or iron.
SULFONAMIDES **Ex: TMP-SMX**	Rash in 3-5%; do not give after 2nd trimester: may develop **kernicterus.** **Sulfa allergy, hemolysis if G6PD deficient.**
METRONIDAZOLE	**Avoid ETOH during and 48h after; Disulfiram-like reaction, neurotoxicity,** metallic taste, possible carcinogenic potential, pancreatitis.
PHOTOSENSITIVITY	Tetracyclines, Fluoroquinolones, Sulfonamides, Trimethoprim-sulfamethoxazole Pyrazinamide.
AUGMENTIN	Augmentin is the penicillin with the highest occurrence of diarrhea.

TETANUS

- ***Clostridium tetani*** (gram-positive rod).
- Transmission: ubiquitous in soil; germinates **especially in puncture & crush wounds**.
- Pathophysiology: neurotoxin **(tetanospasmin) blocks neuron inhibition** by blocking the release of the inhibitory neurotransmitters GABA & glycine. This leads to **severe muscle spasm.**

CLINICAL MANIFESTATIONS

3-21 day incubation period.

- **Generalized:** pain & tingling at the inoculation site. Early symptoms: **local muscle spasms, neck or jaw stiffness, trismus (lockjaw) is the most common presenting symptom,** dysphagia, hyperirritability followed by drooling, **risus sardonicus** (facial contractions), opisthotonus (arched back), muscle rigidity in descending fashion (hands & feet usually spared). These spasms **may affect the respiratory muscles. Spasm with minor stimulation, increased deep tendon reflexes.** Autonomic dysfunction can lead to tachycardia, hyperpyrexia & hypertension (though bradycardia and hypotension may also be seen). **Spatula test** - reflex spasms of the masseter muscles instead of normal gag reflex when the posterior pharynx is touched with a tongue blade or spatula.
- Neonatal: usually transferred from a non-immunized mother or unsanitary practices (such as using a soiled instrument in cutting of the umbilical cord).
- Localized: uncommon variant - just the local muscles around the wound are affected.
- Cephalic: cranial nerve involvement only.

MANAGEMENT

- **Metronidazole +** IM **Tetanus immune globulin** (eg, **5,000 units**).
- Benzodiazepines to reduce spasms (eg, **Diazepam**). IV Magnesium has been shown to prevent muscle spasm.
- Respiratory support if needed. Debridement of the wound will control the source of toxin production.

PROPHYLAXIS

- **Previously vaccinated: Tdap (preferred)** or Td vaccine booster **every 10 years** (also given for major or dirty wounds occurring >5y since last booster).
- **Never vaccinated: Tetanus immune globulin 250u + initiation of tetanus toxoid vaccine**, second dose between 4-8 weeks & third dose given between 6-12 months after the second.

PREVENTION

- **DTaP schedule:** 5 doses given at 2, 4 & 6 months of age, between 15-18 months & between 4-6 years of age.
- **Tdap booster:** at 11-12 years of age. Also given to pregnant mothers and those around them. Also given at 10 year intervals after 11-22 years of age or after a major injury if the last booster was 5 years ago or longer (now preferred over Td).
- Tetanus vaccine recommended for every pregnancy.

GAS GANGRENE (MYONECROSIS)

- Clostridial myonecrosis (life-threatening muscle infection).

ETIOLOGIES

- ***Clostridium perfringens*** **most common cause of traumatic gas gangrene.**

- *Clostridium septicum* most common cause of spontaneous gas gangrene (hematogenous spread from the GI tract with muscle seeding).

RISK FACTORS

- Anaerobic conditions (eg, traumatic injuries, punctures, IV drug injection) or postoperative (eg, recent GI or biliary surgery).

CLINICAL MANIFESTATIONS

- **Sudden onset of edema and extreme muscle pain** in an area of wound contamination + **skin discoloration** (pallor that is followed by bronze color followed by violaceous or erythematous discoloration).

- **Bullae with blood-tinged exudates** overlying the affected area.

- **Crepitus (gas) in the tissues on palpation.**

- **Systemic toxicity** (eg, fever, chills, tachycardia, shock).

DIAGNOSIS

- Radiographs: **air in the soft tissues.** CT/MRI gives more detail. Muscle involvement seen.

- Culture or smear of exudates: **gram-positive bacilli with few leukocytes**. Blood cultures.

MANAGEMENT

- **Emergent and aggressive surgical debridement (may need fasciotomy) + antibiotics (IV Penicillin plus Clindamycin).**

- Hyperbaric oxygen therapy can be added to improve survival in some patients.

- Clindamycin alone can be used in Penicillin-allergic patients. Tetracycline & Metronidazole alternatives.

BOTULISM

- ***Clostridium botulinum*** **-** anaerobic, gram-positive, spore-forming rod.

- Pathophysiology: neurotoxin **inhibits acetylcholine release at the neuromuscular junction,** leading to weakness, flaccid paralysis, & respiratory arrest.

TRANSMISSION
- **Adult:** ingestion of preformed toxin in **canned, smoked, & vacuum-packed foods.**

- **Infant:** **ingestion of honey** or dust-containing spores cause active toxin production in the gut.

- Wound: rare. Most common after traumatic injury (eg, puncture wounds, deep infections) or in **IV drug users**.

CLINICAL MANIFESTATIONS
- Symptoms occur 12-36 hours after ingestion (6-8 hours if <1 year old).

- Foodborne: prodromal GI symptoms (nausea, vomiting, abdominal pain, diarrhea) followed by sudden onset of **8 Ds:** Diplopia, Dysphagia, Dry mouth, **Dilated, fixed pupils,** Dysarthria, Dysphonia, **Descending Decreased muscle strength** (flaccid paralysis), & decreased deep tendon reflexes. Bilateral cranial nerve palsies.

- Infantile: **"floppy baby syndrome"** - neonates presenting initially with constipation followed lethargy, weakness, feeding difficulties, flaccid paralysis, hypotonia, & weak cry.

- Wound: weakness that may be associated with fever and leukocytosis and lack of prodromal GI symptoms.

DIAGNOSIS
- Primary a clinical diagnosis.

- Can be confirmed by toxin assays from stool, wound, or serum.

MANAGEMENT OF FOODBORNE:
- **Antitoxins first-line therapy**
  - If > 1 years of age, use equine-derived heptavalent antitoxin.
  - If <1 years of age, human-derived botulism immune globulin.

- Intubation if respiratory failure.

- **No antibiotics in foodborne or infantile** (may worsen disease via toxin release from lysis of bacteria).

MANAGEMENT OF WOUND:
- **Antitoxin + antibiotics (Penicillin G first line).**

- Metronidazole if Penicillin allergic.

- Wound debridement if needed.

RESPIRATORY DIPHTHERIA

- Infectious disease caused by ***Corynebacterium diphtheriae,*** a gram-positive bacillus.

- Vaccination has dramatically decreased incidence in the US. It may still occur in children & vaccinated adults.

TRANSMISSION
- Inhalation of respiratory secretions. Exotoxin induces an inflammatory response.

CLINICAL MANIFESTATIONS
- **Tonsillopharyngitis or Laryngitis: classic presentation.** 1-7 day incubation period. Sore throat, fever, malaise, and nasopharyngeal symptoms. May develop neuropathy.

- **Myocarditis:** arrhythmias or heart failure (exotoxin-induced inflammatory response).

- May be associated with an asymptomatic carrier state.

PHYSICAL EXAMINATION
- **Pseudomembrane - friable, gray to white membrane on the pharynx** that bleeds if scraped. Pseudomembranes are composed of WBCs, RBCs, fibrin, epithelial cells, & organisms.

- **Cervical lymphadenopathy:** neck swelling due to lymphadenopathy sometimes referred to as a bull neck.

DIAGNOSIS
- Clinical diagnosis with culture confirmation (using Loffler medium or tellurite agar).

MANAGEMENT
- **Diphtheria antitoxin (horse serum) most important + either Erythromycin or Penicillin** x 2 weeks. Antitoxin reduces sequelae & increase recovery time while antibiotics are used to prevent the spread of Diphtheria. Airway management if needed.

- Place the patient on **respiratory droplet isolation** until 2 consecutive cultures 24 hours apart are negative. Serial ECGs and cardiac enzymes to assess for Myocarditis.

- Clindamycin or Rifampin are alternatives.

- Endocarditis: Penicillin + Aminoglycoside

PROPHYLAXIS FOR CLOSE CONTACTS
- **Erythromycin** x 7- 10 days or **Penicillin benzathine G** x 1 dose.

PREVENTION
- **DTaP schedule:** 5 doses given at 2, 4, & 6 months of age, between 15-18 months, & between 4-6 years of age.

- **Tdap booster:** at 11-12 years of age. Also given to pregnant mothers and those around them. Also given at 10 year intervals after 11-22 years of age or after a major injury if the last booster was 5 years ago or longer (now preferred over Td).

METHICILLIN-RESISTANT STAPHYLOCCUS AUREUS (MRSA)

ORAL MANAGEMENT
- Doxycycline, Clindamycin, Trimethoprim-Sulfamethoxazole or Linezolid
- IV: Vancomycin, Ceftaroline, Daptomycin or Linezolid.

GONOCOCCAL INFECTIONS

- ***Neisseria gonorrhoeae* (gram-negative diplococci).** 2-8 day incubation period.

CLINICAL MANIFESTATIONS
- Urethritis and Cervicitis: **discharge** (anal, vaginal, penile, or pharyngeal), Pelvic inflammatory disease, Epididymitis, Prostatitis.

DISSEMINATION
- **Triad of dermatitis, polyathralgias, & tenosynovitis** - rash (maculopapular, petechial), arthralgia (joint pain), tenderness along the tendon sheath. Often associated with fever, chills, & malaise.

- **Purulent gonococcal septic arthritis (especially the knee).** In women, it occurs more frequently during menses.

DIAGNOSIS
- **Nucleic acid amplification most sensitive & specific for *C. trachomatis, N. gonorrhoeae,* &** *M. genitalium* (recommended over culture).
  - First-void or first-catch urine ideal if urethritis.
  - If disseminated, samples are taken at multiple sites (eg, urethral, rectal, pharyngeal, cervical).

- Gram stain: 2 or more WBCs/hpf. No organisms seen is suggestive of Nongonococcal urethritis (eg, *Chlamydia trachomatis*). Gram-negative diplococci = *N. gonorrhoeae.* Urethral swab.

- Urinalysis or dipstick: positive leukocyte esterase on dipstick or 10 or more WBCs/hpf (pyuria) on microscopy suggestive.

- **Synovial fluid:** nucleic acid amplification testing (NAAT) or culture on chocolate agar or Thayer-Martin medium.

- **Nucleic acid amplification tests** taken at multiple sites (eg, urethral, rectal, pharyngeal, cervical).

- Blood cultures.

MANAGEMENT:
- Gonococcal arthritis: **IV Ceftriaxone is the first-line treatment**.

- Urethritis & Cervicitis: **Ceftriaxone 250mg IM plus either Doxycycline or Azithromycin** (for additional coverage for Gonorrhea as well as to cover possible Chlamydia).

CHLAMYDIA

- ***Chlamydia trachomatis* is the most common overall bacterial cause of STIs in the US.**

CLINICAL MANIFESTATIONS
- Urethritis: purulent or mucopurulent discharge, pruritus, dysuria, dyspareunia (pain with intercourse), hematuria. Up to 40% asymptomatic (especially men).

- Pelvic inflammatory disease: abdominal pain, ⊕ **cervical motion tenderness.**

- Reactive arthritis: **urethritis, uveitis, arthritis** (reactive arthritis is an autoimmune reaction). ⊕ HLA-B27.

- Lymphogranuloma venereum: genital/rectal lesion with softening, suppuration & lymphadenopathy.

DIAGNOSIS
- **Nucleic acid amplification most sensitive & specific for *C. trachomatis, N. gonorrhoeae,*** & *M. genitalium* (vaginal swab or first-catch urine preferred).

- Genetic probe methods, culture, antigen detection.

MANAGEMENT
- **Azithromycin** (1 gram x1 dose) or **Doxycycline** 100mg bid for 10 days. Re-test in 3 weeks to ensure clearance of the organism.
- Also treat for Gonorrhea (Ceftriaxone 250mg IM x 1 dose).

LYMPHOGRANULOMA VENEREUM

- Genital ulcer disease cause by L1, L2 & L3 serovars of ***Chlamydia trachomatis.***
- Most commonly seen in tropical & subtropical areas of the world.
- Pathophysiology: extension from the infection site to the draining lymph nodes.

CLINICAL MANIFESTATIONS
- **Painless genital ulcer at the site of inoculation.**

- The secondary stage appears 2-6 weeks later – **painful inguinal &/or femoral lymphadenopathy (buboes).**

- May develop proctocolitis (rectal discharge, anal pain, constipation, fever and/or tenesmus).

DIAGNOSIS
- Often clinical.
- Cultures and serologic testing have low yield. Nucleic acid amplification testing.

MANAGEMENT
- **Doxycycline 100 bid x 21 days treatment of choice.**
- Azithromycin 1g orally once weekly x 3 weeks.
- Buboes may need needle aspiration or incision & drainage to avoid rupture or sinus tract formation.
- All patients should be tested for other STIs including HIV.

ACUTE RHEUMATIC FEVER

- Acute autoimmune inflammatory multi-systemic illness mainly affecting **children 5-15 years old.**

PATHOPHYSIOLOGY

- Symptomatic or asymptomatic **infection with Group A *Streptococcus*** (aka **Strep pyogenes)** stimulates antibody production to host tissues & damages organs directly.
- The infection usually precedes the onset of Rheumatic fever by 2-6 weeks.

CLINICAL MANIFESTATIONS

- **Polyarthritis:** (75%) **2 or more joints affected** (simultaneous more diagnostic) **or migratory** (lower ⇨ upper joints). Medium/large joints most commonly affected (knees, hips, wrists, elbows, shoulders). **Heat, redness, swelling, & severe joint tenderness must be present.** Joint pain (arthralgia) without other symptoms doesn't classify as major. Usually lasts 3-4 weeks.
- **Active carditis:** (40-60%) can affect valves (especially mitral & aortic), myocardium (myocarditis) &/or pericardium (pericarditis). **Carditis confers great morbidity & mortality.**
- Sydenham's chorea: (<10%) "Saint Vitus dance" may occur 1- 8 months after initial infection. Manifestations include sudden involuntary, jerky, non-rhythmic, purposeless movements especially involving the head/arms. Usually resolves spontaneously. Most common in females.
- **Erythema marginatum:** often accompanies carditis. Macular, erythematous, non-pruritic annular rash with rounded, sharply demarcated borders (may have central clearing). Most commonly seen on the trunk & extremities (not the face). Crops last hours-days before disappearing.
- Subcutaneous nodules *rare.* Seen over joints (extensor surfaces), scalp, & spinal column.
- Other findings not associated with Jones criteria: abdominal pain, facial tics/grimaces, epistaxis.

DIAGNOSIS

JONES CRITERIA FOR RHEUMATIC FEVER	(2 Major OR 1 major + 2 minor)
MAJOR CRITERIA	**MINOR CRITERIA**
1. Joint (migratory polyarthritis)	CLINICAL
2. Oh my heart **(active carditis)**	Fever (≥101.3° F/≥ 38.5° C)
3. **Nodules** (subcutaneous)	Arthralgia (joint pain)
4. Erythema marginatum	LABORATORY
5. Sydenham's chorea	↑acute phase reactants (↑ESR, CRP, leukocytosis)
	ECG: prolonged PR interval

PLUS

Supporting evidence of a recent group A streptococcal infection:
- Positive throat culture for GAS or
- Rapid streptococcal antigen or
- Elevated/increased streptococcal Ab titers (eg, antideoxynuclease B or antistreptolysin O)

MANAGEMENT

- **Anti-inflammatory: Aspirin** (2-6 weeks with taper); ± Corticosteroids in severe cases & carditis.

- **Penicillin G antibiotic of choice (or Erythromycin if PCN-allergic)** both in acute phase & after acute episode. Prevention is the most important therapeutic course. Therefore all patients (even if presenting with Acute rheumatic fever) should be treated with antibiotics.

COMPLICATIONS

- **Rheumatic valvular disease - mitral (75-80%), aortic** (30%); tricuspid & pulmonic (5%).

SCARLET FEVER (SCARLATINA)

- Diffuse skin eruption that occurs in the setting of **Group A *Streptococcus*** (***S. pyogenes***) infection.

PATHOPHYSIOLOGY
- Type IV (delayed) hypersensitivity reaction to a pyrogenic strain (erythrogenic toxin A, B, or C).

CLINICAL MANIFESTATIONS
- Fever, chills, **pharyngitis**
- Rash: **diffuse erythema** that blanches with pressure + multiple small (1-2 mm) papular elevations with a **sandpaper texture.** The rash usually starts in the axillae and groin and then spreads to the trunk and extremities (usually spares the palms and soles).
- Flushed face with **circumoral pallor & strawberry tongue.**
- Pastia's lines: linear petechial lesions seen at pressure points, axillary, antecubital, abdominal or inguinal areas.

DIAGNOSIS
- Clinical or testing for GABHS (eg, rapid strep, anti-streptolysin titer, throat culture).

MANAGEMENT
- **Penicillin G or VK first-line.** Amoxicillin. **Macrolides if penicillin-allergic.** Clindamycin, Cephalosporins. Children may return to school 24 hours after antibiotic administration.

ROCKY MOUNTAIN SPOTTED FEVER

- Potentially fatal but curable tick-borne disease caused by ***Rickettsia rickettsii.***
- Pathophysiology: *Rickettsia rickettsii* – gram-negative, obligate intracellular bacterium with an affinity for vascular endothelial cells, leading to **vascular injury,** microhemorrhages, & microinfarcts.
- Vectors: ***Dermacentor andersoni*** & ***variabilis*** **(wood & dog tick** respectively).
- Most common in Southcentral & Southeastern United States (especially in the spring & summer).

CLINICAL MANIFESTATIONS
- Rash: 2-14 days after tick bite. **Headache, fever,** chills, malaise, myalgias, arthralgias, nausea, vomiting, lethargy, seizures followed by a **blanching, erythematous macular rash <u>first on wrists & ankles</u> (palms & soles** involvement common) then spreads to the trunk. The rash starts as faint macules and become papular & **petechial.** 10% will not develop a rash.
- Associated symptoms: periorbital or pedal edema (especially in children), conjunctivitis, retinal abnormalities, encephalitis, ARDS, cardiac, or bleeding disorders.

DIAGNOSIS
- **<u>Clinical diagnosis</u> (don't wait for serologies):** fever + rash + history of tick exposure.
- Serologies: indirect immunofluorescent antibody test for IgM and IgG antibodies.
- May develop thrombocytopenia, pancytopenia, or hyponatremia.
- CSF: low glucose & pleocytosis (increased cell count). Skin biopsy.

MANAGEMENT
- **Doxycycline first-line treatment for non-pregnant adults and children (even if < 8 years of age)** x 5-14 days.
- Chloramphenicol second line. **Chloramphenicol treatment of choice in pregnancy.** Third trimester usage of Chloramphenicol associated with gray baby syndrome.
- Ideally, treatment should begin ideally within 5 days of symptom onset to reduce mortality.

ANTIFUNGAL MEDICATIONS

POLYENE ANTIFUNGALS Nystatin (topical, oral); Amphotericin B

MOA: *binds to cell membrane sterols* (increasing the permeability/fragility of the cell membrane).

AMPHOTERICIN B

- INDICATIONS: **antifungal of choice** for most **invasive or life-threatening fungal infections.**
- ADVERSE EFFECTS: **fever/chills during infusion,** electrolyte abnormalities (**↓K,** ↓Mg), **nephrotoxicity** & hematologic toxicity (anemia), azotemia (↑BUN/creatinine), cardiac arrhythmias.
- **Lipid-based Ampho B:** - advantages: high tissue concentrations, decreased infusion-related reactions, marked ***decrease in nephrotoxicity*** but VERY expensive.

NYSTATIN

- **Indications:** used primarily topically (vaginal) & local treatment: **oral candidiasis (thrush).**
- Because of poor oral bioavailability, there are no significant drug interactions.

"AZOLES" ANTIFUNGALS

- Imidazoles: **Clotrimazole** (Lotrimin), **Ketoconazole** (Nizoral), **Econazole, Miconazole**
- Triazoles: **Fluconazole** (Diflucan), **Itraconazole, Voriconazole, Posaconazole**

MOA: inhibits ergosterol synthesis (ergosterols are essential for fungal cell membrane stability).

INDICATIONS: Candidiasis, Cryptococcus, Histoplasmosis, Coccidioidomycosis, Tinea (topical).

- **Fluconazole** – **drug of choice for noninvasive Candida & Cryptococcal infections,** water soluble, **good for urine & CSF infections.** Fluconazole is eliminated by the kidney.
- **Voriconazole** EXTENDED spectrum (covers Aspergillus). **Voriconazole drug of choice for invasive Aspergillus.** Does not cover Mucorales species well.
- **Itraconazole**: EXTENDED spectrum (covers Aspergillus). **Drug of choice for noninvasive Histoplasmosis, Blastomycosis, & Coccidioidomycosis** (Adverse effect: may cause CHF).
- **Ketoconazole & Itraconazole** - lipid soluble, **poor CSF penetration**, inhibits CP450.

ADVERSE EFFECTS

- **Fluconazole: hepatitis,** nausea, rash, alopecia, headache.
- **Ketoconazole: suppression of testosterone & cortisol** (used to treat refractory Cushing's). **↑LFTs**

ALLYLAMINES Terbinafine (Lamisil); Butenafine (Mentax)

MOA: inhibits ergosterol synthesis (by inhibiting squalene epoxidase).

INDICATIONS: *dermatophyte infections:*

- Onychomycosis: Terbinafine PO. Tinea (Corporis, Pedis, Cruris): Terbinafine or Butenafine topical

GRISEOFULVIN

MOA: **inhibits fungal cell mitosis preventing proliferation & function.**

INDICATIONS: Tinea infection: capitis, cruris, pedis, unguium.

Give with fatty meals to increase absorption.

S/E: **Hepatitis, teratogenic:** (including males – males must avoid attempting to conceive for 6 months after treatment).

CASPOFUNGIN, ANIDULAFUNGIN, MICAFUNGIN

MOA: **Inhibits cell wall glucan synthesis.** Echinocandins.

INDICATIONS: includes azole- & AmB-resistant strains of Aspergillus & Candidiasis.

Adverse effects: fever, thrombophlebitis, headache, ↑LFTs, rash, flushing. only IV - very expensive.

CANDIDIASIS

- ***Candida albicans*** is part of the normal GI & GU flora but **most common opportunistic pathogen.**

CLINICAL MANIFESTATIONS

- **Esophagitis:** substernal odynophagia, gastroesophageal reflux, epigastric pain, nausea, vomiting.
  - Endoscopy: white linear plaques/erosions.
  - Management: **oral Fluconazole** first-line treatment.

- **Oropharyngeal (Thrush): friable white plaques (± leave erythema if scraped).**
  Management: **Nystatin** swish & swallow or Clotrimazole troches.

- **Vulvovaginal candidiasis:** vulvar pruritus, burning, vaginal discharge **(white, thick curd-like).**
  Management: **Miconazole, Clotrimazole, Fluconazole.** Fluconazole weekly if persistent vaginitis

- **Intertrigo:** cutaneous infection most common in moist, macerated areas. **Pruritic rash beefy red erythema** with **distinct, scalloped borders & satellite lesions.**
  Management: **Clotrimazole topical,** keep area dry.

- **Fungemia, Endocarditis:** seen in immunocompromised patients, ±indwelling catheters.
  Management: **IV Amphotericin B.** Caspofungin if severe. ±IV Fluconazole if mild.

DIAGNOSIS

- Potassium Hydroxide (KOH) smear: **budding yeast & pseudohyphae.** Clinical diagnosis.

CRYPTOCOCCOSIS

- ETIOLOGY: ***Cryptococcus neoformans*** or *C. gattii* (encapsulated budding round yeast).
- TRANSMISSION: inhalation of **pigeon & bird droppings.**
- RISK FACTORS: **most common in immunocompromised** (eg, HIV with CD4 count ≤100 cells/μL).

CLINICAL MANIFESTATIONS

- **Meningoencephalitis: most common cause of fungal meningitis.** Presents with headache & meningeal signs (neck stiffness, nausea, vomiting, photophobia). Meningeal signs uncommon in patients with HIV.
- **Pulmonary: Pneumonia** (cough, pleuritic chest pain, dyspnea), nodules, abscess, or pleural effusions.
- Skin lesions may be seen if disseminated.

DIAGNOSIS

- Lumbar puncture: **Fungal CSF pattern - increased WBC (lymphocytes), decreased glucose,** & increased protein. Lumbar puncture is performed even if pulmonary or dermatologic symptoms.
- CSF evaluation: **Cryptococcal antigen in CSF** (via latex agglutination or ELISA) or visualization of **encapsulated yeast** on **India ink staining.**
- May have positive blood cultures in patients with HIV.

MANAGEMENT

- **Meningoencephalitis: Amphotericin B plus Flucytosine** x 2 weeks **followed by oral Fluconazole** x 10 weeks.
- Pneumonia if immunocompetent: Fluconazole or Itraconazole x 3-6 months.

PROPHYLAXIS IN HIV

Cryptococcus considered an AIDS defining illness. Routine prophylaxis is usually not indicated but in select persons, *Fluconazole* may be given *if CD4 ≤100* cells/μL.

HISTOPLASMOSIS

- ***Histoplasma capsulatum*** - dimorphic oval yeast (not encapsulated despite its name).
- Transmission: inhalation of moist **soil containing bird & bat feces** in the **Mississippi & Ohio river valleys.** Also seen with demolition, people who explore caves (spelunkers), or excavators in those areas.
- Pathophysiology: once inhaled, *H. capsulatum* are ingested by alveolar macrophages. *H. capsulatum* grows within the phagosome, where they remain viable in macrophages & can disseminate via the macrophages.
- Risk factors: immunocompromised states - AIDS-defining illness especially if CD4+ is ≤*150* cells/μL.

CLINICAL MANIFESTATIONS
- **Asymptomatic: most patients** (flu-like symptoms if they become symptomatic).
- **Pneumonia** (atypical). Fever, nonproductive cough, myalgias. **Can mimic Tuberculosis.**
- Dissemination: if immunocompromised: hepatosplenomegaly, fever, oropharyngeal ulcers, bloody diarrhea, adrenal insufficiency.

DIAGNOSIS
- Labs: increased alkaline phosphatase & LDH. Pancytopenia
- Chest radiographs: pulmonary infiltrates, hilar or mediastinal lymphadenopathy.
- **Antigen testing via sputum (PCR) or urine highly specific.**
- **Cultures: most specific test.** Sputum. Blood culture positivity if disseminated/HIV.

MANAGEMENT
- **Asymptomatic: no treatment required** (eg, patients with pulmonary symptoms < 4 weeks).
- **Mild-moderate disease: Itraconazole first line treatment.**
- **Severe disease: Amphotericin B.** Also used if Itraconazole therapy is ineffective.

BLASTOMYCOSIS

- *Blastomyces dermatitidis* - pyogranulomatous fungal infection. It is a fungus in nature, mold in tissues.
- RISK FACTORS: occurs most commonly in **immunocompetent men involved in outdoor activities (around soil or decaying wood) in close proximity to waterways in Central & Eastern US** (eg, Mississippi & Ohio river basins or Great Lakes). HIV.

CLINICAL MANIFESTATIONS
- **Pulmonary:** most common site of involvement. **Many are asymptomatic**. Chronic disease: **flu-like symptoms** - cough with or without sputum production, dyspnea, headache, fever. **Pneumonia** - high fever, chest pain, productive cough.
- **Cutaneous:** papules progressing to **verrucous, crusted or ulcerated lesions** which expand (may leave a central scar when healed). Skin most common site of extrapulmonary disease.
- Disseminated: **most common in the lungs, skin, bone** (ribs or vertebral pain), & **genitourinary system** (prostatitis or epididymitis).

DIAGNOSIS
- Cultures: sputum, discharge or urine - round **broad-based budding yeast** with thick, refractile double walls. Potassium hydroxide wet preparation or Calcofluor-white staining used on the specimens.
- CXR: **alveolar infiltrates or a mass lesion** (can mimic bronchogenic carcinoma), ± pleural effusions.

MANAGEMENT
- Mild-moderate: **Itraconazole first line treatment of choice.**
- Severe: Amphotericin B if rapidly progressive, AIDS-related or CNS disease (eg, meningitis).

ASPERGILLOSIS

- *Aspergillus fumigatus* is a fungus that **most commonly affects the lungs, sinuses, & the CNS.**

TRANSMISSION
- Via inhalation. Commonly found in **garden and houseplant soil & compost.**

CLINICAL MANIFESTATIONS
- **Allergic bronchopulmonary aspergillosis:** **type I hypersensitivity reaction** occurring almost exclusively in patients with **Asthma, Bronchiectasis, or Cystic fibrosis.** Classically presents with refractory asthma, fever, malaise, & intermittent **expectoration of brownish mucus plugs** in the sputum.

- **Aspergilloma:** the fungus colonizes a preexisting pulmonary cavitary lesion. Can be an asymptomatic incidental finding on CXR or patient may complain of cough or **hemoptysis.**

- Acute invasive Aspergillosis: fever, headache, toothache, epistaxis, **invasive chronic sinusitis.** Commonly involves the lungs - **hemoptysis, pleuritic chest pain**, dyspnea. Increased LDH. Often fatal. Usually occurs in severely immunocompromised patients (eg, neutropenia, leukemia).

DIAGNOSIS
- **Allergic:** **increased IgE,** eosinophilia, *Aspergillus* skin test positivity or detectable IgE levels vs. *Aspergillus fumigatus.*

- Invasive: Galactomannan levels (found in the cell walls of Aspergillus - specific), beta-D glucan assay, PCR, & culture.

- Biopsy: tissue appears **dusky & necrotic** (eg, nose).
  Septate hyphae with regular branching at acute (45 degree) angles.

RADIOGRAPH FINDINGS
- Allergic: changes of bronchiectasis, parenchymal opacities (especially in the upper lobes) or atelectasis.

- Invasive Aspergillosis: single or multiple nodules with a halo sign (rim of ground glass opacity) with or without cavitation, patchy or segmental consolidation, peribronchial infiltrates.

- Aspergilloma: air crescent sign - radiopaque structure "fungal ball" that moves when the patient changes position.

MANAGEMENT
- **Allergic Bronchopulmonary Aspergillosis:** **tapered oral corticosteroids** + chest physiotherapy first-line. **Itraconazole** added in some cases.

- Severe/Invasive Aspergillus or Sinusitis: **Voriconazole drug of choice,** Isavuconazole, or Caspofungin. Amphotericin B may be adjunctive to Voriconazole. Surgical debridement if refractory.

- Aspergilloma:
  - **Symptomatic: surgical resection.**
  - **Asymptomatic: observation.**

COCCIDIOIDOMYCOSIS "Valley fever"

- ***Coccidioides immitis*** grows in **soil in arid/desert regions in Southwestern US** (eg, New Mexico, Southern California), Mexico, Central & South America.

TRANSMISSION
- Inhalation of spores when the soil is disrupted.

CLINICAL MANIFESTATIONS
- Primary pulmonary disease: 60-65% asymptomatic.
  Mild flu-like illness - fever, chills, nasopharyngitis, headache, cough, pleuritic chest pain.

- **Valley fever: fever, arthralgias (pain & swelling of the knees & ankles common), & skin involvement (erythema nodosum, erythema multiforme,** or maculopapular rash).

- Disseminated or persistent: **CNS** (eg, **Meningitis**) in 50%. Can affect any organ especially the lungs, skin, soft tissue, lymph nodes, & joints.

DIAGNOSIS
- **Early: serologies** - enzyme-linked immunoassays for **IgM & IgG antibodies usually the first test ordered** with immunodiffusion tests conducted only if the EIA is positive.

- **Cultures most definitive.** PCR, skin testing.

- Histology: **spherules** (thick-walled spherical structure containing endospores) seen in tissues.

- Meningitis: CSF complement fixing antibodies, Fungal CSF pattern (lymphocytosis & decreased glucose).

- Pulmonary: CXR: persistent cavitations, miliary pneumonia, abscesses, & nodules.

MANAGEMENT
- **Most cases asymptomatic/mild & are self-limited** & require no treatment. Localized lung disease is treated symptomatically in most cases.

- **CNS disease: Fluconazole or Itraconazole**.

- Amphotericin B reserved for severe disease or pregnancy in the first trimester.

MYCOBACTERIAL DISEASES

MYCOBACTERIUM AVIUM COMPLEX

- *Mycobacterium avium* & *intracellulare*, etc.
- TRANSMISSION: present in soil & water (not person to person).

RISK FACTORS
- Symptoms seen in patients with **underlying pulmonary disease** (eg, Bronchiectasis, COPD).
- Immunocompromised patients (eg, **HIV with CD4 count ≤ 50** cells/μL).
- Symptoms rarely occur in immunocompetent patients without underlying lung disease.

CLINICAL MANIFESTATIONS
- **Pulmonary:** presents similar to Tuberculosis (eg, cough, chest pain, fever, weight loss, upper lobe infiltrates & cavities).
- **Disseminated: fever of unknown origin** (most common), sweating, weight loss, fatigue, diarrhea, dyspnea, RUQ pain, hepatosplenomegaly. **Most commonly seen with HIV.**
- **Lymphadenitis in children**: cervical, submandibular, & maxillary.

DIAGNOSIS
- Acid fast bacillus staining & culture.

MANAGEMENT
- **Clarithromycin plus Ethambutol plus a Rifamycin** (eg, Rifabutin or Rifampin).
- Parenteral aminoglycoside may be added to the above regimen in life-threatening disease.
- Second-line: Ethambutol + a Rifamycin (eg, Rifabutin) plus Aminoglycoside.
- Surgical excision of infected lymph nodes is curative in 90% of patients with lymphadenitis.

PROPHYLAXIS IN HIV
- **Clarithromycin or Azithromycin if CD4 count ≤ 50** cells/μL.

MYCOBACTERIUM MARINUM "Fish tank Granuloma"

- Atypical *Mycobacterium* found in fresh & salt water.

TRANSMISSION
- Inoculation of a **break in the skin barrier** (laceration abrasion, puncture, etc.) **with exposure to** contaminated **fresh or salt water, including aquariums, marine organisms, & swimming pools**.
- **Occupational hazard** of aquarium handlers, marine workers, fisherman, & seafood handlers.

CLINICAL MANIFESTATIONS
- Localized cutaneous disease: **erythematous bluish papule or nodule at the site of trauma** that can ulcerate (history of exposure to non-chlorinated water 2 – 3 weeks earlier).
- **Subsequent lesions may occur along the path of lymphatic drainage** over a period of months.

DIAGNOSIS: culture

MANAGEMENT
- No consensus on the regimen or duration of therapy.
- **Rifampin** has been shown to be efficacious.
- Doxycycline, Moxifloxacin have also been used.

LEPROSY (HANSEN's DISEASE)

- Chronic disease cause by ***Mycobacterium leprae & lepromatosis*** that primarily affects superficial tissues (especially the **skin & peripheral nerves**).
- Endemic in subtropical areas. Requires long exposure (few months to 20-50 years incubation period).

CLINICAL MANIFESTATIONS

- **Lepromatous: nodular, plaque, or papular skin lesions (lepromas)** with poorly defined borders. Hypopigmented lesions can be seen especially in cooler areas of the body: face (leonine), ears, wrists, elbows, buttocks, & knees. Loss of eyebrows & eyelashes. Slowly evolving **SYMMETRIC nerve involvement (sensation preserved). Paresthesias in the affected peripheral nerves.** Most commonly seen in immunocompromised patients.

- **Tuberculoid: limited disease:** sharply demarcated **hypopigmented macular lesions numb to the touch (loss of sensation)** with sudden onset of **asymmetric** nerve involvement. Most common in immunocompetent patients (immune system reaction in the nerves causes the loss of sensation).

- Mononeuritis multiplex: nerve damage: posterior tibial nerve, median & ulnar involvement (clawing), common peroneal nerve (foot drop). Vibratory & proprioception preserved.

DIAGNOSIS

- Acid fast bacillus smear performed on tissue obtained from a skin biopsy.

MANAGEMENT

- Lepromatous: Dapsone, Rifampin, Clofazimine x 2-3 years.
- Tuberculoid: Dapsone + Rifampin 6-12 months followed by Dapsone x 2 years.

PARASITIC DISEASES

ENTEROBIASIS (PINWORM)

- Nematode infection caused by ***Enterobius vermicularis* (pinworm).**
- Most common helminthic infection in the US

TRANSMISSION

- Via hand-mouth contact with contaminated fomites, autoinoculation, **fecal-oral contamination** (especially **school-aged children** 5-10 years).

CLINICAL MANIFESTATIONS

- **Perianal itching, especially nocturnal** (eggs are laid at night).
- In severe cases, it may be associated with abdominal pain, nausea, & vomiting.

DIAGNOSIS

- **⊕ Cellophane tape test or pinworm paddle test** early in AM to look for **eggs under a microscope.**

MANAGEMENT

- **Albendazole, Mebendazole, or Pyrantel.**
- If treatment is needed during pregnancy, Pyrantel is preferred.
- Simultaneous treatment of the entire household can help to reduce reinfection.
- Hand washing, trimming of fingernails, and taking a bath early in the morning daily to reduce egg contamination is recommended.

ASCARIASIS

- Giant roundworm infection caused by ***Ascaris lumbricoides*** that parasitizes the human intestine.
- Most common intestinal helminth worldwide.
- TRANSMISSION: ingestion of food or water contaminated with *Ascaris* eggs. Contaminated soil.

PATHOPHYSIOLOGY
- Once ingested, the eggs hatch in the small intestine and the organisms migrates hematogenously to the lungs, where the larvae mature. The larvae migrate caudally to the trachea and are then swallowed, after which they mature, mate, and produce eggs that pass into the stool.

CLINICAL MANIFESTATIONS
- Small worm load: asymptomatic.
- Larger load: vague abdominal symptoms (eg, anorexia, nausea, vomiting, abdominal discomfort).
- High load: intestinal obstruction (most common), hepatic or biliary manifestations. Early stage may develop pulmonary symptoms.

DIAGNOSIS
- **Stool ova and parasite:** examination for ova or visual examination of adult worms. Eosinophilia

MANAGEMENT
- **Albendazole or Mebendazole.**
- Pyrantel if pregnant (given after first trimester)

TRICHINOSIS

- Parasitic roundworm infection cause by *Trichinella* species (especially ***T. spiralis***).

TRANSMISSION: **raw or undercooked meat (especially pork, wild boar, or bear).**

PATHOPHYSIOLOGY
- Larvae cysts are ingested then go to the duodenum and jejunum to grow into adults & replicate.
- Adults are excreted in the stool & larva penetrate intestinal wall & **encapsulate in striated muscle tissue.** Severity of disease correlates with the number of ingested larvae.

CLINICAL MANIFESTATIONS
- **GI phase:** abdominal pain, nausea, diarrhea, & vomiting with progression to muscle phase.
- **Muscle phase: myositis:** muscle pain, tenderness, swelling, and weakness with high fever. Eye: **palpebral or circumorbital edema,** retinal hemorrhages, conjunctival hemorrhages. **Subungual splinter hemorrhages**; macular or urticarial rash, dyspnea, dysphagia.
- Cardiac: **myocarditis** (due to eosinophilia). CNS: encephalitis or meningitis. Pulmonary: pneumonia.

DIAGNOSIS
- Usually a clinical diagnosis confirmed with serologies: consider in any patient with **periorbital edema, myositis, & eosinophilia**.
- **Eosinophilia hallmark; increased creatine kinase & LDH** (due to muscle involvement).

MANAGEMENT
- Mild cases: most cases are mild and self-limited & require only symptomatic treatment (analgesia and antipyretics).
- CNS, cardiac, or pulmonary: **Albendazole** or Mebendazole (antiparasitic) plus Corticosteroids. Albendazole & Mebendazole are contraindicated in children 2 years or younger & in pregnancy.

HOOKWORM

- ***Ancylostoma duodenale*** (human hookworm) in the tropics or subtropics *or* ***Necator americanus*** (N. or S. America, Central Africa, South Pacific, and India). Occasional cases occur in the United States (Southeast). *Ancylostoma ceylanicum* (India & SE Asia).

- 25% of the world is infected.

- **Common in countries with poor access to adequate water, sanitation, and hygiene.**

TRANSMISSION
- 3 conditions needed – **human fecal contamination of soil,** favorable soil conditions for larvae growth (moisture, warmth, shade) and **contact of human skin with contaminated soil** (eg, barefoot or open footwear).

PATHOPHYSIOLOGY
- The larvae penetrate the skin & migrate to the pulmonary capillaries. They are carried to the mouth via the mucociliary escalator & swallowed, where they enter the small bowel and suck blood (whole cycle about ~4 weeks).

CLINICAL MANIFESTATIONS: 4 phases
- Phase 1 (skin): very **pruritic erythematous maculopapular dermatitis** at the site of larvae entry (eg, feet and ankles). Usually resolves within a few days.

- Phase 2 (transpulmonary): **usually asymptomatic**. Mild cough or pharyngeal irritation if symptomatic. Loeffler syndrome = pulmonary symptoms (low grade fever sputum, wheezing, cough) + increased IgE + eosinophilia (rarely seen).

- Phase 3 (GI): nausea, vomiting, diarrhea, mid-epigastric pain (especially postprandial) mimicking peptic ulcers. GI bleeding rare.

- Phase 4 (chronic nutritional impairment): **major impact of hookworm infection.** Hookworms cause blood loss by lacerating capillaries and ingesting blood, leading to **daily loss of blood, iron, and albumin**.

DIAGNOSIS
- Stool examination: Kato-Katz technique for ova and parasites. Not helpful for skin or pulmonary phase. Serial exams may be necessary if negative.

- **Eosinophilia,** increased IgE. Chronic blood loss: **iron deficiency anemia** (hypochromic microcytic anemia) and positive guaiac.

MANAGEMENT
- **Albendazole** or Mebendazole, Pyrantel.

- Supportive: iron supplementation, multivitamins.

CHAGAS DISEASE

- Disease caused by ***Trypanosoma cruzi,*** a protozoan parasite, that is characterized by **dilated cardiomyopathy and GI disease**. **Leading cause of CHF in Latin America.**
- TRANSMISSION: vector is the assassin bug (bites in the evening). Prevalent in Latin America northward to Texas. Congenital, consumption of contaminated food or drink.

ACUTE
- Most are asymptomatic. Symptoms most common in children and are nonspecific (eg, malaise, fever anorexia). Acute illness can last 3 weeks to 3 months.
- Physical examination: **Chagoma:** swelling or inflammation at the bite site. **Romaña sign: unilateral periorbital swelling**. Fever, lymphadenopathy, hepatosplenomegaly.

CHRONIC
- Indeterminate form is associated with positive serologies but no GI or cardiac disease & normal ECG.
- Determinate form associated with destruction of nerve cell ganglia, cardiac, and/or GI complications.
- Cardiac: **dilated cardiomyopathy, CHF,** arrhythmias.
- GI complications: **megacolon** (progressive constipation, colicky abdominal pain & bloating) & **megaesophagus** (progressive dysphagia & regurgitation of food).

DIAGNOSIS
- Acute phase: peripheral blood smear: trypomastigote (flagellated motile form) seen. PCR
- Chronic phase: serology (ELISA)
- ECG: may show arrhythmias (eg, AV blocks)
- Echocardiogram: **cardiomegaly with apical atrophy or aneurysm.**

MANAGEMENT
- Benznidazole or Nifurtimox for 90-120 days depending on age (obtained from CDC). Indications include acute phase and patients without significant cardiac and/or GI disease.

HUMAN AFRICAN TRYPANOSOMIASIS

- Protozoa ***Trypanosoma brucei*** *(rhodesiense & gambiense)*. "African sleeping sickness".
- Transmission: vector is the **Tsetse fly.** Prevalent in Sub-Saharan Africa as well as South & Central America.

CLINICAL MANIFESTATIONS: 2 stages
- Early hemolymphatic stage: **painless chancre at the bite site** 2-3 days after bite, increasing in size, resolving in 2-3 weeks. Intermittent ever, general malaise, headaches, joint pains, & itching. **Generalized or regional lymphadenopathy** (often extremely large).
  Winterbottom sign – posterior cervical lymphadenopathy. Transient rash.
- Late CNS stage: persistent headache, **daytime sleepiness followed by nighttime insomnia** (tryptophol released by *T. brucei* induces sleep), behavioral changes, wasting syndrome, seizures in children.

DIAGNOSIS: Peripheral blood smear or aspiration of an affected lymph node.

MANAGEMENT
- Infectious disease consult.
- *T. brucei gambiense:* Early stage: Pentamidine. Late stage: Eflornithine & Nifurtimox.
- *T. brucei rhodesiense:* Early stage: Suramin. Late stage: Melarsoprol (may add Nifurtimox).

MALARIA

- Mosquito-borne **red blood cell disease caused by *Plasmodium spp*** (*falciparum, vivax, ovale, malariae*). **Falciparum most dangerous type.**
- Distribution: throughout most of the tropics, especially in Sub-Saharan Africa.
- Sickle cell trait & thalassemia trait are protective vs. Malaria.
- Pathophysiology: *Plasmodium spp.* infects red blood cells causing RBC lysis, leading to cyclical fever.

TRANSMISSION

- Protozoa that are transmitted via the **female *Anopheles* mosquito** (especially at dusk & dawn).

CLINICAL MANIFESTATIONS

- **Cyclical fever** (cold stage/chills followed by hot stage/fever followed by diaphoretic stage every other or third day), headache, fatigue, myalgias, GI symptoms. Splenomegaly. Cyclical fever every 48 hours (*P. vivax & P. ovale*) & 72 hours (*P. malariae*). Irregular fever with *P. falciparum*.

- **P. falciparum: cerebral malaria** (AMS, delirium, seizures, coma), **blackwater fever** = severe hemolysis + hemoglobinuria (dark urine) + renal failure.

DIAGNOSIS

- Clinical diagnosis – suspect in patients with fever who traveled to endemic area + parasitic diagnosis.

- **Giemsa-stained blood smear: (thin & thick)** - parasites (trophozoites & schizonts) in RBCs with light microscopy. Thick smear for detection, thin smear for speciation. Schuffner's dots (small brick-red granules throughout the erythrocyte cytoplasm) seen with *P. vivax & ovale.*

- Rapid diagnostic tests: antigen or antibody. Can pick up very low parasitemia.

- **Leukopenia, hemolytic anemia, thrombocytopenia.**

MANAGEMENT

- **Chloroquine first-line treatment of uncomplicated *P. falciparum* in sensitive regions.** Hydroxychloroquine is an alternative.
- Primaquine is an add-on agent used to kill latent hypnozoites in *P. vivax & P. ovale* infections to prevent recurrence (test for G6PD prior to use).

Chloroquine resistant *P. falciparum*:

- **Artemisinin combination therapy** (eg, Artemether-lumefantrine) or **Atovaquone-proguanil.**
- Second-line: Quinine sulfate plus either Doxycycline, Tetracycline, or Clindamycin.

Chloroquine resistant *P. vivax*:

- Quinine sulfate plus Doxycycline or Tetracycline + Primaquine
- Atovaquone-proguanil plus Primaquine
- Mefloquine plus Primaquine

Life threatening infection

- IV Quinidine gluconate

Prophylaxis

- Options include Atovaquone/Proguanil, Mefloquine, Doxycycline, and Tafenoquine.

BABESIOSIS

- Infectious disease caused by Malaria-like protozoa of the *Babesia spp* (eg, ***Babesia microti***).

TRANSMISSION:
- Tick vectors (eg, ***Ixodes scapularis,*** the same tick for Lyme disease).
- Rarely, transmission can occur via blood transfusion, congenitally or via transplantation.

RISK FACTORS
- Location: endemic to upper Midwest & **Northeast US** (eg, Long Island, Massachusetts).
- **Elderly, asplenia, and immunocompromised.**

PATHOPHYSIOLOGY
- Similar to Malaria, the *Babesia* protozoa **infect and lyse red blood cells, leading to hemolysis.**

CLINICAL MANIFESTATIONS
- **Malaria-like symptoms** - fever, chills, fatigue, sweats, headache, myalgia, jaundice, arthralgia, and anorexia.

DIAGNOSIS
- Peripheral blood smear with Giemsa or Wright stain – parasites within RBCs especially in **pathognomonic tetrads** (Maltese cross appearance). **Intraerythrocytic ring forms** with central pallor. Best initial test.
- CBC: **mild to severe hemolytic anemia** (decreased haptoglobin, increased reticulocytes), lymphopenia, thrombocytopenia. Increased transaminases.
- PCR: for detection of *Babesia* DNA. Most accurate test. Serologies.

MANAGEMENT
- Atovaquone + Azithromycin OR
- Quinine + Clindamycin

LEISHMANIASIS

- Caused by *Leishmania* protozoan **transmitted via the female Sand fly.**
- Prevalent in Mediterranean, Central & South America, Africa, & Asia.

CLINICAL MANIFESTATIONS
- **Localized cutaneous: ❶ small erythematous papule** that enlarges into a nodule, leading to painless **ulceration** with an indurated border OR **❷ dry, indurated plaque** with **satellite pustules** that develops at the bite site weeks to months after infection. May crust over in the center **leaving a raised, bordered scar.** May become painful later but **not painful initially.** May be multiple if diffuse. **Regional lymphadenopathy.**
- **Mucocutaneous: ulcers of the skin, mouth, and nose** (especially cartilaginous areas).
- **Visceral:** fulminant disease if organism migrates liver, spleen, & bone marrow (***hepatosplenomegaly***).

DIAGNOSIS
- Demonstration of the parasite in a clinical specimen (often the skin) by culture, histology or PCR.
- Disseminated: direct visualization of aspirates from the liver, spleen, or marrow if visceral (*Leishmania donovani* has a higher incidence of causing visceral infection).

MANAGEMENT
- Infectious disease consult. Sores usually heal spontaneously.

TOXOPLASMOSIS

- Infection due to ***Toxoplasma gondii*** (intracellular **protozoa**).
- Most common CNS infection in patients with AIDS not receiving appropriate prophylaxis or not on HAART.

TRANSMISSION

- Ingestion of infectious oocysts, usually from **soil or cat litter contaminated with feline feces** or undercooked meat from an infected animal.

CLINICAL MANIFESTATIONS

- Primary infection: usually asymptomatic infection in immunocompetent patients. May develop a Mono-like illness with cervical lymphadenopathy if symptomatic.

Reactivation associated with Encephalitis & Chorioretinitis.

- **Encephalitis:** headache, neurologic symptoms, fever, AMS, focal neurologic deficits. Seen especially seen with **CD4 count ≤ 100 cells/microL**. May have cervical lymphadenopathy.
- **Chorioretinitis:** posterior uveitis – eye pain and decreased visual acuity.
- Pneumonitis: fever, dyspnea, & nonproductive cough (similar to PCP pneumonia).

DIAGNOSIS

- Clinical diagnosis: presumptive diagnosis of CD4 ≤ 100 cells/microL not on prophylaxis, compatible symptoms, positive *T. gondii* IgG antibody, MRI imaging consistent (eg, multiple ring-enhancing lesions).
- Serologies: **anti-toxoplasma IgG antibodies** via ELISA.
- Neuroimaging: **multiple ring-enhancing lesions** (nonspecific as they may also be seen with CNS lymphoma). MRI preferred > head CT.
- CSF: mononuclear pleocytosis, increased protein, may have reduced CSF glucose. CSF PCR.

MANAGEMENT

- **Sulfadiazine** (or Clindamycin) + **Pyrimethamine (with folinic acid/Leucovorin** to prevent folic acid depletion).
- Spiramycin if pregnant.

PROPHYLAXIS:

- **Trimethoprim-sulfamethoxazole is first-line prophylaxis when CD4 count is ≤ 100.**
- Second-line: Dapsone + Pyrimethamine & Leucovorin.

CONGENITAL TOXOPLASMA INFECTION

- Associated with the **triad of chorioretinitis, hydrocephalus, and intracranial calcifications.**
- Other findings include seizures, jaundice, hepatosplenomegaly, lymphadenopathy, and thrombocytopenia.
- Most congenital infections are asymptomatic with subclinical disease.
- Congenital Toxoplasma infection is part of ToRCH syndrome: Toxoplasmosis, Other (Syphilis), Rubella, CMV, HSV.

DIAGNOSIS

- Serologies: **anti-toxoplasma IgM antibodies** best initial test. PCR for Toxoplasmosis most accurate.

MANAGEMENT

- **Sulfadiazine + Pyrimethamine**

CAT SCRATCH DISEASE

- Etiology: ***Bartonella henselae*** transmitted from the **scratch or bite from an infected cat or exposure to cat fleas** (2-4 week incubation period).
- Risk factors: most common in children and young adults.

CLINICAL MANIFESTATIONS
- Brown or red **papule or ulcer at the inoculation site**.
- 1-7 weeks later, the development of **fever,** headache, malaise followed by **lymphadenopathy** (erythema & warmth of the overlying skin) lasting 2-4 months.

DIAGNOSIS
Based on clinical presentation & lab studies
- **Serologic: most common test used** - via ELISA or indirect immunofluorescence assay. **A negative test does not rule out CSD.** Empiric treatment usually given in those with a presumed diagnosis.
- Biopsy: of skin lesions or lymph node – may perform PCR to detect bacterial DNA, Warthin-Starry silver staining & histology on the sample (neutrophilic infiltrate & granulomatous changes). Biopsy not usually required.

MANAGEMENT
- **Mild: symptomatic treatment (usually self-limited)** - antipyretics, analgesics, warm compresses.
- Moderate: **Azithromycin first line. Doxycycline.**
- Severe: Rifampin, Gentamicin, Ciprofloxacin.
- Doxycycline (or Azithromycin) + Rifampin preferred if ocular, neurologic disease or hepatosplenomegaly.

CHANCROID

- Sexually transmitted infection leading to genital ulcers, lymphadenopathy, and bubo formation.
- Etiology: ***Haemophilus ducreyi*** transmitted after a break in the skin. Gram-negative fastidious coccobacillus.
- Incubation period 3-7 days.
- Risk factors: most common in children and young adults.
- 10% coinfection with HSV or Syphilis in the US (rare in US).

CLINICAL MANIFESTATIONS
- One or more **painful genital ulcers** at the inoculation site (well-defined irregular borders that are sometimes undermined on an erythematous base & may be covered with a gray or yellow purulent exudate) followed by **painful inguinal lymphadenopathy,** which can liquefy and become fluctuant (**bubo formation**).

DIAGNOSIS
- Usually a clinical diagnosis (difficult to culture).
- PCR or immunochromatography.
- Must rule out HSV by (PCR or culture) and rule out Syphilis.

MANAGEMENT
- **Azithromycin** 1g x 1 dose.
- Ceftriaxone 250mg IM x 1; Erythromycin 500mg tid x 7 days; Ciprofloxacin.

PRENATAL TRANSMISSION OF DISORDERS

CONGENITAL VARICELLA SYNDROME

- Occurs if **mothers develop Varicella (chickenpox) between 8 and 20 weeks' gestation**.

CLINICAL MANIFESTATIONS

- Scarring skin lesions, abnormalities of the limb (eg, hypoplasia of bone and muscle)
- Ocular abnormalities (eg, cataracts, chorioretinitis, microphthalmos)
- CNS abnormalities (seizures, cognitive deficits)

PREVENTION

Varicella Immune globulin (VZIG) reduces the severity of infection after exposure to Varicella virus in patients at high risk for severe infection and complications including:

- **Newborns of mothers with Varicella 5 days before to 2 days after delivery**.
- Premature infants at or greater than 28 weeks' gestation who are exposed and whose mother has no evidence of immunity.
- Premature infants < 28 weeks' gestation or who weigh <1000 g at birth and were exposed during hospitalization.
- Pregnant women who lack evidence of immunity to VZV

NEONATAL HERPES SIMPLEX VIRUS

PERINATALLY-ACQUIRED INFECTION

- Majority of neonatal HSV infection are acquired perinatally, via an infected maternal genital tract.

CLINICAL MANIFESTATIONS

- Localized to the skin, mouth, and eyes – classic vesicular lesions; ulcerations of the mouth, tongue, and palate; conjunctivitis & excessive tearing.
- Localized CNS disease: seizures, irritability, tremors, lethargy, poor feeding.
- Disseminated disease: temperature instability, which can lead to jaundice, hypotension, respiratory distress, DIC, & septic shock. May have skin & CNS involvement.

DIAGNOSIS

- Viral culture, PCR, viral antigens using direct immunofluorescence assays. Serologies not helpful.
  - Collected specimens: swabs/scrapings of skin lesions for viral culture. Surface swabs (mouth, conjunctivae, nasopharynx, rectum) for viral culture or HSV PCR. CSF for PCR. Blood or plasma for PCR (HSV DNA).

MANAGEMENT

- IV Acyclovir x 14 days followed by oral suppressive Acyclovir for 6 months. Topical ophthalmic solution (eg, Trifluridine, Idoxuridine, Ganciclovir) added if ocular involvement.

CONGENITAL (IN UTERO) INFECTION

Rare.

- Intrauterine infection due to maternal viremia: occurs due to primary HSV infection during pregnancy.
  - Clinical manifestations: triad of skin vesicles, ulcerations, or scarring + severe CNS involvement (eg, hydrancephaly, microcephaly) + ocular damage.

- Intrauterine infection due to ascending infection: occurs in mothers with active HSV infection after prolonged rupture of membranes.
  - Clinical manifestations: cutaneous skin lesions, cutaneous scarring, signs of disseminated disease, or fatal neonatal pneumonitis.

ZIKA VIRUS

- Arthropod-borne flavivirus transmitted by ***Aedes* mosquito (eg, *A. aegypti*).**

TRANSMISSION
- **Bite of an infected mosquito, sex** (oral, vaginal, and anal), **maternal-fetal,** blood product transfusion, organ transplantation, and laboratory exposure.

RISK FACTORS
- Residence in or travel to an area where mosquito-borne transmission of Zika virus infection has been reported or unprotected sexual intercourse with a person who meets these criteria (common in Central & South America, the Caribbean, & the Pacific).

ASSOCIATED CONDITIONS
- Guillain-Barré syndrome or permanent neurological damage.
- **Congenital Zika syndrome: microcephaly, intracranial cerebral malformation**, ocular lesions, congenital contractures, and hypertonia.

CLINICAL MANIFESTATIONS
- **Most are asymptomatic**.
- Self-limited symptoms in 20% include low-grade fever, maculopapular pruritic rash (trunk followed by extremities), arthralgias (especially small joints of hands and feet), or conjunctivitis (nonpurulent).
- Hematospermia in males.

DIAGNOSIS
- **Serum or urine Zika virus IgM initial test of choice**.
- Reverse-transcriptase PCR of the serum or urine. Can be used as screening in pregnant women (in the first & second trimester) with risk factors.

MANAGEMENT
- Supportive care: hydration, acetaminophen for fever and arthritis.
- Aspirin should not be used until Dengue fever has been ruled out and not used in children (increased risk of Reye syndrome).

PREVENTION
- CDC recommendation (August 2018) – **men with relevant history should wait at least 3 months** after Zika virus onset (if symptomatic) or last possible exposure (if asymptomatic) before having unprotected sex.
- **Women** (whether symptomatic or not) should wait **at least 8 weeks** after symptom onset (if symptomatic) or last possible exposure (if asymptomatic) before having unprotected sex.
- Relevant exposure = residence in or travel to an area where mosquito-borne transmission of Zika virus infection has been reported or unprotected sexual intercourse with a person who meets these criteria.
- Pregnant women should avoid or consider postponing travel to areas below 6,500 feet where mosquito transmission is ongoing.

CONGENITAL ZIKA SYNDROME
- **Characterized by 5 main features: severe microcephaly, decreased brain tissue** (including subcortical calcifications), **eye damage** (macular and retinal changes), **congenital contractures** (eg, clubfoot or arthrogryposis), & **hypertonia** restricting body movement after birth.

PERINATAL OR PRENATAL HPV INFECTION

- Perinatal or prenatal Human papillomavirus infection can occur via ascension of the infection into the uterus and via hematogenous spread.
- Clinical manifestations: perianal warts

CONGENITAL RUBELLA SYNDROME

- Rubella infection is teratogenic, **especially in the first trimester.**
- Part of the ToRCH syndrome

CLINICAL MANIFESTATIONS
- Most are asymptomatic at birth. Neonates may have growth retardation, radiolucent bone disease, hepatosplenomegaly, purpuric skin lesions **"blueberry muffin" rash** (due to Thrombotic thrombocytopenic purpura and extramedullary hematopoiesis).
- **Triad of cardiac defects, eye defects, and auditory defects.**
- Auditory: sensorineural deafness.
- Cardiac defects: **patent ductus arteriosus most common,** pulmonary artery stenosis.
- Eye defects: cataracts, glaucoma, retinopathy.
- Neurologic: developmental delays, meningoencephalitis,
- Endocrine: Diabetes mellitus, thyroid dysfunction, liver dysfunction, hyperbilirubinemia.

DIAGNOSIS
- RV-IgG antibodies in neonatal serum using ELISA.

MANAGEMENT
- Supportive

PREVENTION
- Maternal screening: with rubella titers in early pregnancy. Laboratory diagnosis if symptoms consistent with Rubella (RV -IgG and IgM titers).

CONGENITAL SYPHILIS

- Congenital infection can lead to stillbirth, prematurity, and hydrops fetalis.
- Part of the ToRCH syndrome

CLINICAL MANIFESTATIONS
- Most are asymptomatic at birth.
- Early < 2 years of age: mucocutaneous (eg, syphilitic rhinitis, rash), hematologic abnormalities, CNS, pulmonary complications.
- Late > 2 years of age: facial abnormalities - **saddle nose deformity, Hutchinson teeth (notched teeth)**, chorioretinitis, sensorineural hearing loss, & developmental delays.

DIAGNOSIS
- Symptoms consistent with congenital Syphilis + VDRL or RPR titer ≥fourfold the maternal titer; Positive darkfield microscopy or fluorescent antibody testing of the umbilical cord, placenta, or body fluids.

MANAGEMENT
- **IV Penicillin** x 10 days.

SPIROCHETAL DISEASES

SYPHILIS

- Chronic infection caused by the spirochete ***Treponema pallidum.***
- Known as "the great imitator" because the rash & disease can present in many different ways similar to other diseases.

TRANSMISSION

- **Direct contact of a mucocutaneous lesion** (eg, **sexual activity**). May also be transmitted to the fetus via the placenta.

PATHOPHYSIOLOGY

- *T. pallidum* enters tissues from direct contact, forming a chancre at the inoculation site and from there, goes to the regional lymph nodes before disseminating.

CLINICAL MANIFESTATIONS

Primary Syphilis

- **Chancre: painless ulcer at or near the inoculation site** with raised indurated edges (usually begins as a papule that ulcerates). Chancres heal spontaneously on average within 3-4 weeks (even without medical management).

- Nontender regional lymphadenopathy near the chancre site lasting 3-4 weeks.

Secondary Syphilis

Symptoms may occur a few weeks - 6 months after the initial symptoms.

- **Maculopapular rash** diffuse bilateral maculopapular lesions **(involvement of the palms & soles common).** Lesions may be pustular in some patients.

- **Condyloma lata:** wart-like, moist lesions involving the mucous membranes & other moist areas. Especially near the chancre site. Highly contagious.

- Systemic symptoms: fever, lymphadenopathy (may be tender), arthritis, meningitis, headache, hepatitis (elevated alkaline phosphatase), alopecia.

Tertiary (late) Syphilis

May occur from 1 to > 20 years after initial infection or after latent infection.

- **Gumma:** noncancerous granulomas on skin & body tissues (eg, bones).

- **Neurosyphilis:** headache, meningitis, dementia, vision/hearing loss, incontinence; **Tabes dorsalis** (demyelination of posterior columns leading to ataxia, areflexia, burning pain, weakness).

- **Argyll-Robertson pupil**: small, irregular pupil that constricts with accommodation but is not reactive to light.

- **Cardiovascular**: **aortitis,** aortic regurgitation, aortic aneurysms.

DIAGNOSIS

Nontreponemal tests (screening):

- **RPR** (Rapid Plasma Reagin). These tests look at titers (eg, a positive test indicates a titer of 1:32 or greater). Because they are nonspecific, a **positive RPR or VDRL test must be confirmed** by specific **treponemal testing (eg, FTA-ABS).** RPR is usually positive 4-6 weeks after infection. Changes in titers also help to determine therapeutic response.

- **VDRL:** Venereal Disease Research Laboratory.

- Nontreponemal tests are nonspecific. False positives can be seen with antiphospholipid syndrome, pregnancy, tuberculosis, *Rickettsial* infections (eg, Rocky Mountain spotted fever).

Treponemal testing (confirmatory):

- **FTA-ABS** (fluorescent treponemal antibody absorption)
- Microhemagglutination test for *T. pallidum* antibodies.

Darkfield microscopy

- Allows for **direct visualization of *T. pallidum*** from **chancre or condyloma lata.**

MANAGEMENT

- **Penicillin is the treatment of choice for all stages of Syphilis.**

Early Syphilis: (primary, secondary & early latent)

- **Penicillin G benzathine 2.4 million units IM x 1 dose.**
- Doxycycline for 14 days if Penicillin-allergic.

Late Syphilis: (tertiary or late latent)

- **Penicillin G benzathine 2.4 million units IM once weekly x 3 weeks.**

Neurosyphilis:

- **IV Penicillin G preferred** (3-4 million units every 4 hours for 10 – 14 days).
- Patients with Penicillin allergy who are pregnant, present with neurosyphilis, have cardiovascular manifestation of late syphilis, or have treatment failure should be tested for Penicillin allergy and desensitized (if immediate-type reaction) or rechallenged (if delayed reaction) with Penicillin.

MONITORING

- All patients with Syphilis should be tested for HIV and other STIs.
- All patients should be reexamined clinically & serologically at 6 months and 12 months after treatment. Patients with HIV may be monitored more frequently.
- A nontreponemal titer should be obtained prior to initiating therapy. A fourfold decline in the nontreponemal titer within 6 months is considered an acceptable response.

JARISCH-HERXHEIMER REACTION

- An **acute, self-limited febrile reaction** that usually occurs **within the first 24 hours after receiving therapy for a spirochetal infection** (eg, Syphilis, Lyme disease).
- It is thought to be due to the release of cytokines and immune complexes from killed organisms.
- It classically presents with **fever, chills, headache, myalgias, hypotension, and worsening of the rash may occur.**

Management

- Is self-limited and usually resolves without intervention in 12 to 24 hours but NSAIDS or antipyretics may be used for symptoms.

LYME DISEASE

- Arthropod-borne disease due to ***Borrelia burgdorferi*** (gram-negative **spirochete**) that is spread by the Deer tick. Most common in the spring & summer (when the nymphs feed).

PATHOPHYSIOLOGY

- Most cases are **transmitted by the *Ixodes scapularis* (deer tick)** in the nymphal phase – most common sources are the white-tailed deer & white-footed mouse.
- The highest likelihood of transmission is if the tick is engorged and/or has been attached for at least 72 hours (minimum of 24 hours needed for transmission).
- **Most common in the Northeast states** (CT, NY, NJ, MA), Midwest, & Mid-Atlantic regions of the US.

CLINICAL MANIFESTATIONS

- **Early localized: erythema migrans** (90%) **– expanding, warm, annular, erythematous rash** that may develop **central clearing (bull's eye or target** appearance) usually within a month of and around the area of the tick bite. May be accompanied by a viral-like syndrome (eg, fatigue, headache, fever, malaise, arthralgias and/or lymphadenopathy).

- Early disseminated: (1-12 weeks) **neurologic**: cranial nerve palsies (**CN VII/Facial nerve palsy most common neurologic manifestation),** headache, meningitis, weakness, neuropathy; **cardiac: AV block most common cardiac manifestation,** pericarditis, & arrhythmias; Multiple erythema migrans lesions.

- Late disease: **intermittent or persistent arthritis most common,** especially of the large joints (**knee most common**), persistent neurological symptoms (eg, subtle cognitive changes, distal paresthesias, spinal radicular pain, & subacute encephalitis).

DIAGNOSIS

- **Clinical: especially in early localized Lyme disease** (eg, **erythema migrans** rash - patients with the rash of EM residing in or who have recently traveled to an endemic area should be treated for Lyme). **Patients with erythema migrans are often seronegative in this early stage.**

- **Serologic testing: ELISA followed by Western Blot if ELISA is positive or equivocal.** IgM &/or IgG antibodies to *B. burgdorferi* are employed as an adjunct to patients with clinical symptoms suggestive of Lyme disease as it only tells if a patient has been infected with the spirochete (does not determine if the person has an active infection). Serologic testing is used in patients who fit all 3 criteria:
  - Reside in or travel to an endemic area PLUS
  - Risk factor for exposure to ticks PLUS
  - Symptoms consistent with early disseminated or late Lyme disease (arthritis, meningitis, cranial nerve palsy, carditis, radiculopathy, or mononeuritis).

  Because serologic testing takes weeks to become positive and does not distinguish acute from past infection, serologic testing is **not** performed in:
  - **Patients with an erythema migrans** rash (patients with the rash of EM residing in or who have recently traveled to an endemic area should be treated for Lyme).
  - Screening of asymptomatic patients living in endemic areas.
  - Patients with non-specific symptoms only.

- False positive ELISA: other spirochetal diseases: syphilis, yaws; viral or bacterial illnesses & other Borrelial species.

MANAGEMENT

Early disease:

- **Doxycycline first-line** bid x 10-21 days for early localized (early disseminated duration 14-28 days).
- Amoxicillin and Cefuroxime are alternatives.
- **Amoxicillin treatment of choice in pregnancy** (14-21 day course). Cefuroxime.
- Azithromycin or Erythromycin.

Late or severe:

- **IV Ceftriaxone if second/third AV heart block, syncope, dyspnea, chest pain**, CNS disease, other than CN VII palsy (eg, **Meningitis)**.

PROPHYLAXIS

- **Prophylaxis for Lyme disease (Doxycycline 200mg x 1 dose)** may be given within 72 hours of tick removal if the tick was present for at least 36 hours (determined by severity of tick engorgement or time of exposure) and there are > 20% of infected ticks in the area where the bite occurred.
- If Doxycycline cannot be used (eg, allergic or contraindicated) no prophylaxis is given.

OTHER DISEASES

TULAREMIA

- ***Francisella tularensis*** – gram negative coccobacillus.
- Transmission: **rabbits important reservoir, ticks, deer flies,** fleas, or handling animal tissues.

CLINICAL MANIFESTATIONS: most are asymptomatic

- **Ulceroglandular most common type.** Fever, headache nausea followed by a **single papule at the site of inoculation,** followed by ulceration of papule with **central eschar formation & tender regional lymphadenopathy.** Ulcers of the hand or arm most common after animal exposure. Ulcers of the head, trunk, or legs most common after tick exposure. Splenomegaly.
- Glandular: tender regional lymphadenopathy without skin lesions (most common in children).
- Oculoglandular: if splashed in the eye with infected material followed by eye pain, photophobia, & tearing + regional lymphadenopathy (preauricular, postauricular, cervical).
- Pharyngeal: fever or sore throat following ingestion of contaminated food or water.
- Typhoidal: ingestion of infected meat (eg, undercooked rabbit meat) followed by fever & GI symptoms (nausea, vomiting, diarrhea).
- Pneumonia, meningitis, pericarditis.

DIAGNOSIS

- **Serologies.** Cultures not usually performed (they produce dangerous spores).

MANAGEMENT

- **Streptomycin drug of choice.** Gentamicin if severe. Fluoroquinolones or Doxycycline.

DISEASES WITH ESCHARS: Tularemia, Anthrax, Leishmaniasis, Coccidioidomycosis, Mucormycosis

BRUCELLOSIS

- ***Brucella spp.*** are gram-negative coccobacilli (*B. melitensis* most common).
- **Endemic in Mediterranean, Mexico & South America.** Rare in US.

TRANSMISSION
- **Ingestion of infected dairy products (eg, unpasteurized milk & cheese),** consumption of undercooked meat.
- Occupational exposure, such as **Veterinarian or farmer or contact with livestock** (eg, goat, sheep, cattle, hogs) or those handling infected tissues.

CLINICAL MANIFESTATIONS
- **Nonspecific symptoms - triad of undulant fever (most common)** + sweating (often described as moldy, wet hay smell) + migratory arthralgia or myalgia.
- Weakness, headache, anorexia, weight loss, easy exhaustion.
- Physical examination: hepatosplenomegaly & lymphadenopathy.

DIAGNOSIS
- Blood culture, bone marrow culture (higher yield), serologies (IgM or IgG), lymphocytosis.

MANAGEMENT
- **Doxycycline + Rifampin first-line.**
- Alternative: Doxycycline plus either Streptomycin, Gentamicin or Trimethoprim-sulfamethoxazole.
- Rifampin + Trimethoprim-sulfamethoxazole in children.

COMPLICATIONS
- Endocarditis most lethal. Meningoencephalitis.
- 20% develop Osteomyelitis (especially of the lumbar spine).

HOT TUB FOLLICULITIS

- Benign self-limited skin lesions caused by ***Pseudomonas aeruginosa.***
- Commonly seen 8-48 hours after exposure to water in a **contaminated spa, swimming pool, or hot tub (especially** if it is **made of wood).**

CLINICAL MANIFESTATIONS
- **Small** (2–10 mm), **tender, pruritic, pink to red papules, papulopustules or nodules** around the hair follicles.
- May have malaise and low grade fever.

MANAGEMENT
- **No treatment needed in most cases** - usually spontaneously resolves within 7–14 days without treatment.
- **Ciprofloxacin orally if persistent.**

Q FEVER

- Zoonotic infection caused by ***Coxiella burnetii.*** Gram-negative.

TRANSMISSION

- Inhalation of spores or ingestion. **Exposure to farm animals** (eg, **sheep, goats, cattle) & their products** (eg, **wool, unpasteurized milk**). Individuals living downwind from farms & contaminated manure, straw, or dust.

CLINICAL MANIFESTATIONS

- **Acute: pneumonia is the main manifestation of acute Q fever.** Influenza-like illness: severe headache, fever (with relative bradycardia), cough, abdominal pain, **hepatitis,** or encephalopathy.
- **Chronic: culture-negative endocarditis main manifestation of chronic Q fever.** Vascular infection of the aorta, persistent low grade fever, rash (septic thromboembolism).

DIAGNOSIS

- Acute: **immunofluorescence IFA most common test used** (Coxiella anti-phase II immunoglobulins). PCR.
- Chronic: Phase I IgG immunoglobulins.
- Leukopenia, increased LFTs. Weil-Felix testing was used prior to IFA.
- All patients with Q fever should have a transthoracic echocardiogram.

MANAGEMENT

- **Doxycycline initial treatment of choice.** Fluoroquinolones, Macrolides, Trimethoprim-sulfamethoxazole.
- Rifampin may be used in chronic disease.

ERYSIPELOID

- Self-limited soft tissue infection caused by *Erysipelothrix rhusiopathiae* (gram-positive bacillus).
- May lead to systemic infection.

TRANSMISSION

- **Occupational disease follows skin abrasion, puncture wound from raw fish, shellfish, raw meat or poultry** (eg, butchers, slaughterhouse workers, fisherman, farmers, & veterinarians).

CLINICAL MANIFESTATIONS

- **Localized cutaneous:** limited to hands, fingers, or web spaces - **red macule at the inoculation site** followed by **non-pitting edema, purplish (violaceous) lesion with sharp irregular raised borders extending peripherally but clearing centrally.**
- Diffuse cutaneous: may be associated with fever, arthralgia + involvement of other areas.
- Generalized: low grade fever. Endocarditis & bacteremia uncommon but serious sequelae.

DIAGNOSIS

- Usually clinical. Culture from material obtained during biopsy.

MANAGEMENT

- **Penicillin first line** (eg, Penicillin VK, **Amoxicillin,** or G benzathine)
- Cephalexin or Clindamycin are alternatives.

PLAGUE

- ***Yersinia pestis*** (gram-negative rod). Incubation period 2-10 days.
- Rare in US (10-15 cases/year in US in states like Arizona, New Mexico, California, Colorado, Utah).

TRANSMISSION
- **Flea bites** (eg, **rodent fleas**). Respiratory droplets from untreated person with pulmonic form.

CLINICAL MANIFESTATIONS
- Rapid onset of fever, chills, weakness, malaise, myalgias, tachycardia, severe headache, & altered mental status. 3 main forms:
- **Bubonic: most common form** (95%) - **acutely swollen, extremely, warm, red, painful nodes (buboes)** 2-10cm in diameter in the **groin, axilla, & cervical regions.** Lymphatic spread may lead to hematogenous spread (can become septicemic or pulmonic).
- **Septicemic:** subsequent, advanced disease characterized by **DIC & gangrene**. Plague without the presence of buboes. **DIC: extensive purpura** 'black death". **Acral gangrene:** distal extremities, nose, or penis. Patients often die from pneumonia or meningitis.
- **Pneumonic:** tachypnea, productive cough, frothy **blood-tinged sputum** "red death", cyanosis. **Most lethal form** (nearly 100% mortality if not treated within 24 hours of symptom onset).

DIAGNOSIS
- Gram stain from tissue: bipolar staining **(safety pin appearance).** Cultures.

MANAGEMENT
- **Streptomycin or Gentamicin first line treatment.** Doxycycline second line.
- Place on strict respiratory isolation for at least 48 hours after initiating antibiotic therapy.
- Post exposure prophylaxis: Doxycycline or Tetracycline. Trimethoprim-sulfamethoxazole is an alternative.

NECROTIZING FASCIITIS (FLESH EATING DISEASE)

- Necrotizing soft tissue infection leading to rapid tissue destruction, systemic toxicity, & high mortality.
- Etiologies: **usually polymicrobial (Group A *Streptococcus*** most common isolate).
- Risk factors: Diabetes mellitus, chronic corticosteroid use, alcohol abuse, IV drug use.

CLINICAL MANIFESTATIONS
- Erythema & **extreme pain out of proportion to physical exam** followed by the development of **blue, hemorrhagic bullae (blisters at site)** followed by **gangrene** followed by septic shock. Crepitus may be elicited.
- **Fournier gangrene**: necrotizing fasciitis of the **perineum, often with scrotal involvement** especially seen with **impaired immunity (eg, Diabetes Mellitus)** or after trauma to the area.

DIAGNOSIS
- **Established via surgical exploration** of the soft tissues in the operating room.

MANAGEMENT
- **Immediate & aggressive surgical debridement mainstay of treatment + broad spectrum antibiotics:**
  - Carbapenem or Piperacillin-Tazobactam PLUS MRSA coverage (Vancomycin or Daptomycin) PLUS Clindamycin (Clindamycin has antitoxin effects on *streptococci* and *staphylococci*).

LISTERIOSIS

- ***Listeria monocytogenes*** non-spore forming, endotoxin-producing, gram-positive bacilli.
- Transmission: most commonly found in contaminated food (eg, **cold deli meats, hot dogs,** & **unpasteurized dairy products, such as soft cheese & milk).**

RISK FACTORS

- Highest in 4 populations: children, the elderly, immunocompromised states, and during pregnancy.

CLINICAL MANIFESTATIONS

- Listeriosis: **bacteremia and/or meningitis** in **infants <2 months, immunocompromised, & elderly.** Third most common cause of neonatal bacterial Meningitis.
- Listerial febrile illness: fever, "flu-like" symptoms & diarrhea. Self-limited (lasts about 48 hours).
- Pregnancy: **third trimester** - febrile illness **associated with premature labor, stillbirth, or infected newborns** (may have brown or cloudy amniotic fluid).

DIAGNOSIS: Cultures: blood or CSF - gram-positive facultative intracellular bacilli

MANAGEMENT

- **IV Ampicillin initial management of choice** (or Penicillin G).
- **Gentamicin** often added for synergy in meningitis, endocarditis & infections in immunocompromised patients. *Listeria is resistant to all Cephalosporins.*
- Meningitis: Ampicillin + Cefotaxime + Gentamicin if < 1 month old. >50 years – Vancomycin + Ceftriaxone + Ampicillin.
- Trimethoprim-sulfamethoxazole in Penicillin-allergic patients.
- Listerial febrile gastroenteritis: oral Amoxicillin in immunocompromised, pregnancy, and older adult patients. Trimethoprim-sulfamethoxazole is an alternative in non-pregnant patients. In all other immunocompetent patients, antibiotics are not usually given since it is self-limited.

AMEBIASIS

- ***Entamoeba histolytica*** – protozoan most commonly transmitted by ingestion of cysts from fecally-contaminated food and/or water. May also be associated with **amebic liver abscess.**
- Not common in the US. Usually occurs in migrants from or travelers to endemic areas.

CLINICAL MANIFESTATIONS

- Most infections are asymptomatic. Liver abscess: fever, RUQ pain, anorexia.
- GI symptoms: 1-3 week subacute onset of a range of **mild diarrhea to severe dysentery** (abdominal pain, diarrhea, bloody stools, mucus in stools, weight loss, fever).

DIAGNOSIS

- Stool microscopy O&P (ova & parasites) – cysts with ingested RBCs. Because cysts are not constantly shed, at least 3 stool samples on different days should be examined.
- Antigen testing (eg, ELISA) – sensitive, easy to perform and rapid.
- Stool PCR – detects parasitic DNA or RNA in the stool. Liver abscess: ultrasound, CT or MRI

MANAGEMENT

- **Colitis: Metronidazole** or Tinidazole followed by an intraluminal parasitic (eg, **Paromomycin,** Diloxanide furoate or Diiodohydroxyquinoline).
- **Liver abscess:** Metronidazole or Tinidazole + intraluminal antiparasitic followed by Chloroquine. May need drainage if no response to medications after 3 days.
- Asymptomatic infections should be treated with an intraluminal agent alone.

ANTHRAX

- ***Bacillus anthracis*** (gram-positive, spore-forming rod) is **naturally found in livestock** (eg, cattle, horses, goats, sheep).

TRANSMISSION
- Inhalation, ingestion of spores or direct contact (eg, **wool, handling animal hide or hair**).

CLINICAL MANIFESTATIONS
- **Cutaneous:** 5-14 days after exposure - erythematous papule at the inoculation site that ulcerates followed by a **painless black eschar** with edematous borders & vesicles. **Most common type.**
- GI: rare in the US. Ingestion of meat with spores lead to ulcerative lesion (eg, GI bleeding, abdominal pain, nausea and vomiting).
- Inhalation: nonspecific flu-like symptoms rapidly progressing to dyspnea (pleural effusions), hypoxia & shock. Rapidly fatal. Inhalation <5%. Called "woolsorter's disease".

DIAGNOSIS
- **Most cases diagnosed clinically** and confirmed with positive serology, culture, or immunochemistry.
- Chest radiograph: **widening of the mediastinum** (due to hemorrhagic lymphadenitis).
- Cultures: boxcar-shaped, encapsulated **gram-positive rods** with a "Medusa head" appearance on microscopy.

MANAGEMENT
- **Cutaneous: Fluoroquinolones first-line** (eg, **Ciprofloxacin,** Levofloxacin, Moxifloxacin). Alternatives include Clindamycin, or Doxycycline.
- **Inhalation: IV Ciprofloxacin + an antitoxin** (Raxibacumab or anthrax immunoglobulin) + supportive care (drainage of pleural effusions).
- Alternatives: Penicillin, Chloramphenicol, Tetracycline, Erythromycin, Streptomycin.
- *B. anthracis* is not susceptible to Cephalosporins or Trimethoprim-sulfamethoxazole.

ACANTHAMOEBA KERATITIS

- Infection of the cornea due to *Acanthamoeba,* a free-living amoeba.
- Present in tap water and swimming pools.
- Risk factors: **most common in contact lens wearers** (eg, **wearing lens for long periods of time,** swimming or showering with contact lens, poor contact lens hygiene).
- Transmission: use of nonsterile tap water in preparation of contact lens solution, or use of infected contact lens solution.

CLINICAL MANIFESTATIONS
- **Keratitis:** ocular pain, photophobia, tearing, blurred vision, conjunctival injection. Physical exam: partial or complete **ring infiltrate of the corneal stroma,** hypopyon, pseudo-dendritic lesions.
- Encephalitis & granulomatous disease seen in immunocompromised patients.

DIAGNOSIS
- Staining of cornea scrapings: trophozoites can visualized using the fluorescent dye calcofluor. Corneal cultures of scrapings. PCR.

MANAGEMENT
- Combination treatment: Polyhexamethylene biguanide or Biguanide-Chlorhexidine in combination with Propamidine or Hexamidine.
- Chronic refractory: corneal transplantation

EHRLICHIOSIS & ANAPLASMOSIS

- **Tick-borne illness** caused by gram-negative intracellular bacteria that **infect & destroy white blood cells.**

ETIOLOGIES: 2 diseases with similar presentations:
- Human granulocytic Anaplasmosis: caused by ***Anaplasma phagocytophilum*** transmitted by the ***Ixodes scapularis*** tick (the same tick associated with Lyme disease & Babesiosis).
- Human monocytic Ehrlichiosis: ***Ehrlichia chaffeensis*** & *canis* transmitted by the **Lone star tick** (*Amblyomma americanum*).

CLINICAL MANIFESTATIONS
- Symptoms usually begin 7-10 days after a tick bite with a prodrome of rigors, malaise, & nausea followed by high fever, chills, myalgia, headache. May have splenomegaly.
- Not usually associated with a rash but if it develops, it can be macular, maculopapular. Petechial rash reflects thrombocytopenia.

DIAGNOSIS
- Serologies: indirect fluorescent antibody test most useful test to support the diagnosis. ELISA, PCR.
- Peripheral smear or **Buffy coat**: **morulae in WBCs** (granulocytes in HGA) and monocytes in HME. Morulae = clusters in the cell vacuoles, forming large **mulberry-shaped aggregates**, especially with HGA (less often with HME).
- **Leukopenia** (reflects the WBC destruction associated with infection), increased LFTs, **thrombocytopenia.**

MANAGEMENT
- **Doxycycline first-line treatment.**
- Second line: Rifampin. Chloramphenicol.

TYPE OF PRECAUTIONS	COMMON DISEASES
AIRBORNE	• Tuberculosis (including N95 mask) • Chicken pox (contact and airborne) • Disseminated Herpes Zoster • Measles
DROPLET	• Influenzae • Neisseria meningitidis & meningitis • Respiratory Diphtheria • Pertussis • Mumps • Rubella • RSV (droplet & contact)
CONTACT	• C. difficile • MRSA, VRE • Localized Herpes Zoster • RSV (droplet & contact) • Adenovirus • Cutaneous Diphtheria • Chicken pox (until all lesions are crusted and healed)

HERPES SIMPLEX VIRUS 1

TRANSMISSION

- Direct contact with contaminated saliva or other infected bodily secretions (eg, mouth to mouth contact, shared drinkware).

PATHOPHYSIOLOGY

- Direct contact at mucosal or skin sites cause viral entry into the epidermis until it reaches the sensory & autonomic nerve endings.

Primary lesions:

- Most primary infections are asymptomatic but may cause **tonsillopharyngitis in adults** and **gingivostomatitis in children**.
- **Herpetic whitlow:** can occur in dentists and health care workers exposed to infected secretions.

Secondary lesions:

- **Herpes labialis (cold sore):** reactivation of latent infection in ganglion neurons characterized by **prodromal symptoms** (pruritus, burning, tingling or pain) within 24 hours followed by the development of **grouped vesicles on an erythematous base** that undergoes crusting prior to healing.

DIAGNOSIS

- **PCR: test of choice (most sensitive and specific).** HSV-1 serology gold standard.
- Viral cultures, direct fluorescent antibody; Tzanck smear (nonspecific finding of multinucleated giant cells).

MANAGEMENT

- Orolabial: oral **Valacyclovir** (2g bid x 1 day). **Acyclovir** is an alternative.
- Chronic suppression may be needed for recurrent outbreaks.

GENITAL HERPES

- **Most cases of recurrent genital herpes are caused by Herpes simplex 2.** HSV-1 less common cause.
- Seen in about 25% of the population in the US.

TRANSMISSION

- Sexually transmitted via direct close contact with infected lesions.
- The virus can enter and stay dormant in the sensory nerve ganglion where it can become activated.

CLINICAL MANIFESTATIONS

- **Painful genital ulcers** often **preceded by prodromal symptoms** (eg, burning, paresthesias, numbness). Dysuria, fever

PHYSICAL EXAMINATION

- **Multiple, shallow, tender ulcers. Grouped vesicles on an erythematous base,** inguinal lymphadenopathy.

DIAGNOSIS

- **PCR is the test of choice (most sensitive and specific).**
- HSV-1 serology gold standard (not as sensitive or specific as PCR). Viral cultures, direct fluorescent antibody.
- Tzanck smear: **multinucleated giant cells** (intranuclear eosinophilic Cowdry A inclusions). Classic but not specific (can be seen with HSV1, HSV 2 and VZV).

MANAGEMENT

- **Acyclovir, Valacyclovir, Famciclovir**

HSV ENCEPHALITIS

- Severe **infection of the brain parenchyma** caused by **HSV-1.**
- **Associated with high mortality** (> 70% if untreated, 20-30% with treatment).
- **HSV-1 the most common cause of Encephalitis** in the US.
- Pathophysiology: virus gains access to the brain along axons of the trigeminal ganglia, leading to **temporal lobe necrosis.**

CLINICAL MANIFESTATIONS

- **Focal neurologic findings: fever +** altered mental status, decreased alertness, hemiparesis, focal cranial nerve deficits, dysphasia, aphasia, focal seizures, or ataxia. Primarily affects the **temporal lobe,** leading to bizarre behavior and focal neurologic deficits.

DIAGNOSIS

- Lumbar puncture: classic viral CSF pattern – **increased lymphocytes + normal glucose,** increased protein. **PCR detection of HSV DNA in CSF gold standard.** Brain biopsy may be indicated in cases refractory to treatment.
- Neuroimaging: **temporal lobe abnormalities.**

MANAGEMENT

- **IV Acyclovir initiated as soon as the diagnosis is considered.**
- Do not delay treatment while waiting for laboratory confirmation. Even with early administration of therapy, many patients have significant residual neurologic deficits.

EPSTEIN-BARR VIRUS (INFECTIOUS MONONUCLEOSIS) - HHV-4

- **Infection due to Epstein-Barr virus** characterized by **fever, lymphadenopathy, and tonsillar pharyngitis.** 80% of adults are seropositive.
- Pathophysiology: Epstein-Barr virus (EBV) infects B cells. EBV is part of the Human herpesvirus family.
- Transmission: **saliva** (known as the kissing disease) especially ages 15-25 years of age.

CLINICAL MANIFESTATIONS

- **Fever, lymphadenopathy (especially posterior cervical).** Can be generalized.
- **Tonsillar pharyngitis** (may be exudative). May have petechiae on the hard palate.
- May be associated with **fatigue,** headache, malaise, **splenomegaly,** hepatomegaly.
- **Rash** seen in ~5%, **especially if given Ampicillin**.

DIAGNOSIS

- **Heterophile antibody** (eg, **Monospot**) **– test of choice** (positive within 4 weeks).
- Rapid Viral Capsid Antigen test. Increased LFTs
- Peripheral smear: lymphocytosis >50% with >10% **atypical lymphocytes.**

MANAGEMENT

- **Supportive mainstay of treatment** - rest, analgesics (eg Acetaminophen, NSAIDs), antipyretics. Symptoms may last for months.
- Corticosteroids used ONLY if airway obstruction due to lymphadenopathy, hemolytic anemia, or severe thrombocytopenia. Strep & EBV can coexist.
- **Avoid trauma & contact sports at least 3-4 weeks** (depending on activity level) if splenomegaly is present **to prevent splenic rupture.**

COMPLICATIONS

- Hodgkin lymphoma, Burkitt lymphoma, CNS lymphoma, Nasopharyngeal carcinoma, Gastric carcinoma

CYTOMEGALOVIRUS (HHV 5)

- CMV – human herpesvirus 5 transmitted via body fluids or vertical transmission.
- CMV is present in most people (70% in the US) with **clinical disease primarily in immunocompromised patients.**
- Primary infection: **most are asymptomatic.** If symptomatic, symptoms are **similar to Mononucleosis** (fever, cough, myalgia, arthralgias) except it is **usually without sore throat or lymphadenopathy.**

REACTIVATION: **most commonly seen in immunocompromised** (eg, HIV, long-term steroid use, chemotherapy, post-transplant).

- **Colitis: most common.** Diarrhea, fever, abdominal pain, bloody stools. Increased risk in HIV with CD4 ≤100 cells/μL.
- **Retinitis:** decreased visual acuity and floaters. Funduscopy - **hemorrhage with yellow-white soft exudates** (scrambled eggs/ketchup or pizza pie appearance). **Most commonly seen when CD4 count is ≤50** cells/μL.
- Esophagitis: odynophagia with **large superficial ulcers on upper endoscopy.**
- Pneumonitis (especially post-transplant).
- Neurologic: Encephalitis, Guillain-Barré syndrome.

DIAGNOSIS

- Serologies (antigen tests, IgM, IgG titers). PCR.
- Labs: lymphocytes with atypical lymphocytosis
- Biopsy of tissues: **owl's eye appearance** (epithelial cells with **enlarged nuclei surrounded by clear zone** & cytoplasmic inclusions).

MANAGEMENT

- **Reactivation: Ganciclovir first-line treatment of choice.**
- Second-line: Foscarnet, Cidofovir. Valacyclovir.
- Primary disease in immunocompetent is mainly supportive therapy.

HIV PROPHYLAXIS

Valganciclovir if CD4 ≤50 cells/μL.

CONGENITAL CMV

- Congenital infection can lead to stillbirth, prematurity, and hydrops fetalis.
- **Most common congenital viral infection.** Part of the ToRCH syndrome.

CLINICAL MANIFESTATIONS

- Most are asymptomatic at birth but neonates may have petechiae, jaundice at birth, hepatosplenomegaly.
- Neurologic: **sensorineural hearing loss most common sequelae**, periventricular calcifications, cerebral palsy, vision impairment (including chorioretinitis), & seizures.

DIAGNOSIS

- Urine or saliva viral titers. Urine or saliva PCR for viral DNA most accurate test.

MANAGEMENT

- Ganciclovir

VARICELLA ZOSTER VIRUS (HHV-3)

CHICKENPOX (VARICELLA)

- **Varicella zoster virus,** part of the Human herpes virus family (HHV-3).
- VZV causes 2 clinically distinct diseases: **Primary – varicella (chickenpox)** and **reactivation**, known as **Herpes zoster (Shingles).**

TRANSMISSION
- **Aerosolized droplets from nasopharyngeal secretions or direct contact** with skin lesions.
- 10-20 day incubation period.

CLINICAL MANIFESTATIONS
- Prodrome fever, malaise, anorexia or pharyngitis followed by generalized vesicular rash, usually within 24 hours.
- Evolution: classic evolution = **erythematous macules that become papules then vesicular then crust over.** The rash begins on the face, then goes to the trunk before spreading to the extremities. Usually **pruritic**.

PHYSICAL EXAMINATION
- **Asynchronous rash in different stages of evolution,** including, macules, papules, clusters of **vesicles on an erythematous base ("dew drops on a rose petal")** & crusted lesions.
- More severe presentation may occur in adults.

DIAGNOSIS
- **Usually a clinical diagnosis.**
- **PCR has the highest yield when testing is needed.** Can be performed on fluid from lesions, skin scrapings or CSF.
- Direct fluorescent antibody staining largely replaced Tzanck smear.
- Tzanck smear – multinucleated giant cells (can also be seen with HSV).
- Serologies: anti-VZV IgM in response to an acute infection. IgG denotes immunity.

MANAGEMENT
- **Previously healthy child 12 years or younger** - **supportive & symptomatic treatment** (eg, Acetaminophen & Calamine lotion). Avoid acetylsalicylic acid (increased risk of Reye syndrome). NSAIDs may increase risk of superinfection.

- **Acyclovir should be given to adolescents (13 years old or older), adults, & immunocompromised patients** because they are susceptible to complications (eg, pneumonia, encephalitis, & hemorrhagic complications). When given within 72 hours of onset, Acyclovir can limit both the severity & duration of Varicella.

- Hospitalized patients should be placed on **contact and airborne precautions.**

- **Chickenpox can be spread from 48 hours prior to the onset of the rash up until all the lesions have crusted over.** During that time frame, patients should avoid contact with pregnant women and unvaccinated individuals.

COMPLICATIONS
- **Bacterial superinfection most common complication in in children.**
- **Varicella pneumonia is the leading cause of mortality & morbidity in adults** (may develop within 3-7 days following the rash).
- Encephalitis. Reye syndrome (rare).

POST EXPOSURE TO VARICELLA

Varicella zoster immune globulin within 96 hours of exposure is recommended in susceptible individuals with high risk of developing Varicella (ideally as soon as possible) if there has been exposure within 10 days.

A second full dose is administered to high-risk patients with additional exposures to Varicella >3 weeks after the first dose.

VZIG reduces the severity of infection after exposure to Varicella virus in patients at high risk for severe infection and complications including:

- **Immunocompromised children & adults who lack evidence of immunity to VZV** (unvaccinated or seronegative).
- **Newborns of mothers with Varicella 5 days before to 2 days after delivery.**
- Premature infants at or greater than 28 weeks' gestation who are exposed and whose mother has no evidence of immunity.
- Premature infants < 28 weeks' gestation or who weigh <1000 g at birth and were exposed during hospitalization.
- Pregnant women who lack evidence of immunity to VZV.

NEONATAL VARICELLA

TRANSMISSION:

- Vertical transmission during pregnancy or delivery or acquired after birth from the environment or infected care providers.
- The risk of mortality is increased when the mother develops symptoms of varicella from 5 days before to 2 days after delivery.

CLINICAL MANIFESTATIONS

- Can range from a mild illness similar to varicella to disseminated disease.

DIAGNOSIS

- Clinical classic rash in different stages. If testing is needed, PCR is the diagnostic test of choice.

POST-EXPOSURE PROPHYLAXIS:

- **Neonates should be provided with Varicella immunoglobulin if maternal infection occurs < 5 days before to 2 days after birth,** preterm infants with gestational age at or greater than 28 weeks born to mothers without immunity & preterm infants <28 weeks. Mothers with active disease must be isolated from other patients, including their neonates.

- **Varicella immunoglobulin is not needed if maternal infection > 5 days before birth** (because maternal antibodies are formed & transferred to the neonate, conferring protection).

- **Acyclovir is given to neonates with active disease** (rash, pneumonia, encephalitis, severe hepatitis, thrombocytopenia).

- Breastfeeding is encouraged in infants exposed to or infected with varicella.

HERPES ZOSTER (SHINGLES)

- Varicella zoster virus causes 2 clinical distinct diseases: **primary – Varicella (chickenpox)** and **reactivation**, known as **Herpes zoster (Shingles).**
- Pathophysiology: after initial infection, the virus becomes latent in the dorsal root ganglia or trigeminal ganglia, where it can reactivate.
- Risk factors: **age > 50 years, immunocompromised** (eg, chemotherapy, HIV)

CLINICAL MANIFESTATIONS
- **Prodrome of fever, malaise, sensory changes** (pain, burning, paresthesias) followed by **painful eruption of vesicles on an erythematous base unilaterally within a single dermatome that does not cross the midline** (eg, **thoracic most common**, cervical, trigeminal, facial nerve, and lumbosacral).

COMPLICATIONS
- Cranial neuropathies, CNS involvement.
- Dissemination: outside of the dermatome or organ involvement (most common in immunocompromised).
- Post-herpetic neuralgia: persistent pain or sensory symptoms >90 days after the onset of Herpes zoster.

DIAGNOSIS
- **Usually a clinical diagnosis.**
- **PCR has the highest yield when testing is needed.** Can be performed on lesions of all stages & CSF.
- Direct fluorescent antibody staining largely replaced Tzanck smear.
- Tzanck smear – multinucleated giant cells (can also be seen with HSV). Viral cultures.

MANAGEMENT
- **Acyclovir, Valacyclovir, Famciclovir.** Analgesics for pain (eg, oral, topical lidocaine, nerve blocks).
- **The patient is no longer infectious once all the lesions crust over** (on average about 7-10 days). During the infectious stage, they should avoid pregnant patients, immunocompromised people, and those who are not immunized against VZV.

POST-EXPOSURE PROPHYLAXIS

Varicella zoster immune globulin is given to people exposed to shingles who are at risk of infection within 72 hours of exposure. Passive immunization via the VZIG is recommended in:
- **Immunocompromised patients** (primary or acquired).
- Persons taking immunosuppressive therapies
- Persons with neoplastic diseases
- Neonates

POST HERPETIC NEURALGIA

- Persistent pain or sensory symptoms >90 days after the onset of Herpes zoster (shingles). Most commonly seen in the elderly.

Risk factors: **age > 50 years, immunocompromised,** greater rash severity.

CLINICAL MANIFESTATIONS
- Pain (eg, burning, stabbing or sharp) or sensory changes (eg, allodynia).
- Most commonly affects the thoracic, cervical and trigeminal nerves.

MANAGEMENT
- **Gabapentin or Pregabalin initial management of choice.**
- Topical Capsaicin in mild to moderate.
- **Tricyclic antidepressants** may be used if unable to tolerate first-line agents.

HERPES ZOSTER OPHTHALMICUS

- Potentially sight-threatening disorder that is a variant of reactivation, Varicella zoster **(shingles).**
- Pathophysiology: after initial infection, Varicella zoster virus becomes latent in the dorsal root ganglia or trigeminal ganglia, where it can reactivate, involving the **ophthalmic division of the Trigeminal (cranial nerve V)**.

CLINICAL MANIFESTATIONS
- Prodrome of headache, malaise and fever.
- Unilateral pain or hypesthesia in the affected eye, forehead or top of the head may precede or occur after the prodrome.
- Eye involvement: Conjunctivitis, Uveitis, Episcleritis. **Keratitis (epithelial or stromal increased risk for vision loss).**

PHYSICAL EXAMINATION
- **Grouped vesicles on an erythematous base on the face,** conjunctivitis, uveitis, episcleritis, and keratitis.
- **Hutchinson sign: vesicles on the side or the tip of the nose** have a high correlation with ocular involvement (due to involvement of the nasociliary branch of CN V), which also innervates the globe.
- Slit lamp examination: **dendritic (branching) uptake of fluorescein** if keratoconjunctivitis is present.

MANAGEMENT
- **Oral antivirals** (eg, **Acyclovir, Valacyclovir or Famciclovir**) to limit VZV replication plus topical Glucocorticoids to blunt the inflammatory response and reduce or prevent immune-mediated Keratitis and Iritis.
- IV Acyclovir if immunocompromised or in cases requiring hospitalization for sight-threatening cases.

HERPES ZOSTER OTICUS

- **AKA (Ramsay-Hunt syndrome)** - reactivation of Varicella zoster virus in the geniculate ganglion of the **facial nerve (CN VII).**

CLINICAL MANIFESTATIONS
- **Triad of ipsilateral facial paralysis + ear pain + vesicles in the auditory canal and/or auricle.**
- In addition, other ipsilateral findings of facial nerve palsy (eg, altered taste perception, decreased hearing tinnitus, hyperacusis, and decreased lacrimation) may be seen.
- May develop **vestibular disturbances** (if CN VIII is involved).

MANAGEMENT
- **Valacyclovir and Prednisone.**
- In severe cases, IV therapy may be initiated with transition to oral antivirals as the condition improves.

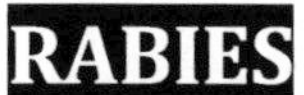

RABIES

- Life-threatening **Rhabdovirus infection** of the CNS (encephalitis of gray matter).

TRANSMISSION

- **Infected saliva from rabid animal bites**. The 4 major animal reservoirs in the US are **bats (most common), raccoons, skunks, & foxes** (dogs cause >90% in developing countries). **Rodents and rabbits are not generally considered at risk** (the only rodent that will survive long enough to transmit it is a woodchuck).

- If a person was **asleep in a room with a bat, they should be given prophylaxis** **even if no visible bat bite** is seen.

PATHOPHYSIOLOGY

- Rhabdovirus goes through axons from the peripheral to the central nervous system via cellular uptake of the virus via acetylcholine receptors.
- Incubation period usually 3-7 weeks (rarely can occur after years).

CLINICAL MANIFESTATIONS

- **Prodrome:** pain, paresthesias, itching at the initial site of the bite is pathognomonic followed by CNS phase.

- **CNS phase:** encephalitis, **hydrophobia** (painful laryngospasm after drinking, seeing or hearing water), numbness, paralysis. Patients may become sensitive to air currents (**aerophobia**) & changes in temperature. May develop rabid rage, hypersalivation (foaming at the mouth) with thick sputum followed by respiratory phase.

- **Respiratory phase:** respiratory muscle paralysis (leading to death).

DIAGNOSIS

- Immunofluorescence: **Negri bodies** in the brain of euthanized animals (especially in the hippocampus).

- **Animal observation 7-10 days** to see if signs or symptoms of Rabies occur if domestic animal (wild animals are usually euthanized if caught).

MANAGEMENT

- **No effective management once symptoms occur** (these patients rarely survive). Coma induction, Amantadine, & Ribavirin.

POST EXPOSURE FIRST EPISODE

- **HDCV (Rabies Vaccine)**
  - **Immunocompetent: days 0, 3, 7, 14 + Rabies Immune Globulin** 20u/kg (half in wound depending on site and the other half IM). Ideally started within 6 days of the exposure.
  - **Immunocompromised add day 28 in the HDCV vaccine schedule** (0, 3, 7, 14, and 28) + RIG

- Post exposure prophylaxis in subsequent exposures: Rabies vaccine day 0 & 3. No immunoglobulin.

HANTAVIRUS (HEMORRHAGIC FEVER)

- Caused by **Hantavirus** associated with 2 syndromes: hemorrhagic fever with renal syndrome & hemorrhagic fever with pulmonary syndrome (Sin Nombre virus).
- Transmission: **inhalation of aerosolized Deer mouse feces, saliva, or urine.**
- **Most common in the SW United States.** 3 week incubation period.
- Risk factors: affects primarily young, healthy adults, especially males.

CLINICAL MANIFESTATIONS

- **Prodromal febrile phase:** the aerosolized virus enters the lung causing a prodromal febrile flu-like syndrome (fever, chills, **severe myalgias especially involving the back & legs**) followed by nausea, vomiting, diarrhea, headache, & weakness.
- **Cardiopulmonary syndrome:** flu-like prodrome 3-6 days with subsequent pulmonary edema & shock (dry cough followed by tachypnea, hypoxia, diffuse rales). May progress to cardiovascular collapse. Generally lasts 2-7 days and recovery is rapid in survivors.
- **Renal syndrome:** flu-like prodrome (**fever**) followed by **hemorrhage** (petechiae, subconjunctival hemorrhage), **hypotension, and oliguric acute kidney injury** followed by a diuretic phase.

DIAGNOSIS

- Mainly a clinical diagnosis. Reverse transcriptase PCR
- Serologies: ELISA for IgM & IgG (four-fold IgG rise distinguishes acute from past infection).
- HPS: increased creatine kinase, decreased serum albumin. Chest radiograph: pleural effusion, **central pulmonary infiltrates**, pericardial haziness (shaggy heart sign).
- HFRS: increased BUN & creatinine, decreased complement 3, hematuria, proteinuria

MANAGEMENT: **supportive** (IV hydration, hemodynamic and respiratory support, ICU admission).

DENGUE FEVER

- Febrile infection caused by one of 4 dengue viruses transmitted by ***Aedes* mosquito** (*aegypti or albopictus*).
- Seen mainly in the tropical & subtropical climates. 7-10 day incubation period.
- Virus replication destroys bone marrow, plasma leakage (increased capillary permeability).

CLINICAL MANIFESTATIONS

- **Biphasic fever phase:** sudden onset of chills, **initial high fever** (3-7 days), followed by remission hours to 2 days followed by **second fever phase** (1-2 days), severe myalgias, "break bone" pain, **headache, retro-orbital or ocular pain**, myalgia, sore throat.
- **Biphasic rash:** erythematous skin mottling, **flushed skin (sensitive & specific)** followed by defervescence with the onset of a **maculopapular rash** (spares palms & soles) followed by **petechiae** on the extensor surface of limbs.
- **Hemorrhagic fever:** ecchymosis, petechiae, gastrointestinal bleeding, menorrhagia, epistaxis. Hemorrhagic fever usually occurs in children in endemic areas. **Positive "tourniquet test":** purpura from the pressure of the tourniquet placed on the arm. **Hepatitis,** pleural effusion, ascites.
- **Hemorrhagic shock:** rapid, weak pulse, narrow pulse pressure, hypotension and cold clammy skin.

DIAGNOSIS:

- Leukopenia, thrombocytopenia, elevated LFTs (hepatitis is common).
- Reverse transcriptase PCR: detection of viral nucleic acid or viral nonstructural protein. Most helpful during the first week. Serologies: IgM, IgG

MANAGEMENT:

- **Supportive care mainstay**: **Acetaminophen** (avoid NSAIDS to reduce bleeding complications and avoid Aspirin to reduce bleeding complications and Reye syndrome). Volume support. Pressors may be needed in shock.

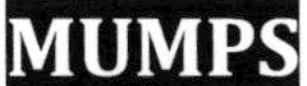

MUMPS

- Parotid gland enlargement cause by **Paramyxovirus.**

TRANSMISSION
- Respiratory droplets, saliva and household fomites.
- ~12-14 day incubation period. Increased incidence in the spring.
- Patients are most infectious 48 hours prior to the onset of parotitis and are infectious around 9 days after the onset of parotitis.

CLINICAL MANIFESTATIONS
- Prodrome of low-grade fever, fatigue, myalgia, malaise, headache, and earache followed by **parotitis (parotid gland pain and swelling) usually bilateral.**
- Physical examination: parotid swelling and tenderness. Erythema and edema of Stensen's duct.

DIAGNOSIS
- Clinical. Serologies. Increased amylase, leukopenia with a relative lymphocytosis.

MANAGEMENT
- **Supportive mainstay of treatment** - antipyretics (eg, Acetaminophen, Ibuprofen), analgesics. Self-limited (symptoms usually lasts 7-10 days).
- If hospitalized, the patient should be placed on droplet precautions and the CDC recommends isolation for at least 5 days after the onset of parotid swelling.

COMPLICATIONS
- **Epididymo-orchitis is the most common complication of Mumps,** especially in postpubertal males (15-30%). May occur 5-10 days after the onset of parotitis. Unilateral in 60-80%.
- Neurologic - aseptic meningitis (most common), encephalitis, deafness.
- Oophoritis, arthritis, infertility.
- Mumps is the most common infectious cause of acute Pancreatitis in children.

PREVENTION
- **MMR vaccine (2 doses): given at 12-15 months of age with a second dose at age 4-6 years of age.** If vaccinated as an adult, 2 doses separated by at least 28 days.

- In 2018, the CDC recommended individuals vaccinated prior with 2 doses of MMR are at increased risk for population outbreak and should receive a third dose (eg, college students).

- MMR is a live attenuated vaccine so it is contraindicated in pregnant women and significant immunosuppression (eg, AIDS, leukemia, lymphoma, chemotherapy). Patients with HIV without severe immunosuppression may receive the vaccine. Women should wait 4 weeks after MMR vaccination to become pregnant.

ROSEOLA INFANTUM (EXANTHEMA SUBITUM)

- **Most commonly caused by human herpesvirus 6** (sometimes HHV-7).
- Also known as **Sixth disease.**
- Transmission: respiratory droplets. ~10 day incubation period.
- 90% occur in children < 2 years of age

CLINICAL MANIFESTATIONS
- Fever prodrome: **high fever** 3-5 days (may exceed 104F) & lymphadenopathy. **Child appears well & alert during febrile phase.** The fever resolves abruptly before the onset of the classic rash.
- Rash: **rose, pink, macular or maculopapular, blanchable** rash **beginning on the trunk and neck before spreading to the face.** Macules 2-5 mm & rash lasts hours up to 2 days.
  Only viral exanthem that starts on the trunk.
- Nagayama spots: erythematous papules on the soft palate and uvula.
- Erythematous tympanic membranes, respiratory symptoms, anorexia.
- 15% risk of febrile seizures.

DIAGNOSIS
- Clinical

MANAGEMENT
- **Supportive: mainstay of treatment (self-limited)** - rest, maintaining fluid intake, antipyretics (eg, Acetaminophen, Ibuprofen).
- Adequate handwashing is important to prevent spread of infection.

RUBELLA (GERMAN MEASLES)

- Caused by the Rubella virus, part of the Togavirus family.
- TRANSMISSION: respiratory droplets. 2-3 week incubation period.

CLINICAL MANIFESTATIONS
- Prodrome: low-grade fever, cough, anorexia, **lymphadenopathy (posterior cervical, posterior auricular**).
- Exanthem: **pink or light-red nonconfluent maculopapular rash** starts on the face and spreads to the trunk and extremities. Rash **lasts 3 days**. Compared to Rubeola, Rubella spreads more rapidly and does not coalesce or darken.
- **Forchheimer spots: small red macules or petechiae on the soft palate** (may also be seen with Scarlet fever).
- Transient photosensitivity & joint pains (especially in young adult women and adolescents).

DIAGNOSIS
- Mainly a clinical diagnosis.
- Rubella-specific IgM antibody via enzyme immunoassay.

MANAGEMENT
- **Supportive mainstay of treatment** (eg, Acetaminophen, Ibuprofen), oral hydration.

PROGNOSIS
- Generally, not associated with complications in children (compared to Rubeola).
- **Teratogenic especially in the first trimester** (Congenital rubella syndrome).

	PRODROME	RASH	MISCELLANEOUS
VARICELLA Chicken Pox	• Flu-like sx: fever, headache, malaise	• ***Rash in DIFFERENT stages simultaneously**** (macules, papules, vesicles, crusted lesions) • Face initially ⇨ extremities.	• ***Vesicles on erythematous base dew drops on a rose petal"****. • Usually does not involve palms/soles
VARIOLA Smallpox	• Flu-like sx: fever, headache, malaise	• ***Lesions appear in the SAME stage simultaneously**** • Vesicles ⇨ pustules ⇨ scarring	• ***Classically involves palms/soles***
RUBEOLA Measles	• URI prodrome: ***3 C's:*** - ***Cough, Coryza, Conjunctivitis***	• ***Maculopapular BRICK-RED* rash beginning @ hair line/face ⇨ extremities. Lasts 7 days.***	• ***KOPLIK SPOTS on buccal mucosa**** • ***Otitis Media MC long term cx****, encephalitis, pneumonia in children
RUBELLA German Measles	• URI prodrome. • ***Post cervical & postauricular lymphadenopathy***	• ***Maculopapular pink-light red* spotted rash on face ⇨ extremities. Lasts 3 days****	• ***Photosensitivity & arthralgias (joint pains) especially in young women*** • Not long term sequelae in children • ***TERATOGENIC in 1st trimester***: (ToRCH)
ROSEOLA Sixth's disease	• 3 days of ***high fevers*** • ***Child appears well during febrile phase.****	• ***Pink maculopapular blanchable rash.*** • ***Only childhood viral exanthema that STARTS ON TRUNK/EXTREMITIES* then goes to face***	• Lasts 1-3 days. • Associated with HHV-6 & HHV-7
ERYTHEMA INFECTIOSUM 5th's disease	• Coryza, fever	• ***Red flushed face "SLAPPED CHEEK APPEARANCE" with CIRCUMORAL PALLOR ⇨ LACY RETICULAR RASH on the body***	• ***Arthropathy in older adults*** • ***Aplastic crisis in Sickle Cell disease**** • ***Increased fetal loss in pregnancy*** • ***Parvovirus B-19***
COXSACKIE A VIRUS Hand Foot Mouth	• Fever, URI symptoms	• ***Vesicular lesions on a reddened base with an erythematous halo in oral cavity ⇨ vesicles on the hands/feet (includes palms & soles)***	• ***Seen especially in summer*** • Affects hands, feet, mouth & genitals
ENDEMIC TYPHUS	• Flu-like sx: fevers, chills, severe headache.	• Maculopapular rash trunk & axilla ⇨ extremities (spares the face, palms & soles)	• ***Flushed face, hearing loss (CN 8 involvement), conjunctivitis***
SCALDED SKIN SYNDROME	• Local S. aureus infection	• Fluid filled blisters with ***positive Nikolsky sign: (sloughing of skin with gentle pressure)*** • ***Painful diffuse red rash begins centrally***	• ***Seen in children <6y*** • ***Due to S. aureus exotoxin***
TOXIC SHOCK SYNDROME	• High fever, watery diarrhea • Sore throat, headache • ***Staph aureus exotoxin***	• ***Red rash (diffuse, maculopapular) with desquamation of palms & soles***	• ***Seen in adults (ex tampon use, nasal packing left in too long) due to*** • **Management: *IV Antibiotics***
ROCKY MOUNTAIN SPOTTED FEVER	• Triad: fever, headache, rash	• ***Red maculopapular rash first on wrists/ankles* ⇨ central (eventually palms & soles). Petechiae***	• *Fever with relative bradycardia*
KAWASAKI	• Fever, conjunctivitis, cervical lymphadenopathy	• ***Strawberry tongue, edema/desquamation of palms & soles.*** Rash can present in different ways	• ***Rare but dreaded complication is myocardial infarction & coronary artery involvement***
SCARLET FEVER		• ***Strawberry tongue, sandpaper rash*, facial flushing with circumoral pallor.*** *Desquamation can occur*	• ***Forchheimer spots***: *small red spots on the soft palate (resolves quickly)*

HUMAN IMMUNODEFICIENCY VIRUS (HIV)

- **HIV**: retrovirus (changes viral RNA into DNA via **reverse transcriptase**).
- HIV-1 (most common) & HIV-2.

CLINICAL MANIFESTATIONS

- Patients may present at any stage and have varied presentations

Acute seroconversion

- 10-60% of individuals with early HIV do not experience symptoms.
- **Flu-like or mononucleosis-like illness (acute retroviral syndrome)** usually within 2-4 weeks of infection - **fever, fatigue, myalgias most common symptoms**; nontender generalized lymphadenopathy (eg, cervical, axillary, occipital nodes), sore throat (usually without tonsillar enlargement or exudates), painful mucocutaneous ulceration, arthralgia, diarrhea, weight loss, headache, malaise, generalized rash. During this stage of early HIV infection, they are highly infectious to others (due to the transient high viral loads).

Opportunistic infections:

- Oral and esophageal Candidiasis is the opportunistic infection most commonly seen in these patients. CMV infection (proctitis, colitis, and hepatitis), PCP pneumonia, cryptosporidiosis.

AIDS:

- **Defined as CD4 count <200** cells/μL. Recurrent severe & potentially life-threatening infections or opportunistic malignancies. AIDS-associated dementia/encephalopathy, HIV wasting syndrome (chronic diarrhea & weight loss idiopathic in nature).

LABS ASSOCIATED WITH EARLY HIV INFECTION

- Viral RNA levels are usually high (> 100,000 copies/mL) often in the millions and CD4+ count can drop transiently.
- Leukocyte count and lymphocytes vary during the acute illness. CD4 counts tend to be lower than CD8 counts.
- Elevation of liver enzymes, mild anemia, and thrombocytopenia.

DIAGNOSIS OF SUSPECTED EARLY HIV INFECTION:

- **Combination antigen/antibody immunoassay (screening) + HIV viral load testing** (eg, RT-PCR).

- If both are negative with high suspicion, repeat both tests within 1-2 weeks.
  - **Negative screening immunoassay + positive virologic tests** suggests early HIV. A second positive virologic test suggests HIV infection.
  - **Positive HIV screening immunoassay + positive virologic test** = early or established infection. **Confirm with a second test (eg, repeat HIV RNA or serologic test) several weeks later.** A positive screening immunoassay should prompt a second antibody-only immunoassay (preferably the HIV-1/HIV-2 differentiation immunoassay).

- **HIV RNA Viral Load: can be positive in the window period** (negative screening immunoassay OR a positive combination antibody/antigen immunoassay with a negative antibody-only immunoassay). Also used to monitor infectivity & treatment effectiveness in patients diagnosed with HIV.

ROUTINE SCREENING FOR HIV INFECTION

- **4th generation antigen/antibody combination HIV-1/2 immunoassay (screening).** It detects both HIV1 and HIV-2 antibodies as well as HIV P24 antigen. **The combination test is better than the antibody only tests because they can detect the HIV P24 antigen** when antibody testing may be negative (eg, window period). P24 antigen is a viral core protein that appears in the blood as the viral RNA level rises following HIV infection. Rapid combination antigen/antibody tests do not appear to be quite as sensitive as the standard combination test. Antibody only test can pick up as early as 3 weeks.

  - **If 4th generation assay is negative,** the person is considered HIV-uninfected and **no further testing needs to be done.**

  - **If 4th generation assay is positive, a confirmatory HIV-1/HIV-2 antibody differentiation immunoassay is performed.**
    - **If confirmatory is positive, a plasma HIV RNA should be obtained** to evaluate for acute infection.
    - **If confirmatory is indeterminate or negative, a plasma HIV RNA should be performed**. HIV RNA is also performed in patients with concern for acute HIV infection.

HIV MANAGEMENT

- Guidelines for HAART initiation: ART should be offered to all HIV-infected patients, including asymptomatic individuals regardless of their immune status (eg, CD4 count). There are more than 25 medications from 6 major classes currently available. Resistance should be tested prior to initiation of therapy.

- **For most treatment-naïve patients, regimen containing 2 different NRTIs plus an INSTI** (eg, Dolutegravir plus Tenofovir/alafenamide-emtricitabine or Bictegravir-Emtricitabine-Tenofovir).
- **Abacavir is contraindicated if the patient is positive for HLA-B*5701 allele**, because of the increased risk of hypersensitivity reaction.
- For most patients unable to take Tenofovir of Abacavir, a combination of Dolutegravir plus Lamivudine plus a boosted PI plus an NSTI OR a boosted PI plus Lamivudine.

HAART REGIMENS FOR TREATMENT NAÏVE PATIENTS:

❶ NNRTI + 2 NRTI's OR	NNRTI = Non-nucleoside Reverse Transcriptase Inhibitor NRTI = Nucleos(t)ide Reverse Transcriptase Inhibitor
❷ PI + 2 NRTI's OR	Protease inhibitor (preferably boosted with Ritonavir)
❸ INSTI + 2 NRTI's	INSTI = Integrase strand transfer inhibitor

NRTI'S Zidovudine Emtricitabine Abacavir Lamivudine Didanosine Zalcitabine Stavudine Tenofovir	MOA: inhibits viral replication by interfering c HIV viral RNA-dependent DNA polymerase Adverse effects: **Zidovudine ⇨ bone marrow suppression;** Peripheral neuropathy, pancreatitis. **Abacavir is contraindicated if the patient is positive for HLA-B*5701 allele,** because of the increased risk of hypersensitivity reaction. Truvada (Emtricitabine/Tenofovir)
NNRTI'S Efavirenz Delavirdine Etravirine Nevirapine Rilpivirine	MOA: inhibits viral replication by interfering with HIV viral RNA-dependent DNA polymerase Adverse effects: **Rash.** Efavirenz causes vivid dreams
PROTEASE INHIBITORS Atazanavir Darunavir Lopinavir & Ritonavir Nelfinavir Indinavir Ritonavir Fosamprenavir Saquinavir	MOA: inhibits HIV protease leading to production of noninfectious, immature HIV particles Adverse effects: GI: N/V/diarrhea, **Lipodystrophy, Hyperlipidemia**
INTI Raltegravir, Dolutegravir	MOA: prevents insertion of a DNA copy of the viral genome into the host DNA Adverse effects: **Hyperlipidemia**, GI symptoms.
FUSION INHIBITORS Enfuvirtide	**MOA:** disrupts the virus from fusing with healthy T cells Adverse effects: **Hyperlipidemia**, GI symptoms
CCR5 ANTAGONISTS	**Maraviroc** MOA: blocks viral entry into WBC's

OPPORTUNISTIC INFECTIONS:

CD4 Count/µL	DISEASE	1ry PROPHYLAXIS	2ry PROPHYLAXIS
700 – 1,500	Normal		
>500	Lymphadenopathy		
500-200	Tuberculosis	INH if latent	Rifampin
	Kaposi Sarcoma, Thrush, Lymphoma, Zoster		
≤ 200 ≤ 150	**Pneumocystis (PCP)**	TMP/SMX	Dapsone, Atovaquone, Pentamidine (aerosolized)
	Histoplasmosis (select)	Itraconazole	Amphotericin B
≤ 100	**Toxoplasmosis**	TMP/SMX	Dapsone + Pyrimethamine + Folinic acid
	Cryptococcus (select)	Fluconazole	Amphotericin B
≤ 50	**MAC**	Azithromycin or Clarithromycin	Rifabutin (must obtain CXR prior to use to rule out active Tuberculosis
	CMV retinitis	Valganciclovir	Ganciclovir + Foscarnet

Others: Diarrhea (Cryptosporidium, Isospora, Microspora), Human Papilloma Virus

CHAPTER 14 - HEMATOLOGIC SYSTEM

ROULEAUX FORMATION

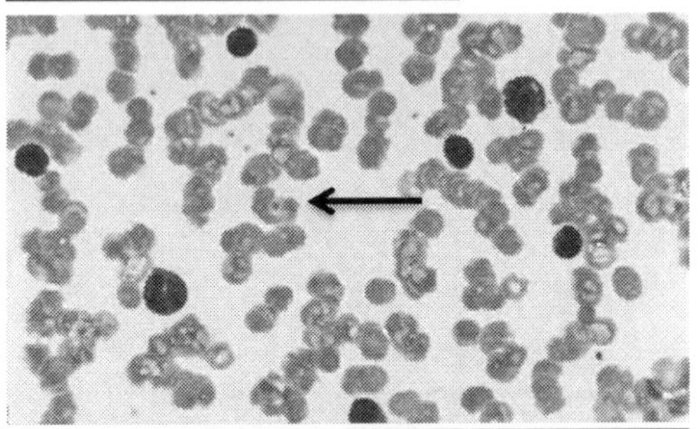

- RBCs stick together like a **"stack of coins"** due to ↑plasma proteins (such as immunoglobulins or fibrinogen).
- The increased density of the RBCs stuck together cause them to settle in the tube faster = ↑**ESR** (Erythrocyte Sedimentation Rate).
- __**Diseases:**__ high protein (**Multiple Myeloma**). disorders with ↑fibrinogen:
  Infections (acute/chronic).

AUTO AGGLUTINATION

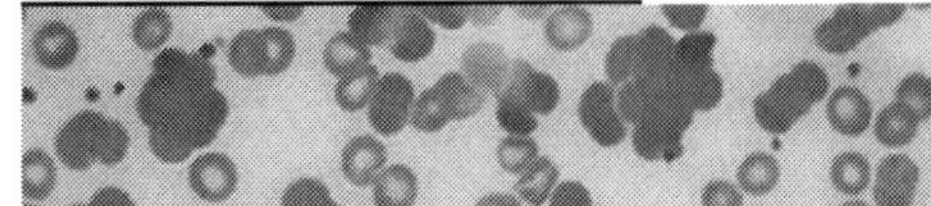

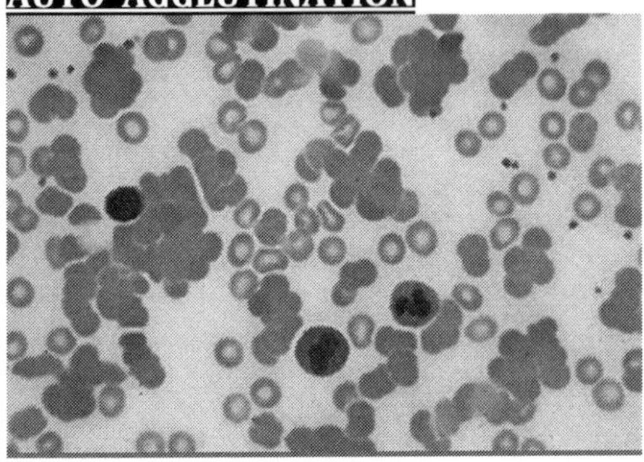

- **Clumping of RBCs** due to IgM auto-antibodies coating the surface of RBCs, leading to ↑RBC destruction by macrophages.
- Cold IgM Ab agglutinins are reactive at colder temperatures (ex 28-31°C).

__**DISEASES**__

- **Cold agglutinin autoimmune hemolytic anemia** (eg, *Mycoplasma pneumoniae*, Epstein-Barr virus)
- Cryoglobulinemia
- Ag-Ab reaction if blood not typed & cross-matched.

HOWELL-JOLLY BODIES

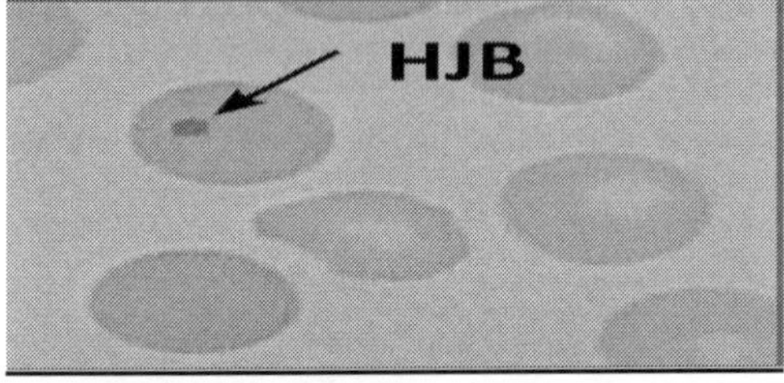

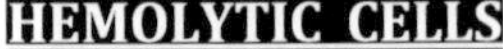

- Small dense basophilic RBC inclusions (usually removed by the spleen).

__**DISEASES**__

- **Decreased splenic function:** autosplenectomy (eg, sickle cell disease), post splenectomy
- Severe hemolytic anemia, megaloblastic anemia

HEMOLYTIC CELLS

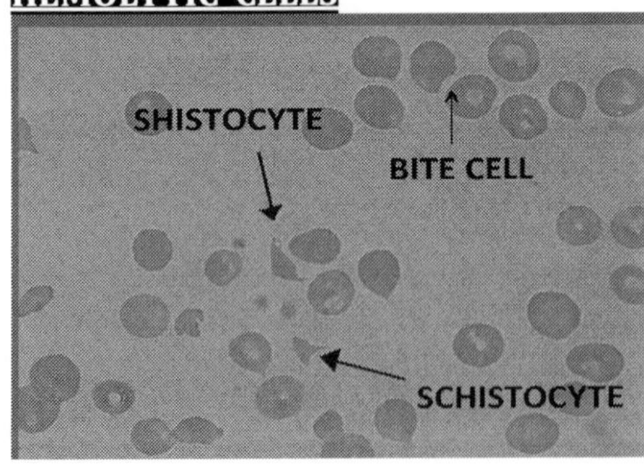

- __**BITE CELLS**__ (degmacyte) = bite-like deformity due to phagocyte removal of denatured Hgb.
  - Thalassemia, G6PD deficiency
- __**SCHISTOCYTES:**__ Fragmented RBCs.
  - Hemolytic anemias, Microangiopathic diseases
- __**KERATOCYTES**__ "Helmet-shaped" RBCs.
  - Mechanical RBC damage in small vessels (microangiopathic diseases - eg, TTP, HUS, DIC, prosthetic valves)

BASOPHILIC STIPPLING

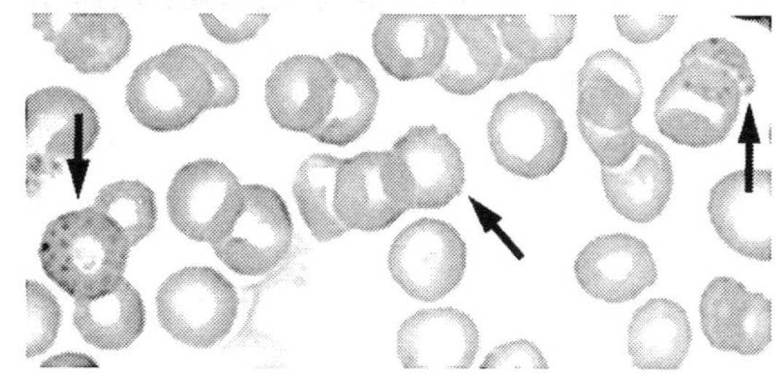

- Coarse blue granules in RBCs (residual RNA in RBCs – looks similar to reticulocytes but **basophilic stippling is evenly distributed throughout the RBC.**

Most commonly acquired:
- **Sideroblastic anemia,** heavy metal poisoning (eg, **lead,** arsenic), TTP
- Hemoglobinopathies: eg, **Thalassemias**
- Myelodysplasia, chronic alcohol use

ECHINOCYTES "Burr cells"

- RBCs with numerous, small, evenly spaced projections due to abnormal cell membrane.

DISEASES
- **Uremia**
- Pyruvate kinase deficiency
- Hypophosphatemia

ACANTHOCYTES "Spur cells"

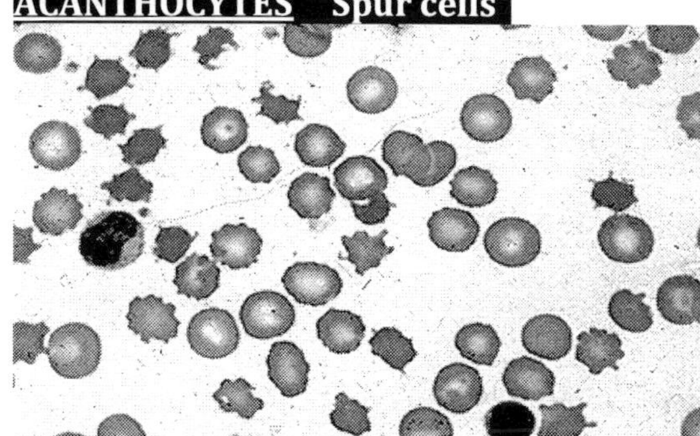

- Few large spiny, irregular projections on the RBC membrane.

DISEASES
- Liver disease (eg, alcoholic cirrhosis)
- Post splenectomy
- Thalassemia
- Autoimmune Hemolytic Anemia
- Renal disease

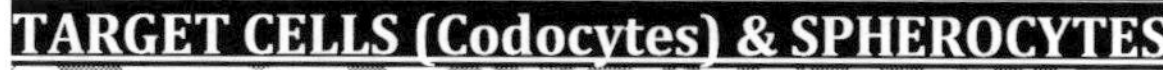

TARGET CELLS (Codocytes) & SPHEROCYTES

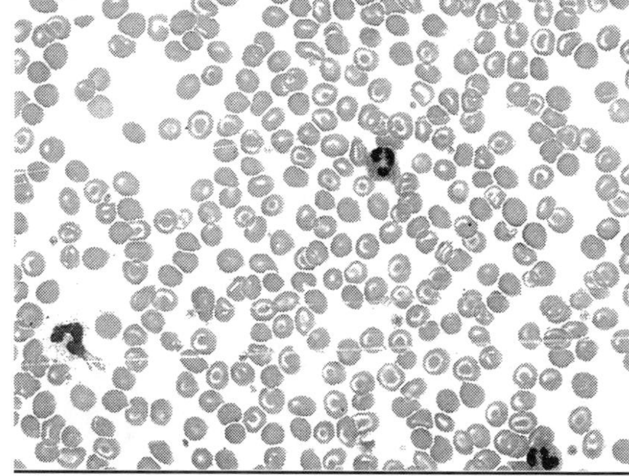

TARGET CELL: hypochromic RBC with round area of central pigment "target-shaped." Seen if there is excess cell membrane in relation to the hemoglobin content.

DISEASES
- **Hemoglobinopathies: sickle cell, Thalassemia,** severe Fe deficiency, asplenia, liver disease.

SPHEROCYTES: usually associated with hyperchromia (often with microcytosis).

DISEASES
- **Hereditary Spherocytosis**
- **Warm Autoimmune Hemolytic Anemia**

HYPERSEGMENTED NEUTROPHILS

- Neutrophils with >5 lobes

DISEASES

- **B_{12} & Folate deficiencies**
  (especially if macrocytosis is present)

AUER RODS

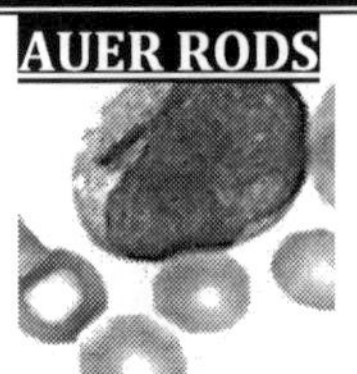

Acute Myelogenous Leukemia:
Seen in promyelocytic variant
Myeloperoxidase positive

REED-STERNBERG CELL

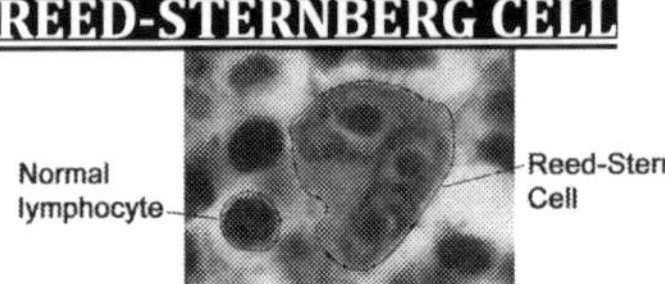

Hodgkin Lymphoma

APPROACH TO ANEMIA

MORPHOLOGIC APPROACH

Normal MCV is 80-100 fL.
Anemia with a low reticulocyte count can be separated (via Mean Corpuscular Volume [MCV]) into Normocytic (80 – 100), Microcytic (<80), or Macrocytic (>100).

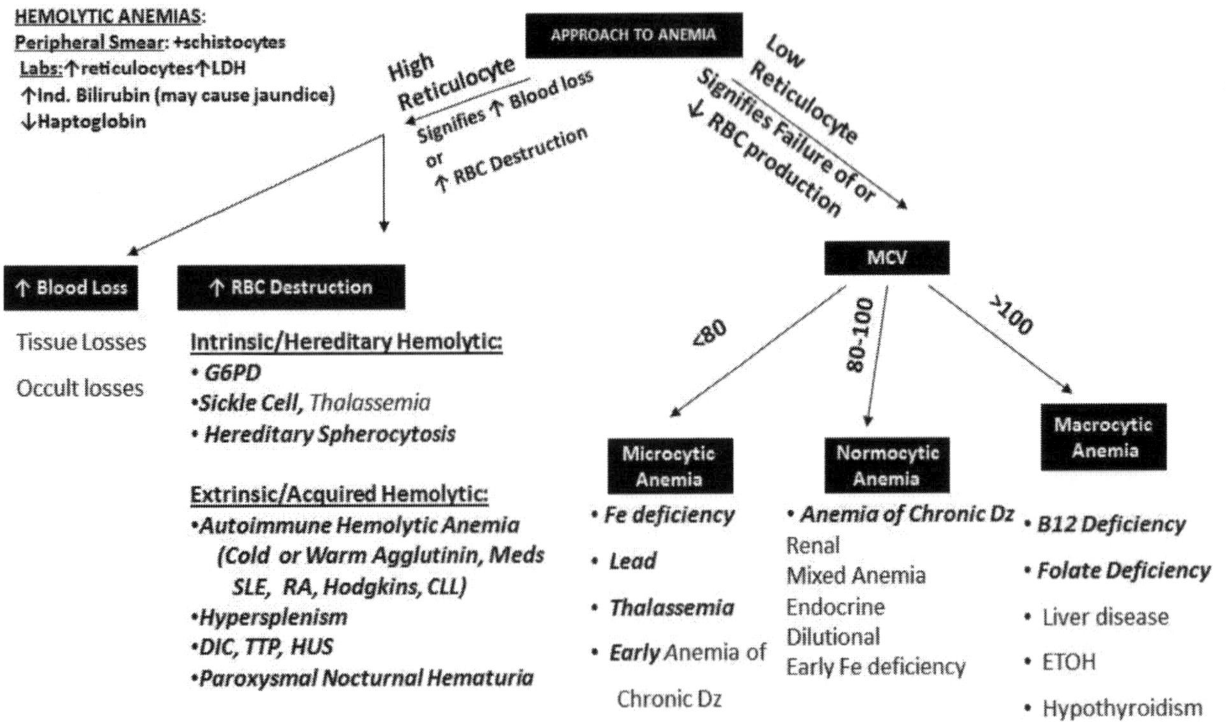

MICROCYTIC ANEMIAS

ETIOLOGIES: 3 most common clinically are **iron deficiency, alpha/beta thalassemia, early anemia of chronic disease (ACD). Lead poisoning is also in the differential.** ❶↓**iron availability**: severe iron deficiency, anemia of chronic disease, copper disease ❷↓**heme production**: lead poisoning, sideroblastic anemia ❸↓**globin production**: thalassemia & hemoglobinopathies (eg, sickle cell, Hgb SC). They all present with **hypochromic, microcytic anemia.**

IRON DEFICIENCY ANEMIA

- **Most common cause of anemia worldwide**.

ETIOLOGIES
- **Chronic blood loss: most common cause in US** - excessive menstruation, occult GI blood loss (eg, **Colon cancer**). Parasitic hookworms most common cause of blood loss-related IDA in resource-poor countries.
- Decreased absorption: **diet (most common cause worldwide),** Celiac, bariatric surgery, *H. pylori.*

RISK FACTORS
- Increased metabolic requirements: children, pregnant, and lactating women.
- Cow milk ingestion in young children: infants fed cow's milk younger than 1 year of age, toddlers fed large volumes of cow's milk.

PATHOPHYSIOLOGY
- Decreased RBC production due to lack of iron & decreased iron stores (decreased ferritin). Normally, iron is stored in ferritin primarily in the bone marrow, liver and spleen.

CLINICAL MANIFESTATIONS
- Classic symptoms of anemia: fatigue, weakness, exercise intolerance, dyspnea.
- CNS: poor concentration, apathy, irritability, poor school performance, cognitive disturbances. Restless legs syndrome.
- **Pagophagia:** craving for ice (specific). **Pica:** appetite for non-food substances (eg, clay, starch).
- Physical examination: **koilonychia** (spooning of the nails), angular cheilitis (inflammation of one or both corners of the mouth), tachycardia, glossitis (smooth tongue), signs of anemia (eg, pallor).

DIAGNOSIS
- CBC: **microcytic hypochromic anemia classic** (may be normocytic, normochromic early on). **Increased RDW** (red cell distribution width), anisocytosis. Decreased reticulocytes. May have thrombocytosis & poikilocytosis.
- Iron studies: **decreased ferritin (pathognomonic), increased TIBC** (transferrin), **decreased transferrin saturation** <20-15%, decreased serum iron.
- Bone marrow: absent iron stores definitive diagnosis (rarely performed).

MANAGEMENT
- **Iron replacement** results in increased reticulocytes (within 5-10 days), correction of anemia (6-8 weeks) & repletion of iron stores (1 to 3 months).
- Preparations: oral (eg, ferrous sulfate), iron-containing formulas in bottle-fed infants. Iron-enriched food and red meats. Parenteral.
- Increased absorption: **take iron replacement with vitamin C (ascorbic acid),** with **water or orange juice & on an empty stomach**. Iron should be given 2 hours before or 4 hours after ingestion of antacids (reduced acidity impairs absorption).
- Adverse effects: GI (eg, nausea, vomiting, constipation, flatulence, diarrhea, dark stool). Gradually increase the dose to reduce GI effects.
- Severe life-threatening anemia: red blood cell transfusion (eg, myocardial ischemia).

LEAD POISONING ANEMIA (PLUMBISM)

PATHOPHYSIOLOGY

- Lead poisons enzymes, causing cell death; it shortens the life span of RBCs; it inhibits multiple enzymes needed for heme synthesis, causing an **acquired sideroblastic anemia.**
- Risk factors: **most common in children** (especially in children <6y) due to increased permeability of the blood-brain barrier as well as iron deficiency (may increase lead absorption).
- Sources: **ingestion or inhalation of environmental lead** (eg, **paint chips or lead dust**) is the primary source of childhood lead poisoning in the US (lead was used in household paints prior to the 1970s). Lead in gasoline and industrialized use of lead.

CLINICAL MANIFESTATIONS

- May be asymptomatic or nonspecific symptoms.
- **Neurologic symptoms: ataxia, fatigue, learning disabilities, difficulty concentrating,** developmental delays, hearing loss. Peripheral neuropathy (eg, **wrist or foot drop**). Encephalopathy: mental status changes, vomiting, seizures, cerebral edema, SIADH.
- **GI:** lead colic - **intermittent abdominal pain, vomiting, loss of appetite, and constipation**.
- Anemia: pallor, shock, coma.
- Renal: glycosuria, proteinuria, chronic interstitial nephritis.
- Burton's line: thin, blue-black line at the base of the gums near the teeth (seen primarily in adults).

DIAGNOSIS

- **Serum lead levels**: > 10 mcg/dL on venous sampling most accurate. Capillary fingerstick sample often the initial test performed.
- Peripheral smear**: microcytic hypochromic anemia** with **basophilic stippling** (dots of denatured RNA seen in RBCs). **Ringed sideroblasts in the bone marrow.**
- Normal or increased serum iron, decreased TIBC.
- Increased erythrocyte protoporphyrin: elevations can be seen in both iron deficiency & lead poisoning but tend to be worse in lead poisoning.
- Radiographs: **"lead lines"** - linear hyperdensities at the metaphyseal plates in children.

MANAGEMENT

- **Removal of the source of lead is the most important component of treatment**.
- Mild 44 mcg/dL or lower: outpatient follow-up and lifestyle modifications.
- Moderate (45-69 mcg/dL): **Succimer first-line** as inpatient (oral chelation). Calcium disodium edetate (CaNa2EDTA) if oral therapy not tolerated. D-penicillamine third-line.
- Severe (70 or higher): without encephalopathy (Succimer + CaNa2EDTA).
  Encephalopathy – Dimercaprol (IM) followed by CaNa2EDTA (IM or IV).

THALASSEMIA OVERVIEW

THALASSEMIA: **decreased production of globin chains.** Distribution of Thalassemia follows Plasmodium falciparum – thought to be **genetic benefit vs. Malaria**). Most adults are heterozygotes.

- **Normally after 6 months of age, adult Hgb is the predominant Hgb produced:**

HgbA (Adult):	2 alphas, 2 betas **(ααββ)**	**95%**
HgbA$_2$:	2 alphas, 2 deltas (αα/δδ)	1.5-3%
HgbF (Fetal):	2 alphas, 2 gammas (ααγγ)	trace amounts

Think Thalassemia if microcytic anemia with normal/↑ serum Fe or no response to Fe treatment.

ALPHA THALASSEMIA

- **Decreased α-globin chain production.** 4 genes determine it.
- **Most common in SE Asians** 68%, Africans 30%, Mediterranean (5-10%).

Disease	Abnormal Alleles	CLINICAL MANIFESTATIONS
Silent Carrier State	1/4	Clinically normal (usually asymptomatic).
Alpha Thalassemia minor (trait)	2/4	Mild microcytic anemia – no treatment needed.
Alpha Thalassemia Intermedia	3/4	**Presents similar to β-Thalassemia major**
Hydrops Fetalis	4/4	Associated with stillbirth or death shortly after birth **Hgb Barts: gamma tetramers (γγγγ)**

Thalassemia should be suspected in any patient with:

- **Microcytic hypochromic anemia**
- **Normal or increased serum iron**
- **Normal or increased ferritin**

Hemoglobin electrophoresis in Alpha Thalassemia:

- 1 & 2 gene deletion: **normal Hb ratios in adults** (distinguishes alpha from beta).
- 3 gene deletion: presence of **HbH (beta chain tetramer) – Heinz bodies.**
- 4 gene deletion: presence of Hb Bart (gamma tetramer).

DNA analysis provides definitive diagnosis.

HEMOGLOBIN H DISEASE (Alpha Thalassemia intermedia)

- **A type of Alpha thalassemia** characterized by decreased alpha-globin chain production.

PATHOPHYSIOLOGY

- **3/4 gene** deletions cause decreased alpha chain production. Excess beta chains form **insoluble beta chain tetramers (Heinz bodies)** with no oxygen-carrying capacity in the RBCs. The presence of Heinz bodies in RBCs lead to their destruction by the spleen (hemolytic anemia). It is characterized by **moderate to severe anemia** (hemoglobin levels of 7-10 g/dL).

CLINICAL MANIFESTATIONS

- Patients usually **symptomatic at birth** (neonatal jaundice & anemia).
- Symptoms of anemia. Hepatosplenomegaly, pigmented gallstones.
- Increased bone marrow hematopoiesis: **frontal bossing,** maxilla overgrowth

DIAGNOSIS

- **Microcytosis, hemolytic anemia** (**schistocytes,** tear drop cells, **increased reticulocytes**), **target cells,** basophilic stippling, **increased RBC count,** decreased hemoglobin (7-10 g/dL).
- ⊕ **Heinz bodies** (HbH).
- Hemolysis (increased indirect bilirubin, decreased haptoglobin).
- Iron overload: **normal or increased serum iron.**
- **Hemoglobin electrophoresis:** presence of **HbH (beta chain tetramer).**

MANAGEMENT

- **Episodic blood transfusions** during periods of increased hemolysis or severe anemia (eg, infection, pregnancy).
- Vitamin C & folate supplementation (substrates for RBC production).
- **Iron chelating agents** (eg, **Deferoxamine,** Deferasirox) prevent iron overload & remove **excess iron** from chronic transfusions. Avoid iron supplementation (patients are iron-overloaded).
- Splenectomy in some cases (stops RBC destruction) may be needed by the second or third decade.
- Bone marrow transplantation definitive treatment in major.

BETA THALASSEMIA

- Genetic hemoglobinopathy characterized by **decreased production of beta-globin chains**, leading to excess alpha chains.
- Risk factors: **most common in Mediterranean** (eg, Greek, Italian), Africans, & Indians.

Disease	Abnormal alleles
β-Thalassemia trait (minor)	½
β-Thalassemia Major (Cooley's Anemia)	$^2/_2$
β-Thalassemia Intermedia	Mild homozygous form

CLINICAL MANIFESTATIONS

- Beta thalassemia minor (trait): **most common type.** Only one gene is defective. Usually asymptomatic but may have mild to moderate anemia.
- Beta thalassemia intermedia: mild homozygous form (anemia, hepatosplenomegaly, bony disease).
- **Beta thalassemia major (Cooley's anemia):** both beta genes are mutated. Deficient beta-chain production leads to excess alpha chains that are not able to form tetramers. This leads to ineffective erythropoiesis & shortened RBC life span.

CLINICAL MANIFESTATIONS OF BETA-THAL MAJOR:

- **Symptoms often occur after 6 months of life** (when fetal hemoglobin begins to diminish).
- Anemia: **severe, chronic anemia:** Pallor, irritability, dyspnea, mental delays. **Hemolytic anemia**: jaundice, **hepatosplenomegaly**.
- Extramedullary hematopoiesis: bony abnormalities, abnormal, delayed skeletal development, extramedullary expansion (frontal bossing, "hair on end" appearance of the skull, Osteoporosis, abnormal ribs).
- Osteoporosis: by age 10, the haematopoietically-active red marrow is replaced by inactive yellow marrow, leading to Osteoporosis, compression fractures, cord compression, scoliosis, & disc degeneration.
- Endocrine abnormalities: (due to iron overload) - hypogonadism, diabetes, growth failure, hypothyroidism
- Enlarged kidneys (due to increased hematopoiesis in the kidney).
- **Cardiac dysfunction:** heart failure (high output), arrhythmias.

HEMOGLOBIN ELECTROPHORESIS

	Hgb F	$HgbA_2$	HgbA
β-Thal trait (minor):	↑	↑	↓ (due to ↓beta chain production).
β-Thal Major (Cooley's):	**↑ up to 90%**	↑	**Little to no HgbA**

- **CBC in Beta thalassemia major:** hypochromic, microcytic anemia (↓MCV), normal or ↑RBC count, normal or ↑serum iron. Hgb usually about 6g/dL.
  - Peripheral smear: **target cells,** teardrop cells, basophilic stippling, nucleated RBCs.

Skull X-rays: bossing with "hair on end appearance" (due to extramedullary hematopoiesis).

MANAGEMENT

- Beta thalassemia minor (trait): no treatment needed. Genetic counseling.
- Moderate disease: folate (if increased reticulocyte count), avoid oxidative stress (eg, Sulfa drugs).

Management of Beta thalassemia major:

- **Often require frequent transfusions** during periods of increased hemolysis or severe anemia.
- **Iron chelating agents** (eg, **Deferoxamine,** Deferasirox) prevent iron overload & remove **excess iron** from chronic transfusions. Patients may develop endocrine deficiencies as a result of iron overload (eg, hypothyroidism, hypoparathyroidism, gonadal failure, diabetes mellitus) or CHF.
- **Vitamin C & folate supplementation** (substrates for RBC production).
- Splenectomy in some cases (stops RBC destruction). Allogeneic hematopoietic cell transplantation.

MACROCYTIC ANEMIAS

B12 (COBALAMIN) DEFICIENCY

- Sources of B12: natural sources **mainly animal in origin** (eg, meats, eggs, dairy products).
- Absorption: B12 is released by the acidity of the stomach & **combines with intrinsic factor, where it is absorbed mainly in the distal ileum.**

- Pathophysiology: B12 deficiency causes **abnormal synthesis of DNA**, nucleic acids, & metabolism of erythroid precursors. B12 needed to convert homocysteine to methionine for DNA synthesis.

ETIOLOGIES

- **Decreased absorption: Pernicious anemia most common cause** (lack of intrinsic factor due to parietal cell antibodies, leading to gastric atrophy). Pancreatic insufficiency, **Crohn disease** (affects the terminal ileum); Ileal resection, gastric bypass, post gastrectomy, gastritis, achlorhydria, tropical sprue, Zollinger-Ellison syndrome, Celiac disease. **Chronic alcohol use.** Meds: **H2 blockers & PPIs** (decreased acidity leads to decreased absorption), decreased nucleic acid synthesis (**Metformin**, Zidovudine, Hydroxyurea), anticonvulsants. Fish tapeworm.

- Decreased intake: **vegans** (lack of consumption of meat and meat products).

CLINICAL MANIFESTATIONS

- Anemia symptoms **similar to folate but associated with neurologic abnormalities.**

- Hematologic: fatigue, exercise intolerance, pallor.

- Epithelial: glossitis, diarrhea, malabsorption.

- **Neurologic symptoms: symmetric paresthesias most common initial symptom** (especially involving the legs), **lateral and posterior spinal cord demyelination & degeneration:** ataxia, weakness, **vibratory, sensory, & proprioception deficits, decreased deep tendon reflexes** (hypotonia), ⊕ Babinski, seizures, psychosis.

DIAGNOSIS

- CBC with peripheral smear: **increased MCV (macrocytic anemia)** + megaloblastic anemia (**hypersegmented neutrophils, macro-ovalocytes,** mild leukopenia and/or thrombocytopenia), low reticulocytes.

- Decreased serum B12 levels, increased LDH, **increased homocysteine.**

- **Increased methylmalonic acid** distinguishes B12 from folate deficiency.

MANAGEMENT

- Routes of administration: oral, sublingual, nasal and intramuscular/deep subcutaneous injection.

- **Symptomatic anemia or neuro findings: start with IM B12**. In adults, IM cyanocobalamin injection weekly until the deficiency is corrected and then once monthly. Patients can be switched to oral therapy after resolution of symptoms. **Patients with Pernicious anemia need lifelong monthly IM therapy** (or high-dose oral therapy).

- Dietary deficiency: oral B12 replacement.

FOLATE DEFICIENCY

- Functions of Folate: folate required for DNA synthesis. Folate deficiency causes **abnormal synthesis of DNA**, nucleic acids, & metabolism of erythroid precursors.
- Folate stores only last for 2 – 4 months.

ETIOLOGIES
- **Inadequate intake: most common cause** (eg, **alcoholics, unbalanced diet**).
- Increased requirements: pregnancy, infancy, hemolytic anemias, malignancy, Psoriasis (increased skin turnover).
- Impaired absorption: Celiac disease, Inflammatory bowel disease, chronic diarrhea, anticonvulsants (eg, Phenytoin, Phenobarbital, Carbamazepine).
- Impaired metabolism: **Methotrexate, Trimethoprim,** Pentamidine, antiseizure agents (eg, Phenytoin, Valproate, Carbamazepine), ethanol.
- Loss: dialysis

CLINICAL MANIFESTATIONS
- Anemia symptoms **similar to B12 deficiency but without neurologic abnormalities.**
- Hematologic: fatigue, exercise intolerance, pallor, chlorosis (pale, faintly green complexion – extremely rare).
- Epithelial: glossitis, aphthous ulcer, diarrhea, malabsorption.

DIAGNOSIS
- CBC with peripheral smear:
  Increased MCV (macrocytic anemia) + megaloblastic anemia (**hypersegmented neutrophils, macro-ovalocytes),** low reticulocytes. May develop pancytopenia.
- Decreased serum folate levels, increased LDH, **increased homocysteine, normal methylmalonic acid** (distinguishes folate from B12 deficiency).

MANAGEMENT
- Oral folic acid. Parenteral in severe folic acid deficiency.
- Replacing folic acid in patients with B12 deficiency may correct anemia but neurologic symptoms will worsen.

- **EXAM TIP**
- B12 & folate (in common): anemia, macrocytosis, macro-ovalocytes, decreased reticulocytes, hypersegmented neutrophils, and increased homocysteine.
- **B12 only: neurologic symptoms, increased methylmalonic acid.**
- Folate only: no neurologic symptoms, normal methylmalonic acid

CAUSES OF MACROCYTIC ANEMIA
- **B12 (Cobalamin) deficiency**
- **Folate deficiency**
- Chronic liver disease
- Alcoholism
- Hypothyroidism
- Myelodysplastic syndrome and acute leukemia

NORMOCYTIC ANEMIAS

ETIOLOGIES:
Anemia of chronic disease (most common), renal, mixed disorders (eg, iron + B_{12} deficiency); endocrine, early iron deficiency, asplenia, dilutional, sickle cell, G6PD.

ANEMIA OF CHRONIC DISEASE

- Anemia due to decreased red blood cell production in the setting of chronic disease.

ETIOLOGIES
- Chronic inflammatory conditions - chronic infection, inflammation, autoimmune disorders, malignancy.

PATHOPHYSIOLOGY
3 main factors decrease serum iron:
- **Increased hepcidin:** hepcidin is an acute phase reactant that blocks the release of iron from macrophages & reduces GI absorption of iron.
- **Increased ferritin:** ferritin is an acute phase reactant that sequesters iron into storage.
- Erythropoietin inhibition via cytokines.

DIAGNOSIS
- CBC: **mild normocytic normochromic anemia (may present with microcytic hypochromic anemia early on).** Hemoglobin usually not < 9-10mg/dL. Decreased reticulocytes, normal to increased RDW.

- Iron studies: **normal to increased ferritin + decreased TIBC + decreased serum iron** (serum ferritin & TIBC may be within normal limits). Normal or low transferrin saturation.

MANAGEMENT
- Treating the underlying disease will help to correct the anemia.

- **Erythropoietin-alpha if renal disease** or low erythropoietin levels.

- **EXAM TIP**
- **Iron deficiency anemia**: microcytic hypochromic anemia, **decreased ferritin** (depleted iron stores), decreased serum iron, increased TIBC.
- **Anemia of chronic disease:** normocytic, normochromic anemia (may be microcytic early on), normal or **increased ferritin, decreased TIBC**, decreased serum iron.
- **Thalassemia**: microcytic hypochromic anemia, normal or increased ferritin, **normal or increased serum iron.**

	SERUM FE	TIBC	FERRITIN
FE DEFICIENCY	↓(<30μg/dL)	↑	↓ (<20μg/dL)
ANEMIA OF CHRONIC DISEASE	↓(<50μg/dL)	↓	↑ or normal

UNDERSTANDING HEMOLYTIC ANEMIAS

- Hemolytic anemia: anemia caused by ↑RBC destruction when the rate of destruction exceeds the bone marrow's ability to replace the destroyed cells. There are two types: intrinsic & extrinsic.
  Intrinsic (inherited disorders):
  Eg, Sickle cell anemia, Thalassemia, G6PD deficiency, Hereditary spherocytosis.

  Extrinsic (acquired disorders): autoimmune hemolytic anemia, DIC, TTP, HUS, Paroxysmal nocturnal hemoglobinuria, Hypersplenism.

DIAGNOSIS

- Peripheral smear: **increased reticulocytes** (immature RBCs). Schistocytes (bite cells) if intravascular hemolysis.

- **Haptoglobin is decreased** because it becomes depleted when it binds the free hemoglobin with continued RBC destruction.

- **Indirect bilirubin is increased** due to increased RBC destruction, which overwhelms the liver's ability to convert it to direct bilirubin.

- **Reticulocyte count increases** in response to increased RBC destruction. The immature RBCs (reticulocytes) attempt to replace the mature RBCs that are being destroyed.

- **LDH increases** because it is an enzyme that is released from destroyed RBCs.

LOOK FOR THE FOLLOWING TO HELP DISTINGUISH BETWEEN THE HEMOLYTIC ANEMIAS:

- Sickle cell anemia: **sickled cells on peripheral smear, Hgb S** on hemoglobin electrophoresis.

- Thalassemia: **microcytic anemia with normal/↑ serum Fe or no response to Fe tx.** Thalassemias are also associated with severe anemia & abnormal peripheral smear for a given hematocrit level.
  Alpha Thalassemia: hemoglobin electrophoresis with **normal Hgb ratios** of HgbA, A_2, & F or **Hemoglobin H**.
  Alpha thalassemia is a diagnosis of exclusion (since the peripheral smear is normal).
  Beta Thalassemia: hemoglobin electrophoresis: ↓**HgbA**, ↑HgbA_2, ↑**HgbF.**

- G6PD deficiency: **EPISODIC hemolytic anemia associated with sulfa drugs, fava beans, infections.**

- Hereditary spherocytosis: **microspherocytes, Coombs NEGATIVE,** ⊕ osmotic fragility test.

- Autoimmune hemolytic anemia: **microspherocytes, Coombs POSITIVE.**

- TTP & HUS: **normal coags** (unable to distinguish between TTP & HUS via labs).
  TTP: Pentad: Thrombocytopenia, hemolytic anemia, kidney damage, neurologic symptoms, fever.
  HUS: Triad: thrombocytopenia, hemolytic anemia, & kidney damage. HUS MC seen in children (especially with diarrhea prodrome). HUS has a higher association with kidney involvement than TTP & does not classically have fever or neurologic symptoms.

- Disseminated intravascular coagulation: abnormal coags (prolonged PT & PTT).

- Paroxysmal nocturnal hemoglobinuria: dark urine (worse in the morning).

AUTOIMMUNE DISORDERS

HEREDITARY SPHEROCYTOSIS (HS)

- Autosomal dominant hereditary intrinsic hemolytic anemia (some recessive forms of as well).
- Most common in Northern Europeans. 1 in 5,000 incidence.

PATHOPHYSIOLOGY

- **Deficiency in RBC membrane & cytoskeleton (spectrin)**, leading to **increased RBC fragility & sphere-shaped RBCs.** These abnormal RBCs are detected & destroyed by the spleen (hemolysis).

CLINICAL MANIFESTATIONS

- Broad spectrum of clinical presentations. Severe cases may present in infancy (eg, neonatal jaundice). Mild cases may present in adulthood.

- **Recurrent episodes of hemolysis (anemia, jaundice, & splenomegaly) hallmark**; pigmented gallstones (calcium bilirubinate).

DIAGNOSIS

- **Peripheral smear:**
  - **hypERchromic microcytosis**, 80% **spherocytes** (round RBCs that lack central pallor).
  - May have a hemolytic smear (schistocytes, increased reticulocytes).
  - **Increased MCHC most reliable** (mean corpuscular hemoglobin concentration). Increased RDW.

- Hemolysis: increased indirect bilirubin, decreased haptoglobin.

- **EMA binding: preferred test (most accurate)**. Flow cytometric analysis of eosin-5'-maleimide-labeled intact red blood cells & acidified glycerol lysis test.

- Osmotic fragility test: RBCs placed in a relatively hypotonic solution rupture easily due to the increased permeability of the RBC membrane.

- **Negative Coombs testing:** Coombs negativity distinguishes Hereditary spherocytosis from Autoimmune hemolytic anemia (which also has spherocytes but is Coombs positive).

MANAGEMENT

- **Folic acid** not curative but helpful to sustain RBC production & DNA synthesis.

- **Splenectomy curative in severe or refractory disease** (stops splenic RBC destruction). It should be delayed in children until at least 4 years of age (after the risk of severe sepsis has peaked). Anti-pneumococcal vaccine should be given prior to splenectomy.

AUTOIMMUNE HEMOLYTIC ANEMIA (AIHA)

- Acquired hemolytic anemia due to autoantibody production against RBCs.

PATHOPHYSIOLOGY

- **Warm: IgG antibodies** activated by protein antigens on the RBC surface at body temperatures, leading to RBC destruction by splenic macrophages or complement 3 activation (eg, Idiopathic, SLE, RA, CLL).

- **Cold: IgM antibodies** against polysaccharides on the RBC surface induce intravascular **complement-mediated RBC lysis,** especially at **colder temperatures** (<39F). IgM molecule binding can lead to agglutination.

ETIOLOGIES

- **Warm agglutinin:** idiopathic (most common), medications (eg, **Penicillin, Cephalosporins,** Methyldopa, Rifampin, Phenytoin), autoimmune (eg, **Systemic lupus erythematosus**), malignancy (eg, CLL, non-Hodgkin lymphoma), viral infections (especially in children), HIV.

- **Cold agglutinin disease (CAD):** infection (eg, ***Mycoplasma pneumoniae*, Epstein-Barr virus,** HIV), malignancy (eg, CLL, lymphoma), Waldenstrom macroglobulinemia.

CLINICAL MANIFESTATIONS

- Anemia (eg, pallor fatigue, weakness, dyspnea), hemolysis (eg, hemoglobinuria, jaundice). Splenomegaly.

- Cold-induced vascular phenonemona in CAD: **acrocyanosis** (numbness or mottling of the fingers, toes, nose, ears) that resolves with warming up of the body parts. Raynaud phenomenon, livedo reticularis (mottling).

DIAGNOSIS

- CBC + peripheral smear: decreased hemoglobin, hemolysis (reticulocytosis), **microspherocytes (especially warm),** may have increased MCHC. Polychromasia. RBC agglutination only in CAD.

- Labs: **hemolysis** (increased indirect bilirubin, increased LDH, decreased haptoglobin).

- ⊕ **Direct Coombs** (antiglobulin) test: **positive – IgG** & C3 positivity **most accurate test in Warm.** Only positive for complement 3 in Cold.

- Cold agglutinin titer most accurate for CAD (> 1:64).

MANAGEMENT

Warm agglutinin AIHA

- First line: **Glucocorticoids first-line if symptomatic.** Transfusion if severe.
- Second-line: **splenectomy or Rituximab** (anti CD20) **if no response to glucocorticoids.**
- Third-line: steroid-sparing agents (eg, Azathioprine, Cyclophosphamide, Cyclosporine).

MANAGEMENT

Cold agglutinin AIHA

- **Avoid of cold temperatures mainstay of treatment**, warm fluids if hospitalized.
- Severe or symptomatic anemia: transfusions, plasmapheresis, IVIG.
- Rituximab-containing regimens or Bortezomib in some patients.

SICKLE CELL DISEASE

- Group of inherited disorders affecting the beta-globin gene, leading to the production of RBCs that sickle, causing hemolysis & vaso-occlusive disease.
- Disorders include Sickle cell disease (homozygous sickle mutation), sickle beta thalassemia, Hemoglobin SC disease, etc.

PATHOPHYSIOLOGY

- Point mutation where **valine substitutes for glutamic acid** on the **beta chain. Sickle hemoglobin (HbS) has decreased solubility under hypoxic conditions,** leading to conformational change of the RBC shape (sickling) with subsequent **vaso-occlusion** (microthrombosis) & hypoxia. Sickled cells are destroyed by the spleen (**hemolytic anemia**).

SICKLE CELL TRAIT:

- **Heterozygous (AS).** 8% of African-Americans. Patients with Sickle cell trait are usually asymptomatic and are not anemic unless exposed to severe hypoxia, extreme physical stress, high altitudes or dehydration. **May develop episodic hematuria or isosthenuria** (due to papillary necrosis).

SICKLE CELL DISEASE:

- **Homozygous sickle mutation (SS).** 0.2% of African-Americans. The main clinical manifestations are due to **hemolytic anemia and vaso-occlusion** (eg, acute or chronic pain, tissue ischemia or infarction).

SICKLE CELL TRAIT

- **Sickle cell trait: heterozygous (AS).**
- 8% of African-Americans, populations where Malaria is endemic.
- Pathophysiology: In sickle cell trait, about 25-45% of their hemoglobin is HbS.

CLINICAL MANIFESTATIONS

- **Patients with Sickle cell trait are usually asymptomatic** and are not anemic unless exposed to severe hypoxia, extreme physical stress, low temperatures, high altitudes, or dehydration.
- **May develop episodic hematuria or isosthenuria** (due to papillary necrosis).
- May develop splenic infarction at high altitude and sudden death with prolonged exercise or physical training.

DIAGNOSIS

- **Hemoglobin electrophoresis:** presence of **both hemoglobin A (HbA) and Hemoglobin S (HbS) with the amount of HbA greater than HbS.** (FAS pattern in neonates).
- Peripheral smear: usually associated with normal hemoglobin, hematocrit, reticulocyte count, and peripheral smear.

MANAGEMENT

- **Sickle cell trait usually does not require treatment.** Painful crisis is not a component of the trait.
- Papillary necrosis: conservative (eg, IV fluids, bed rest and pain management).

SICKLE CELL DISEASE

- Group of inherited disorders affecting the beta globin gene, leading to production of RBCs that sickle, causing hemolysis & vaso-occlusive disease.

CLINICAL MANIFESTATIONS

- Symptoms **begin as early as 6 months** (when HbSS replaces fetal hemoglobin).
- **Dactylitis most common initial presentation.** Delayed growth & development, fever, infections.

- Infections:
  - **Functional asplenia** & autosplenectomy (from repeated splenic infarctions) often by 1.5 – 3 years of age lead to **increased risk of infection with encapsulated organisms** (eg, *S. pneumoniae, H. influenzae, N. meningitidis*, Group B *Streptococcus, Klebsiella, Salmonella*).
  - **Osteomyelitis:** ***Salmonella spp.*** common organism in patients with Sickle cell disease.
  - **Aplastic crisis** associated with **Parvovirus B19 infections.**

- Splenic sequestration crisis: vaso-occlusion in the spleen & RBC pooling in the spleen leads to **acute splenomegaly and rapid decrease in hemoglobin.** Often occurs in children.

- Hemolytic anemia: jaundice, gallstones (pigmented).

- Painful vaso-occlusive "crisis": triggered by hypoxia, cold weather, infection, dehydration, ETOH, & pregnancy. Associated with abrupt onset of pain **(acute chest syndrome, back, abdominal, bone pain).** Renal or hepatic dysfunction. **Priapism common.**

- Acute chest syndrome: fever, cough, tachypnea, oxygen desaturation, chest pain.

- Bony vaso-occlusion: **avascular (ischemic) necrosis of bones (eg, femoral or humeral head), "H"-shaped vertebrae** (central endplate depression with normal anterior & posterior margins).

- Skin Ulcers: especially on the tibia.

- Chronic hypoxia: pulmonary hypertension, congestive heart failure, symptoms of fatigue, dyspnea.

- **Stroke** (25% have one by age 45y, 25% children have silent episode).

DIAGNOSIS

Peripheral smear: best initial test

- Target cells, **sickled erythrocytes,** decreased hemoglobin (baseline 8-10 g/dL but decreased in crisis), decreased hematocrit.

- **Howell-jolly bodies** indicates functional asplenia.

Hemoglobin electrophoresis:

- **Sickle cell disease: HbS, little to no HbA, increased HbF.**

- Sickle cell trait: HbS, decreased HbA.

DNA analysis definitive.

MANAGEMENT

- **Pain control: IV hydration & oxygen first step in the management of pain crisis** (reverses & prevents sickling). Meperidine is not recommended in patients with SCD (may lead to seizures & renal failure at high doses).

- Folic acid supplementation needed for RBC production & DNA synthesis.

- RBC transfusion therapy may be needed in some crises (eg, acute chest syndrome, splenic sequestration, preoperative transfusion).

- Exchange transfusion therapy is used if there is severe vasoocclusive crisis (eg, acute chest syndrome, stroke, priapism, retinal infarction leading to visual changes).

- Allogeneic stem cell transplant: only potentially curative treatment for Sickle cell disease but has significant side effects.

REDUCTION OF EPISODES:

HYDROXYUREA

Mechanism of action:

- **Increases production of HbF** (which does not sickle and has a higher affinity for oxygen), increases RBC water, **reduces RBC sickling**, alters RBC adhesion to the endothelium. Inhibits ribonucleotide reductase.

Indications:

- **Mainstay of treatment** in SCD - **reduces the frequency and severity of pain episodes, decreases hospitalization rates, and prolongs survival.**
- Because it takes weeks to months to take full effect, it is not used for acute episodes.

Uses:

- Sickle cell disease, Polycythemia vera, Essential thrombocythemia.
- The combination of Hydroxyurea and L-glutamine can have additive benefits.

Adverse effects:

- Myelosuppression, GI (anorexia, nausea).

INFECTION PREVENTION IN CHILDREN

- In patients with Sickle cell disease, functional asplenia & autosplenectomy (from repeated splenic infarctions) often by 1.5 – 3 years of age lead to increased risk of infection with encapsulated organisms (eg, *S. pneumoniae, H. influenzae, N. meningitidis*, Group B Streptococcus, Klebsiella, Salmonella). Salmonella Osteomyelitis is usually associated with Sickle cell disease.
- **Prophylactic Penicillin is given as early as 2-3 months of age until at least 5 years of age to prevent infectious complications.**
- Pneumococcal and Influenza vaccines also help to reduce mortality.

- **EXAM TIP**
- **Aplastic crisis vs. Splenic sequestration:**
- Seen in both: rapid drop in hemoglobin, thrombocytopenia. Both may be caused by Parvovirus B19 infections.
- Aplastic crisis: drop in reticulocytes, mild neutropenia
- Splenic sequestration crisis: reticulocytosis, rapidly enlarging spleen, hypovolemia, thrombocytopenia.

PAROXYSMAL NOCTURNAL HEMOGLOBINURIA

- Rare, acquired stem cell mutation – **RBCs become deficient in GPI anchor surface proteins** (CD55 & CD59).

PATHOPHYSIOLOGY
- CD55 & CD59 normally protect RBCs from complement destruction. Deficiency in these proteins lead to **increased complement activation & intravascular RBC destruction.**

- This hemolysis can be dramatically increased during a viral or bacterial infection due to antigen-antibody reactions.

CLINICAL MANIFESTATIONS
- **Triad of hemolytic anemia (hemoglobinuria) + pancytopenia + unexplained thrombosis in atypical veins.**

- Hemolytic anemia: **dark, cola-colored urine during the night or early in the morning** with partial clearing during the day.

- Venous thrombosis of large vessels: due to haptoglobin and nitric oxide depletion. **Thrombosis in unusual veins** (eg, hepatic, cerebral, abdominal, subdermal veins). Abdominal or back pain, erectile dysfunction, chest pain. Thrombosis usually the cause of death.

- Pancytopenia: protein deficiency seen in RBCs, WBCs, & platelets derived from stem cells, causing bone marrow failure. Often occur after bone marrow injury. **Hypercoagulability despite pancytopenia hallmark.**

DIAGNOSIS
- Hemolysis: (eg, increased indirect bilirubin & LDH, decreased haptoglobin), hemoglobinuria. Increased reticulocytes. Hemosiderinuria.

- **Flow cytometry test: best test to look for PNH** – CD55/CD59-deficient RBCs.

- RBC fragility: sucrose test (cells lyse in hypotonic sucrose solution) & Osmotic fragility test. Increased RDW & Coombs negativity.

MANAGEMENT
- **Complement inhibitors**
  Eculizumab –anti-complement antibody targeting the C5 complement component.
  Ravulizumab (longer half-life).

- Folic acid supplementation.

- Allogeneic hematopoietic cell transplantation only potential for cure.

HEMOSTASIS

The process to stop bleeding (prevents exsanguination during injuries). 2 phases:

PRIMARY HEMOSTASIS: PLATELETS form a plug at the site of vascular injury: **platelet adhesion, activation, & aggregation**. Platelets adhere to site of the injury becoming activated, sending out ADP & Thromboxane A_2, which attract other platelets to aggregate, **forming a platelet plug.**

- **Disease examples:** thrombocytopenia (ITP, TTP, HUS, DIC, von Willebrand deficiency).
- **Disorders that affect platelets will affect primary hemostasis,** bleeding time (eg, immediate bleeding after surgery) but **PT & PTT are usually unaffected** (clotting factors are unaffected).
- These diseases classically cause **petechiae & mucocutaneous bleeding** (oral, GI, menorrhagia).

SECONDARY HEMOSTASIS: CLOTTING FACTORS (proteins) respond in a cascade to form **fibrin strands which strengthens the platelet plug** (that was formed during primary hemostasis).

- **Disease examples:** Hemophilia, DIC & von Willebrand disease.
- Disorders that affect the extrinsic pathway (prolongs PT) and intrinsic pathway (prolongs PTT).
- These diseases classically cause **deep delayed bleeding (eg, hemarthrosis = bleeding into the joints & muscles)** or **delayed bleeding after surgery.**

PRIMARY HEMOSTASIS
PLATELET adhesion, activation, aggregation.

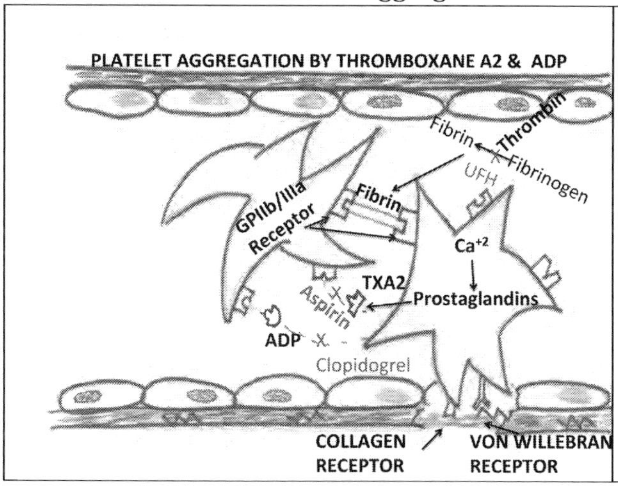

SECONDARY HEMOSTASIS
CLOTTING FACTORS leading to fibrin formation.

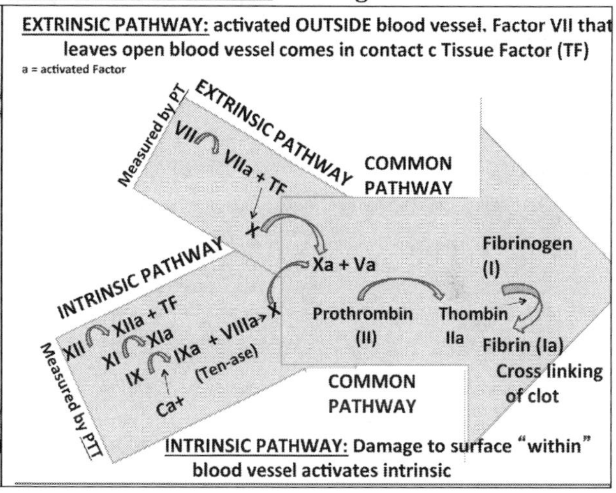

PTT (Partial Thromboplastin Time): measures efficacy of the **INTRINSIC** & common coagulation pathway. Normal PTT times require the presence of Factors I, II, V, **VIII, IX**, X, **XI**, and **XII**.
Factors 1, 2, 5, **8, 9**, **11, & 12.**

Prolonged PTT: Heparin, DIC, vWD, Hemophilia A & B & antiphospholipid antibody syndrome (which paradoxically ↑'es thrombogenicity).
Heparin overdose antidote: Protamine sulfate.

PT (Prothrombin Time):
Measures the **EXTRINSIC (tissue factor) pathway** & common pathway.
Normal PT times primarily require the presence of Factors I, II, V, **VII**, & **X** (1, 2, 5, **7 & 10**).

Prolonged PT: Warfarin therapy, Vitamin K deficiency, DIC.
Warfarin overdose antidote: Vitamin K.

THROMBOTIC THROMBOCYTOPENIC PURPURA (TTP)

- Thrombotic microangiopathy resulting from ADAMTS13 deficiency.

PATHOPHYSIOLOGY
- ADAMTS13 is a von Willebrand factor-cleaving protease.
- **ADAMTS 13 deficiency leads to large vWF multimers that cause small vessel thrombosis.**

ETIOLOGIES
- Primary: idiopathic (autoimmune) – antibodies against ADAMTS13.
- Secondary: malignancy, bone marrow transplantation, estrogen, **Systemic lupus erythematosus,** pregnancy, HIV1, medications (eg, Quinidine, Ticlopidine, Clopidogrel, Cyclosporine).

CLINICAL MANIFESTATIONS: **pentad:**
- **Thrombocytopenia: mucocutaneous bleeding** - epistaxis, bleeding gums, petechiae, purpura, bruising, menorrhagia.

- **Microangiopathic hemolytic anemia:** anemia, jaundice, fragmented RBCs (schistocytes on peripheral smear). **Splenomegaly.**

- **Neurologic symptoms**: headache, visual changes, confusion, seizures, CVA.

- **Fever** (rare). Since plasma exchange therapy, it is rare for patients to present with all 5 simultaneously.
- **Kidney failure or uremia** (not as common).

DIAGNOSIS
- Labs: **thrombocytopenia with normal coagulation studies** (seen in both TTP & HUS). Normal coagulation studies (PT & PTT) helps to distinguish TTP and HUS from DIC.

- **Hemolysis:** peripheral smear – schistocytes (helmet cells), bite or fragmented cells, reticulocytes. Increased LDH & bilirubin, decreased haptoglobin.

- Decreased ADAMTS13 levels. Coombs negative. Increased bleeding time.

MANAGEMENT
- **Plasmapheresis: initial treatment of choice.** Plasmapheresis removes antibodies vs. ADAMTS13 & adds ADAMTS13 to serum - Monitor LDH/platelets until normal x 2 days.

- Immunosuppression: **glucocorticoids and/or Rituximab if no response to Plasmapheresis,** Cyclophosphamide etc.

- Platelet transfusions not usually indicated (may potentiate thrombi formation).

- Splenectomy an option in patients refractory to plasma exchange and immunosuppressants.

HEMOLYTIC UREMIC SYNDROME

- Thrombotic microangiopathy due to **platelet activation by exotoxins**.

- **Triad of <u>thrombocytopenia, hemolytic anemia & renal dysfunction</u> (uremia).** Fever and neurologic symptoms (seen in TTP) are often absent in HUS.

<u>RISK FACTORS</u>

- **Predominantly seen in children with a recent history of gastroenteritis.**

- In adults, it is associated with HIV, SLE, antiphospholipid syndrome or chemotherapy (eg, Mitomycin, Bleomycin, Cisplatin Gemcitabine).

<u>PATHOPHYSIOLOGY</u>

- **<u>D+ HUS (classic):</u> associated with diarrhea prodrome**. Exotoxins (eg, Shigella toxin & Shiga-like toxin in ***Enterohemorrhagic E. coli* 0157:H7**) enters the blood where it **damages vascular endothelium, activating platelets (microthrombi formation),** eventually depleting platelets. The toxins preferentially damage the kidney, leading to **uremia.**

- <u>D- HUS (atypical):</u> not associated with diarrhea. Not common.

- <u>P-HUS:</u> *Streptococcus pneumoniae* releases neuraminidase, which initiates an inflammatory reaction.

<u>CLINICAL MANIFESTATIONS</u>

- May have prodromal diarrheal illness 5-10 days prior (**abdominal pain, bloody diarrhea**, nausea, vomiting). Renal involvement (eg, **oliguria & hematuria**).

- <u>Physical examination:</u> pallor (anemia), jaundice (hemolysis), hepatosplenomegaly. Petechiae & purpura are uncommon.

<u>DIAGNOSIS</u>

Labs are the same in TTP and HUS

- <u>Labs:</u> **thrombocytopenia with normal coagulation studies** (seen in both TTP & HUS). Normal coagulation studies (PT & PTT) helps to distinguish TTP and HUS from DIC.

- **<u>Hemolysis:</u>** peripheral smear – **schistocytes (helmet cells),** bite or fragmented cells, reticulocytes. Increased LDH & bilirubin, decreased haptoglobin.

- **Increased BUN and creatinine.** Coombs negative. Increased bleeding time.

<u>MANAGEMENT</u>

- **<u>Supportive therapy</u> initial management of choice** (eg, fluid & electrolyte replacement, dialysis, discontinuing any nephrotoxic medications, RBC transfusion if severe anemia).

- **Plasmapheresis** (with or without fresh frozen plasma) **if severe**, neurologic complications, & non-renal complications.

- **Antibiotics and anti-motility agents are usually avoided because they may worsen the condition.**

DISSEMINATED INTRAVASCULAR COAGULATION (DIC)

- **Pathological activation of the coagulation system.**

PATHOPHYSIOLOGY
- Uncontrolled fibrin production due to tissue factor activation leads to **widespread microthrombi,** which consumes coagulation proteins (V, VIII, fibrinogen) & platelets. Consumption then leads to **severe thrombocytopenia,** manifested by **diffuse bleeding** from the skin, respiratory tract & GI tract. Microthrombi lead to organ ischemia.

ETIOLOGIES
- **Infections (eg, gram-negative sepsis most common),** Rocky Mountain spotted fever, viral.
- **Malignancies:** Acute myelogenous leukemia; Lung, GI or prostate malignancies.
- **Obstetric:** pre-eclampsia; ~50% of patients with Abruptio placentae or amniotic fluid embolism have evidence of DIC, septic abortion.
- Massive tissue injury & trauma: burns, liver disease, aortic aneurysm, ARDS.

CLINICAL MANIFESTATIONS
- **Bleeding: oozing from venipuncture sites, catheters, drains,** extensive bruising.
- **Thrombosis:** arterial and/or venous – **gangrene** or multi-organ failure (eg, renal, hepatic).

DIAGNOSIS
- Increased thrombin formation: **decreased fibrinogen** (from consumption).
- Bleeding: **increased PT, PTT, & INR. Thrombocytopenia.**
- Increased fibrinolysis: **increased D-dimer** (D-dimer is a fibrin degradation product).
- Peripheral smear: fragmented RBCs, schistocytes.

MANAGEMENT
- **Treating the underlying cause is the mainstay of treatment.**
- Platelet transfusion if platelet count <20,000/microL if not actively bleeding.
- Fresh frozen plasma if severe bleeding (replaces coagulation factors)
- Cryoprecipitate (replaces fibrinogen in patients with severely low levels).
- Heparin for thrombosis in some patients.

DISORDERS	PT	PTT	BLEEDING TIME	PLATELET count
THROMBOCYTOPENIA	Unaffected	Unaffected	**Prolonged**	Decreased
HEMOPHILIA	Unaffected	**Prolonged**	Unaffected (normal platelets)	Unaffected
VON WILLEBRAND DISEASE	Unaffected	**Prolonged**	**Prolonged (especially with aspirin challenge).**	Unaffected
VITAMIN K DEFICIENCY (EG, WARFARIN)	**Prolonged**	Normal or minor prolongation.	Unaffected	Unaffected
DIC	**Prolonged**	**Prolonged**	**Prolonged**	**Decreased**

IMMUNE THROMBOCYTOPENIC PURPURA (ITP)

- Acquired, immune-mediated **isolated thrombocytopenia** (low platelet count).

PATHOPHYSIOLOGY

- **Autoantibodies against platelets, leading to splenic destruction of platelets.** The autoantibodies develop against the GP IIb/IIIa receptor on platelets.

TYPES

- Primary ITP: idiopathic. **Most common after viral infection (self-limited).**

- Secondary ITP: immune-mediated but **associated with underlying disorders** (eg, SLE, **HIV, HCV**, antiphospholipid syndrome). Most common in adults & is usually recurrent.

CLINICAL MANIFESTATIONS

- Often asymptomatic.
- **Mucocutaneous bleeding:** eg, epistaxis, bleeding gums, petechiae, purpura, bruising, menorrhagia.
- Severe bleeding: not common - intracranial hemorrhage, GI bleeding, hematuria.
- **Not associated with splenomegaly.**

DIAGNOSIS

- **Isolated thrombocytopenia** with **normal coagulation studies (PT, PTT, INR),** normal WBC count, normal hematocrit. Peripheral smear usually normal.

- Bleeding time may be elevated (as with other causes of thrombocytopenia)
- Bone marrow: **Megakaryocytes** (large-sized platelets) may be seen. Marrow testing usually reserved for older patients or non-responsive patients.

MANAGEMENT IN ADULTS

Mild bleeding + platelet < 30,000:

- **Glucocorticoids first-line therapy** (blunts the immune response).
- **Intravenous immunoglobulin (IVIG) second-line** therapy or if rapid rise in platelet counts required.
- Refractory: **Rituximab or Splenectomy.**

Severe bleeding (GI/CNS) + platelets < 30,000:

- Platelet transfusion + IVIG + high-dose glucocorticoids.

No bleeding + platelet > 30,000:

- Observation.

MANAGEMENT IN CHILDREN

- No bleeding or mild bleeding not at risk: **observation.**

- **Intravenous immunoglobulin (IVIG) if rapid rise in platelet counts required.**

- **Glucocorticoids** if increased risk of bleeding but rapid rise in platelets not needed.

- Life-threatening bleeding: IV Glucocorticoids plus IVIG.

	ITP	TTP	HUS	DIC
Pathophysiology	• ***Autoimmune-Antibody reaction vs. platelets**** with splenic platelet destruction ⇨ consumptive thrombocytopenia	• ***Auto-Ab vs. ADAMTS13**** (vWF-cleaving protease) ⇨ unusual large vWF multimers ⇨ micro thrombosis of small vessels ⇨ ***thrombocytopenia (consumptive) & hemolytic anemia.***	• ***Exotoxins*** (Shiga-like & Shiga toxins) damages vascular endothelium*, activating platelets ⇨ ***microthrombosis of small vessels*** ⇨ *consumptive* ***thrombocytopenia and hemolytic anemia.*** • ADAMTS13 normal	• ***Pathologic clotting cascade activation*** ⇨ ***widespread thrombi*** ⇨ consumption of platelets ⇨ ***diffuse bleeding***
Incidence	• ***Predominantly young children*** 2-4y. Often ***1-3 weeks following acute viral infection.**** Often self-limited in children. • **Adult:** young women <40y idiopathic. Often recurrent	• ***Young adults*** *20-50y* • ***MC women***	• ***Predominantly seen in children with diarrhea prodrome*: Enterohem. E coli O157:H7 (80%). Shigella, Salmonella,*** • Adults: seen with HIV, SLE, Anti phospholipid syndrome.	• ***MC in young or elderly*** • ***MC gram negative sepsis**** • *OB emergencies* • *Malignancy* • *Massive tissue trauma.*
Clinical Manifestations	• Often asymptomatic. • ***↑mucocutaneous bleeding: petechiae, bruising, purpura, bullae,*** bleeding of tooth & gums, menorrhagia. • ***NO SPLENOMEGALY****	**PENTAD*** 1. ***Thrombocytopenia***: bruising, purpura, bleeding. 2. ***Microangiopathic hemolytic anemia***: anemia, jaundice. 3. *Kidney failure/uremia*: (*not as common as in HUS.* 4. ***Neuro sx:**** headache, CVA, AMS 5. ***Fever***	**TRIAD*** 1. ***Thrombocytopenia***: bruising, purpura, bleeding 2. ***Microangiopathic hemolytic anemia***: anemia, jaundice 3. ***Kidney failure/uremia***: ***predominant feature.**** *Suspect HUS if renal failure in children with diarrhea prodrome*.*	• **Diffuse hemorrhage:** ***venipuncture sites, mouth, nose; extensive bruising.*** • **Thrombosis:** ***renal failure, gangrene*** (as clots block circulation). • Patients usually acutely ill
Diagnosis	• ***ISOLATED THROMBOCYTOPENIA**** • Normal coag tests (PT, PTT)	• ***Thrombocytopenia*** **Hemolytic anemia:** • Peripheral smear: ↑*reticulocytes, schistocytes* ("bite or fragmented cells) • ***LFTs: ↑Ind bili; ↓haptoglobin*** • Normal coag tests (PT, PTT)	• Labs & peripheral smear in TTP & HUS look the same. • ***↑BUN/Creatinine**** (Renal failure) • Normal coags (PT, PTT) distinguish TTP & HUS from DIC*	**Hemolytic anemia:** • Peripheral smear: ↑*reticulocytes, schistocytes* ("bite or fragmented cells) • ***LFTs: ↑Ind bili; ↓haptoglobin*** • ***ABNORMAL COAG TESTS*:*** ***↓fibrinogen, ↑D-dimer, ↑PT, PTT. severe thrombocytopenia.***
Management	• **CHILDREN**: ***observation*** *~80% resolve without tx within 6 months.* ***±Intravenous immunoglobulin.*** • **ADULTS:** ***CORTICOSTEROIDS**** (blunts the immune response) ⇨ ***IVIG*** ⇨ ***SPLENECTOMY IN REFRACTORY CASES.****	• ***PLASMAPHERESIS mainstay**** (↓es mortality). Removes Ab & adds ADAMTS13 • **Immunosuppression**: ***steroids,*** Cyclophosphamides etc.	• ***Observation in most children (usually self-limited).*** • *Plasmapheresis* • ±FFP if severe, • ***NO antibiotics**** - *may worsen the disease (↑toxin release).*	• ***Reversal of the underlying cause mainstay of tx**** • ±Platelet transfusion (if <20,000) • ±Fresh frozen plasma • ±Heparin in select cases.

HEMOPHILIA A (Factor VIII 8 Deficiency)

- **X-linked recessive** disorder **occurring almost exclusively in males** (rarely in homozygous females). Can also be caused by spontaneous mutation.
- **Most common type of Hemophilia.** First episode usually <18 years of age.
- **Lack of Factor VIII** affects the clotting cascade, leading to **failure of hematoma formation.**

CLINICAL MANIFESTATIONS

- **Hemarthrosis** (80%): **delayed bleeding or swelling in weight-bearing joints** (eg, **ankles,** knees, elbows), soft tissues, & muscles (eg, forehead hematoma).
- **Excessive hemorrhage due to trauma & surgery or incisional bleeding** (eg, tooth extraction).
- Epistaxis, bruising. GI or urinary tract hemorrhage.
- Hemophilias less commonly present with purpura, petechiae (because platelet function is normal) or spontaneous hemorrhage (except in the severe form).

DIAGNOSIS

- CBC & coagulation studies: **Prolonged aPTT.** Normal PT, fibrinogen, **platelet levels** (bleeding time).
- Mixing studies: **PTT corrects with mixing studies** (factor deficiency). **Low Factor VIII** - most sensitive.

MANAGEMENT

- **Factor VIII infusion first-line therapy** to increase levels 25-100% (depending on severity). Can be given in response to an **acute bleeding episode or prophylaxis** (eg, prior to surgery, after trauma).
- **Desmopressin (DDAVP):** transiently increases **Factor VIII & vWF** release from endothelial stores. May be used prior to procedures to **prevent bleeding in mild disease**.

HEMOPHILIA B (Christmas Disease) (Factor IX/9 Deficiency)

- **X-linked recessive** disorder **occurring almost exclusively in males** (rarely in homozygous females).
- Also known as Christmas disease. Clinically indistinguishable from Hemophilia A.
- **Lack of Factor IX** affects the clotting cascade, leading to **failure of hematoma formation.**

CLINICAL MANIFESTATIONS

- **Hemarthrosis** (80%): **delayed bleeding or swelling in weight-bearing joints** (eg, **ankles,** knees, elbows), soft tissues & muscles (eg, forehead hematoma).
- **Excessive hemorrhage in response to trauma & surgery or incisional bleeding** (eg, tooth extraction). Epistaxis, bruising. GI or urinary tract hemorrhage.
- Hemophilias less commonly present with purpura, petechiae (because platelet function is normal) or spontaneous hemorrhage (except in the severe form).

DIAGNOSIS

- CBC & coagulation studies: **Prolonged aPTT.** Normal PT, fibrinogen, & platelets (bleeding time).
- Mixing studies: **PTT corrects with mixing studies** (indicating a factor deficiency).
- **Low Factor IX** - most sensitive.

MANAGEMENT

- **Factor IX infusion first-line therapy** to increase levels 25-100% (depending on severity). Can be given in response to an **acute bleeding episode or prophylaxis** (eg, prior to surgery).
- Unlike Hemophilia A, **Desmopressin is not useful.**

VON WILLEBRAND DISEASE

- Autosomal dominant disorder associated with **ineffective platelet adhesion** due to **deficient or defective von Willebrand Factor.**
- **Most common hereditary bleeding disorder** (1% of population). May also be acquired.

FUNCTION OF VWF:
- Von Willebrand factor (VWF) promotes platelet adhesion by crosslinking the GP1b receptor on platelets with exposed collagen on damaged epithelium. VWF also prevents Factor VIII degradation.

CLINICAL MANIFESTATIONS
- **Mucocutaneous bleeding:** eg, epistaxis, bleeding gums, petechiae, purpura, bruising, menorrhagia, prolonged bleeding after minor cuts.
- Incisional bleeding less common in VWD than in Hemophilia.

INITIAL LABS
- Coagulation studies: **prolonged PTT** (corrects with mixing study).
  PTT & bleeding time prolongation worse with Aspirin.
- Platelet count is usually normal (except in 2B which is associated with mild thrombocytopenia).

SCREENING TESTS
- Plasma VWF antigen – **decreased VWF antigen or VWF activity** 30 IU or less is diagnostic.
- Plasma VWF activity (**Ristocetin cofactor activity** and VWF collagen binding). No platelet aggregation with Ristocetin in VWD.
- Factor VIII activity: may be decreased.

SPECIALIZED ASSAYS: helps to determine the type of VWD.
- VWF multimer distribution using gel electrophoresis.
- Ristocetin-induced platelet aggregation (gold standard).

MANAGEMENT

Type I: quantitative deficiency. Most common type (75%).
- **Mild to moderate bleeding: DDAVP (Desmopressin).**

- Severe: **VWF-containing product** (eg, **factor VIII concentrates**, purified VWF concentrates, recombinant VWF).

- **Minor procedures: Desmopressin used in type I and 2A** for minor trauma, dental, and minor surgical procedures. Desmopressin stimulates release of vWF and factor VIII from endothelial cells.

- **Major procedures: VWF containing products** (eg, human derived Factor VIII concentrates).

Type II (qualitative deficiency):
- **DDAVP** for most. VWF or DDAVP prior to procedures.

Type III (severe, absent VWF):
- VWF-containing product (eg, human-derived factor VIII concentrates, purified VWF concentrates, recombinant VWF).

FACTOR V LEIDEN MUTATION

- **Most common inherited cause of hypercoagulability (thrombophilia).**
- 5% of the US population.

PATHOPHYSIOLOGY

- **Mutated factor V is resistant to breakdown by activated protein C**, leading to increased hypercoagulability.

CLINICAL MANIFESTATIONS

- **Increased incidence of DVT, PE, hepatic vein, or cerebral vein thrombosis**. Increased risk of miscarriages during pregnancy.
- Not associated with increased risk of myocardial infarctions or CVA.

DIAGNOSIS

- Activated protein C resistance assay. If positive, confirm with DNA testing.
- DNA testing mutation analysis. Used in patients with a family history of Factor V Leiden mutation or for members of a thrombophilic family.
- Normal PT and PTT.

MANAGEMENT

- High-risk: **indefinite anticoagulation.** May need thrombophylaxis with low molecular weight heparin during pregnancy to prevent miscarriages.
- Moderate-risk: (eg, 1 thrombotic event with a prothrombotic stimulus or asymptomatic) prophylaxis during high-risk procedures.

PROTEIN C or S DEFICIENCY

PATHOPHYSIOLOGY

- **Proteins C & S are vitamin K-dependent anticoagulant proteins** produced by the liver that stimulate fibrinolysis and inactivate factors V and VIII.
- **Decreased protein C or S levels lead to hypercoagulability.**

ETIOLOGIES

- Inherited: both are autosomal-dominant inherited hypercoagulable disorders (C more common).
- Acquired: end-stage liver disease, severe liver disease with synthetic dysfunction, early Warfarin administration (vitamin K antagonist).

CLINICAL MANIFESTATIONS

- **Increased incidence of DVT & PE.**
- **Warfarin-induced skin necrosis.**
- Purpura fulminans in newborns – red purpuric lesions at pressure points, progresses to painful black eschars.

DIAGNOSIS

- Protein C and S functional assay, plasma protein C and S antigen levels.
- Genetic testing not routinely performed

MANAGEMENT

- Thrombosis: protein C concentrate. Indefinite anticoagulation.
- Warfarin-induced necrosis: immediately discontinue Warfarin, administer IV Vitamin K, heparin, protein C concentrate, or fresh frozen plasma.

ANTITHROMBIN III DEFICIENCY

- Decreased levels of antithrombin III, leading to hypercoagulability.

PATHOPHYSIOLOGY
- Normally, antithrombin III inhibits coagulation by neutralizing the activity of thrombin (factors IIa, IXa, and Xa). Decreased levels lead to increased risk of clotting.

ETIOLOGIES
- Inherited: autosomal-dominant.
- Acquired: liver disease, nephrotic syndrome, DIC, chemotherapy

CLINICAL MANIFESTATIONS
- **Increased incidence of DVT & PE.**

DIAGNOSIS
- Antithrombin III assays

MANAGEMENT
- Asymptomatic: anticoagulation only before surgical procedures.
- Thrombosis: high-dose IV heparin followed by oral anticoagulation therapy indefinitely.

HEPARIN INDUCED THROMBOCYTOPENIA

- Acquired thrombocytopenia especially **within the first 5-10 days of the initiation of Heparin.**

RISK FACTORS
- Unfractionated > low molecular weight, surgical > medical, female > male.

PATHOPHYSIOLOGY
- **Autoantibody formation to the hapten of Heparin + platelet factor 4** causes platelet activation & consumption, leading to simultaneous **thrombocytopenia & thrombosis**.

CLINICAL MANIFESTATIONS
- Thrombocytopenia - bleeding
- Thrombosis: venous thrombosis, gangrene, organ infarction and skin necrosis.

DIAGNOSIS
- 4 Ts: thrombocytopenia, timing of platelet drop, thrombosis, absence of other sequelae.
- HIT antibody testing: 14-C-serotonin release assay gold standard, ELISA, functional assays.

MANAGEMENT
- **Immediate discontinuation of all Heparin + initiation of non-Heparin anticoagulants.**

- Non-Heparin anticoagulants: **direct thrombin inhibitors** (eg, **Argatroban & Lepirudin**), Fondaparinux, direct oral anticoagulants (eg, Apixaban, Edoxaban, Rivaroxaban or Dabigatran).

- Long-term anticoagulation with Warfarin can only be started after other non-Heparin anticoagulation has been started & the thrombosis has decreased because of the initial prothrombotic state normally associated with the first 5 days of the initiation of Warfarin therapy.

APLASTIC ANEMIA

- **Pancytopenia with bone marrow hypocellularity.**

PATHOPHYSIOLOGY
- T cells attack hematopoietic stem cells (autoimmunity) or direct stem cell damage leads to bone marrow failure, including replacement of marrow with fat.

ETIOLOGIES
- Idiopathic most common cause. Radiation exposure.

- Infections: seronegative viral hepatitis (non A through G), **Parvovirus B19** in patients with baseline hemolytic anemias (eg, Sickle cell disease, G6PD deficiency) other viruses.

- Medications: antibiotics (eg, **Chloramphenicol, Sulfa drugs),** chemotherapy (anticipated effect), Benzene, **anti-epileptics** (eg, **Carbamazepine**, Phenytoin), Quinine, NSAIDs, anti-thyroid medications.

- B12 & Folate deficiency can cause pancytopenia.

CLINICAL MANIFESTATIONS

Symptoms of pancytopenia - easy bruising, bleeding, frequent infections, & fatigue.
- Thrombocytopenia: **mucocutaneous bleeding** (eg, epistaxis, bleeding gums, petechiae, purpura, bruising, menorrhagia).

- Anemia: weakness, fatigue, dyspnea.

- Leukopenia: recurrent or frequent infections, fever.

DIAGNOSIS
- CBC with peripheral smear: **at least 2 cytopenias -** few or absent reticulocytes, thrombocytopenia, neutropenia, anemia (nucleated RBCs if marrow fibrosis is present).

- Bone marrow biopsy: **most accurate test - hypocellular, fatty bone marrow** (fat cells & fibrotic stroma replace normal marrow).

- Often a diagnosis of exclusion in the setting of bone marrow failure (PNH & myelodysplastic syndrome may present similar).

MANAGEMENT
- **Supportive management initial treatment of choice** (eg, infection prophylaxis with broad-spectrum antibiotics, PRBC transfusion for hemoglobin < 7 mg/dL, or platelets for counts <10,000 or active bleeding).

- Severe AA in otherwise healthy patients < 50 years: **Allogeneic hematopoietic stem cell transplantation treatment of choice.**

- **Immunosuppressive therapy: patients > 50 years of age** or in younger patients without matched donor: Eltrombopag, anti-thymocyte globulin (ATG), Cyclosporine, Prednisone.

HEREDITARY HEMOCHROMATOSIS

- Autosomal recessive disorder characterized by **excess iron deposition** in the parenchymal cells of the **heart, liver, pancreas, & endocrine organs.**

- Associated with **C282Y HFE genotype** (increased in N. Europeans).

PATHOPHYSIOLOGY

- Mutation in the HFE protein leads to decreased hepcidin, the iron regulatory hormone.

- **Decreased hepcidin leads to increased intestinal iron absorption,** leading to organ dysfunction from iron deposition in the parenchymal cells.

CLINICAL MANIFESTATIONS

- May be asymptomatic in the early stages. Symptoms usually begin after 40 years of age.
- Liver: abdominal pain, **cirrhosis,** fatigue, weakness, hepatomegaly.
- Endocrine: **Diabetes** from pancreatic beta cell damage. Hypothyroidism.
- Heart: **restrictive or dilated cardiomyopathy, arrhythmias**, heart failure, heart blocks.
- Reproductive: **hypogonadism, erectile dysfunction,** testicular atrophy.
- Joints: arthralgias, arthritis, synovitis.
- Skin: **metallic or bronze skin** (from iron deposition) "bronze diabetes".
- Increased susceptibility to bacteria that feed on iron (eg, *Yersinia enterocolitica, Vibrio vulnificus*).

DIAGNOSIS

- Iron studies: initial test of choice - **increased serum iron, ferritin, & transferrin saturation.** Normal or decreased TIBC. May have abnormal LFTs.

- Genetic testing for the HFE gene (C282Y and H63D) + Abdominal MRI. Performed if iron studies are abnormal.

- Liver biopsy: **most accurate test - increased hemosiderin** in the liver parenchyma with Prussian blue staining. May be performed if genetic testing + MRI are negative.

MANAGEMENT

- **Phlebotomy mainstay of treatment.** May be performed weekly until ferritin decreases < 50 mcg/dL, decrease in transferrin saturation, or until a mild anemia occurs. May need maintenance phlebotomy therapy (eg, 3-4 times a year for life).

- Iron chelating agents in patients who are unable to undergo phlebotomy. More effective in patients with erythropoietic hemochromatosis. Deferoxamine, Deferasirox, Deferiprone.

- Treat the underlying cause. Avoid iron supplementation, vitamin C and alcohol intake.

WALDENSTRÖM MACROGLOBULINEMIA

- **Lymphoplasmacytic B-cell lymphoma** that **produces excess IgM.**
- Considered an indolent type of non-Hodgkin Lymphoma (incurable but treatable).
- Pathophysiology: **clonal B cell IgM production** (postgerminal center IgM memory B cell that has failed to switch isotype class).

CLINICAL MANIFESTATIONS
- Often asymptomatic (aka smoldering).
- If symptomatic, associated with "OVA" **Organomegaly, Viscosity, Anemia.**
- **Hyperviscosity syndrome:** large IgM molecules increase serum viscosity, slowing the passage of blood through the capillaries, leading to blurred vision, **engorged retinal veins**, papilledema, headache, vertigo, nystagmus, dizziness, tinnitus, diplopia, ataxia, stupor, or coma.
- **Anemia:** due to bone marrow failure - weakness, fatigue, weight loss, pallor.
- **Chronic, oozing blood from nose & gums:** IgM interaction with platelets & inhibition of fibrin.
- **Peripheral neuropathy** (10%) especially due to IgM acting as an autoantibody vs. myelin-associated glycoproteins in nerves & other nerve components.
- **Organomegaly:** lymphadenopathy, splenomegaly, hepatomegaly (30-40%).
- **Cryoglobulinemia:** IgM precipitates out of the serum in cold temperatures results in symptoms. **Raynaud phenomenon**, urticaria, acral cyanosis, and/or tissue necrosis.

DIAGNOSIS
- Serum protein electrophoresis: **IgM monoclonal spike** (macroglobulinemia).
- Bone marrow biopsy: **>10% lymphoplasmacytic infiltrate** (must exclude CLL). Dutcher bodies.
- Anemia, thrombocytopenia, neutropenia. Elevated beta-2 microglobulin level.

MANAGEMENT
- Observation can be done in asymptomatic cases. Highly responsive to chemotherapy (rarely curative).
- Rituximab + Bendamustine first-line medical management.
- Failure or relapse: Bortezomib, Cyclophosphamide, or Ibrutinib.
- **Plasmapheresis used to treat severe hyperviscosity** syndrome with complications.

MONOCLONAL GAMMOPATHY OF UNDERTERMINED SIGNIFICANCE (MGUS)

- **Clinically asymptomatic** premalignant clonal lymphoplasmacytic or plasma cell proliferative disease, leading to **increased immunoglobulins.**
- 1% of adults, 3% of adults >70y. 1% yearly risk of developing Multiple myeloma or lymphoma
- **IgG most common** (69%), IgM (17%), IgA (11%), IgD, kappa light chains (62%), lambda light chains (38%)
- May be associated with other diseases, infection, autoimmune disorders (eg, SLE, ITP).

CLINICAL MANIFESTATIONS: **asymptomatic by definition** - often incidental finding.

DIAGNOSIS
- Serum protein electrophoresis: IgG monoclonal spike (elevated but usually <3g/dL). Monoclonal spike is usually stable over time (usually does not progress).
- Bone marrow: **<10% plasmacytoid or plasma cells.**
- Urine protein electrophoresis: none (or stable) amounts of Bence-Jones proteins.
- Absence of the symptoms of multiple myeloma (eg, hypercalcemia, anemia, renal failure, lytic bone lesions).

MANAGEMENT
- Conservative or observation: low malignant potential risk.

MULTIPLE MYELOMA (PLASMACYTOMA)

- Cancer associated with proliferation of a single clone of **plasma cells,** leading to increased production of ineffective monoclonal antibodies (especially IgG & IgA). IgM.
- **Most common primary bone malignancy in adults.**
- Risk factors: **elderly >65y, African-Americans, men,** benzene exposure.
- Pathophysiology: plasma cells accumulate in the bone marrow, interrupting bone marrow's normal cell production. Protein accumulation causes kidney injury.

CLINICAL MANIFESTATIONS: "BREAK" your bones in Multiple Myeloma

- **Bone pain:** **most common symptom. Vertebral involvement most common, ribs.** Due to **osteolytic lesions**, pathogenic osteopenic fractures**,** spinal cord compression, radiculopathy (plasma cells can form soft tissue tumor). Neurologic involvement.
- Recurrent infections: due to leukopenia & ineffective Ig production. Hyperviscosity (esp. with IgM).
- **Elevated calcium:** due to osteoclast activating factor from plasma cells, leading to bone destruction.
- Anemia: fatigue, pallor, weakness, weight loss, hepatosplenomegaly.
- **Kidney injury:** due to light chain protein antibody deposition in kidneys. Increased BUN & creatinine.

DIAGNOSIS

- Serum protein electrophoresis: **monoclonal protein spike** – **IgG most common** 60%, IgA (20%).
- Urine protein electrophoresis: **Bence-Jones proteins** (composed of **kappa or lambda light chains**). 15% have light chains only.
- CBC: **Rouleaux formation -** RBCs with a "stack of coins" appearance due to increased plasma protein (**increased ESR**).
- Skull radiographs: **"punched-out" lytic lesions.** Bone scans NOT helpful.
- Bone marrow aspiration: **plasmacytosis >10% definitive diagnosis.**

MANAGEMENT

- **Autologous stem cell transplant most effective therapy** - may be preceded by induction chemotherapy (eg, Dexamethasone with Lenalidomide, Bortezomib).
- Chemotherapy usually controls symptoms temporarily.
- Radiation therapy, local treatment, Bisphosphonates

SECONDARY ERYTHROCYTOSIS

- Major cause of ↑RBC mass. Most common in obese, history of cigarette smoking.
- **Secondary erythrocytosis = ↑hematocrit as a response to another process.**

ETIOLOGIES *3 major causes:*

- Reactive (physiologic): due to **hypoxia** - eg, **pulmonary disease (COPD),** high altitude, tobacco smokers, cyanotic heart disease. **Reactive most common type.**
- Pathologic: no underlying tissue hypoxia. Renal disease (eg, renal cell CA), fibroids, hepatoma.
- Relative polycythemia: normal RBC mass in the setting of ↓plasma volume, dehydration.

CLINICAL MANIFESTATIONS

- Symptoms related to the underlying precipitating cause (eg, COPD, renal disease, cyanosis etc).
- Physical Exam: cyanosis, clubbing, hypertension, hepatosplenomegaly, ±heart murmur.

DIAGNOSIS:

- **↑RBCs/hematocrit with normal WBC & platelets,** normal erythropoietin levels (RBC mass normal in reactive polycythemia due to ↓ plasma volume).

MANAGEMENT: treat underlying disorder. Smoking cessation.

POLYCYTHEMIA VERA (PRIMARY ERYTHROCYTOSIS)

- Acquired myeloproliferative disorder with autonomous bone marrow **overproduction of all 3 myeloid stem cell lines (primarily increased RBCs,** but associated with increased granulocytic WBCs and platelets).
- Pathophysiology: **JAK2 mutation** leads to Primary erythrocytosis (increased hematocrit in the absence of hypoxia).
- Risk factors: **peaks 50-60 years of age. Most common in men** (60%).

CLINICAL MANIFESTATIONS

- Symptoms due to increased **RBC mass (hyperviscosity or thrombosis).**
- Hyperviscosity: headache, dizziness, tinnitus, blurred vision, weakness, fatigue, **pruritus, especially after a hot bath or shower** (due to histamine release from basophils), epistaxis.
- Thrombosis: erythromelalgia (episodic burning or throbbing of hands & feet with edema, cyanosis or pallor), TIA.
- Physical examination: **hepatosplenomegaly, facial plethora (flushed face)**, engorged retinal veins.

DIAGNOSIS

- All 3 major or first 2 major + 1 minor
- Major: **increased RBC mass (increased hemoglobin, increased hematocrit** >54% in men or 51% in women), bone marrow biopsy: hypercellularity (eg, erythroid, granulocytic & megakaryocyte proliferation), and JAK2 mutation presence.
- Minor criterion: **decreased serum erythropoietin levels,** Normal O2 saturation. **Increased leukocyte alkaline phosphatase,** increased granulocytic WBCs, platelets, and B12. Iron deficiency despite polycythemia.

MANAGEMENT

- Low-risk (< 60 years & no thrombosis): **phlebotomy first-line until hematocrit <45%. Low-dose Aspirin** to prevent thrombosis.
- High-risk (60 years or older and/or thrombosis): **all the above + Hydroxyurea** (decreased cell count). Interferon-alfa second-line. **Ruxolitinib (JAK inhibitor)** if no response to Hydroxyurea.
- Symptomatic: Antihistamines for pruritus. Allopurinol if hyperuricemia.
- Avoid iron supplementation. Avoid alkylating agents (increased risk of myelofibrosis & progression to AML).

- **EXAM TIP**
- Primary vs. Secondary erythrocytosis.
- Primary erythrocytosis (PV): normal O2 saturation, decreased erythropoietin, increased WBCs & platelets.
- Secondary erythrocytosis (eg, hypoxemia): decreased O2 saturation, increased erythropoietin, normal WBCs & platelets.

MYELODYSPLASTIC SYNDROME

- Heterogenous **preleukemic disorders** characterized by **abnormal differentiation of cells of the myeloid cell line** (hypercellular bone marrow), resulting in ineffective hematopoiesis in the bone marrow (**pancytopenia**).

RISK FACTORS

- **>65 years of age**, radiation therapy, chemotherapy, Benzene exposure, tobacco smoke, mercury or lead exposure.

CLINICAL MANIFESTATIONS

- May present as asymptomatic pancytopenia on routine CBC.

- **Symptoms of pancytopenia** - **easy bruising, bleeding, frequent infections, & fatigue.**

DIAGNOSIS

- CBC with peripheral smear:
  - **Decreased number of one or more myeloid cell lines** - platelets, neutrophils, or RBCs (may be nucleated).
  - Hyposegmented neutrophils, normocytic or macrocytic anemia.

- Bone marrow biopsy:
  - Normal or hypercellular.
  - 20% associated with hypocellularity.
  - **Dysplastic bone marrow is the hallmark** - **increased myeloblasts but < 20%,** ringed sideroblasts, **pseudo-Pelger-Huet cells** (hyposegmented and hypogranulated neutrophils).

MANAGEMENT

- Goals are symptomatic improvement, to improve survival, and to decrease progression to Acute myelogenous leukemia (AML).

- Supportive management: not all patients require management but some may need intermittent blood or platelet transfusions. Erythropoietin.

- Systemic: Pyrimidine analogs (eg, 5-Azacitidine, Decitabine), Lenalidomide (if 5q deletion present).

- Allogeneic stem cell transplantation only effective cure but difficult in patients > 50 years of age.

ACUTE LYMPHOCYTIC LEUKEMIA (ALL)

- Malignancy arising from immature lymphoid stem cells in the bone marrow.
- B cell (most common), T cell, or null type (non B or T cell).
- **Most common childhood malignancy** (25%) - **peak 2-5 years of age**, boys > girls, Down syndrome.
- PATHOPHYSIOLOGY: overpopulation of immature WBCs (blasts) overtake normal hematopoiesis, resulting in pancytopenia.

CLINICAL MANIFESTATIONS
- Nonspecific symptoms associated with pancytopenia.
- **Pancytopenia: fever & infections** (leukopenia), **bleeding** from thrombocytopenia (eg, petechiae, purpura), & **anemia** (eg, pallor, fatigue).
- CNS symptoms: headache, stiff neck, visual changes, vomiting. METS most common to CNS & testes.
- Physical examination: **hepatomegaly or splenomegaly most common clinical findings** - may manifest as anorexia, weight loss, abdominal distention or abdominal pain. **Lymphadenopathy**.

DIAGNOSIS
- CBC + peripheral smear: WBC 5,000 - 100,000, anemia, thrombocytopenia.
- Bone marrow aspiration: **hypercellular with >20% blasts** (definitive diagnosis).
- Flow cytometry test: most accurate test to distinguish subtypes of Leukemia.

MANAGEMENT
- **Highly responsive to combination chemotherapy** (remission >85%). Induction chemotherapy includes Anthracyclines, Vincristine, and Corticosteroids. Maintenance therapy includes 6-MP and Methotrexate. Imatinib used if Philadelphia chromosome positive. Relapsing: stem cell transplant.
- **CNS disease or CNS preventative: intrathecal Methotrexate.**

TUMOR LYSIS SYNDROME

- Oncologic emergency occurring with the treatment of neoplastic disorders due to **rapid tumor cell lysis after initiation of chemotherapy,** releasing massive amounts of potassium, phosphate, and nucleic acids into the circulation.

RISK FACTORS
- High tumor burden (eg, initial WBC count > 20,000/microL), dehydration, & volume depletion.
- Large proliferation rate (eg, Acute lymphoblastic leukemia) and high-grade Lymphomas (eg, Burkitt).

CLINICAL MANIFESTATIONS
- Related to the metabolic derangements, including, muscle cramps, tetany, nausea, vomiting, lethargy, heart failure, kidney injury, & arrhythmias.

LABORATORY FINDINGS:
- **Hyperphosphatemia, hypocalcemia, hyperuricemia, hyperkalemia,** and **acute kidney injury** (including uric acid nephropathy).

MANAGEMENT
- **Treatment of electrolyte abnormalities, IV fluids** (may add loop diuretic to promote excretion)
- Rasburicase.

PROPHYLAXIS
- **Rasburicase (or Allopurinol) PLUS aggressive IV fluid hydration.** Hemodialysis if severe.
- Rasburicase: recombinant uricase that catalyzes oxidation of uric acid to a stable compound. May be more effective than Allopurinol. Contraindicated if G6PD deficiency.
- Allopurinol: xanthine oxidase inhibitor, leading to decrease uric acid production.

CHRONIC LYMPHOCYTIC LEUKEMIA (CLL) (B Cell)

- **Mature B cell clonal malignancy** (considered same disease as Small cell lymphocytic lymphoma).

- **Most common form of Leukemia in adults.**

- Risk factors: **increasing age** (70 years of age median age), men.

CLINICAL MANIFESTATIONS

- **Usually asymptomatic** (incidental finding of lymphocytosis).

- **Pancytopenia:** anemia symptoms (eg, **fatigue most common**, dyspnea), increased infections (neutropenia), mucocutaneous bleeding (thrombocytopenia).

- May have typical "B" symptoms of lymphoma (10%).

- Physical examination: **lymphadenopathy most common physical exam finding** (cervical, supraclavicular axillary or generalized). The lymph nodes are usually firm, round, nontender and freely mobile. **Splenomegaly second most common finding** (25-55%) and is usually painless and nontender to palpation. Hepatomegaly. Skin lesions (leukemia cutis).

DIAGNOSIS

- CBC with peripheral smear: **absolute lymphocytosis** >5,000/microL – **small, well-differentiated, normal-appearing lymphocytes** with scattered **"smudge cells"** (lab artifact when the fragile B cells become crushed by the cover slip during slide preparation). Neutropenia.

- **Hypogammaglobulinemia.** Increased incidence of Autoimmune hemolytic anemia. May have evidence of ITP.

- Immunophenotypic analysis (flow cytometry) - expression of B cell-associated antigens CD19, CD20, & CD23. CD5 (B cell maturity).

- Bone marrow aspirate and biopsy not required.

MANAGEMENT

- Indolent, asymptomatic, stage I and II: observation. Radiation.

- Symptomatic, progressive, III, and IV: chemotherapy (eg, **Fludarabine,** Rituximab, Cyclophosphamide, Chlorambucil).

- Acute blast crisis: treat similar to AML.

- Allogeneic stem cell transplant curative.

- Poorer prognosis: ZAP-70 +, del(17p), del(11q).

ACUTE MYELOID LEUKEMIA (AML)

- Group of hematopoietic neoplasms characterized by clonal proliferation of myeloid precursors with decreased ability to differentiate into more mature cells.
- **Most common acute leukemia in adults** (80% of cases). Median onset 65 years of age.
- PATHOPHYSIOLOGY: **accumulation of leukemic blasts (immature WBCs)** in the bone marrow, peripheral blood or occasionally other tissues. Increased production leads to pancytopenia.

3 MAJOR SUBTYPES:
- **Acute promyelocytic leukemia (APL or M3):** t(15;17) associated with **DIC, presence of Auer rods, & myeloperoxidase positivity.**
- Acute megakaryoblastic leukemia: most common in children < 5 years of age with Down syndrome.
- Acute monocytic leukemia: associated with **infiltration of the gums (gingival hyperplasia).**

CLINICAL MANIFESTATIONS
- **Pancytopenia:** anemia (eg, **general fatigue most common presenting symptom,** dyspnea, weakness), thrombocytopenia (mucocutaneous bleeding), and neutropenia (increased infections & fever).
- Leukostasis. Uncommon symptoms include lymphadenopathy and hepatosplenomegaly.

DIAGNOSIS
- CBC with peripheral smear: **best initial test** - normocytic normochromic anemia with normal or decreased reticulocyte count. Thrombocytopenia. May have circulating **myeloblasts.**
- Bone marrow biopsy: **gold standard. >20% myeloblasts** (immature cells with prominent nucleoli). **Auer rods** (pink/red rod-like granular structures in the cytoplasm) with APL.
- Immunophenotyping: flow cytometry helps to characterize the types with FISH analysis – most accurate test. May have **myeloperoxidase positivity** with APL.

MANAGEMENT
- **Combination chemotherapy** (eg, Cytarabine, Doxorubicin).
- **All-trans-retinoic acid can be added to M3 (promyelocytic leukemia).**
- Hematopoietic stem cell transplant curative.

LEUKOSTASIS REACTION

- Symptomatic hyperleukocytosis most commonly seen in Acute myeloid leukemia or Chronic myeloid leukemia in blast crisis.
- **Medical emergency** due to decreased tissue perfusion from leukostasis.
- Pathophysiology: leukostasis leads to increased blood viscosity and **white cell plugs in the microvasculature**, impeding blood flow in addition to causing local hypoxemia due to high metabolic activity of the rapidly dividing blasts.

CLINICAL MANIFESTATIONS
- Pulmonary: dyspnea, hypoxemia with or without diffuse alveolar or interstitial infiltrate formation.
- Neurologic: headache, dizziness, visual changes, tinnitus, gait instability, confusion, somnolence, coma. Other: priapism, bowel infarction, myocardial ischemia.

DIAGNOSIS
- **Hyperleukocytosis** (WBC > 100,000/microL) **+ symptoms due to tissue hypoxia** (eg, lung, CNS).

MANAGEMENT
- Cytoreduction: **leukapheresis (first-line because associated with rapid improvement),** chemotherapy (eg, Hydroxyurea), or induction chemotherapy.
- Prophylaxis for tumor lysis syndrome should also be initiated.

CHRONIC MYELOGENOUS LEUKEMIA (CML)

- Myeloproliferative disorder of **uncontrolled production of mature and maturing granulocytes** with fairly normal differentiation (**predominately neutrophils** but also basophils & eosinophils).

PATHOPHYSIOLOGY

- Fusion of 2 genes: BCR (on chromosome 22) and ABL1 (on chromosome 9), resulting in the **BCR-ABL1 fusion gene**. **Translocation between chromosomes 9 and 22 = Philadelphia chromosome** (abnormal chromosome 22 which harbors the BCR-ABL1 gene).

CLINICAL MANIFESTATIONS

- Fatigue, night sweats, malaise, weight loss, fever. **Splenomegaly most common finding.**

- **Pruritus after hot baths/showers** (histamine release from Basophils).

- Chronic phase: 70% asymptomatic – usually detected incidentally on CBC (well-differentiated WBCs – granulocyte proliferation).

- Accelerated phase: neutrophil differentiation becomes progressively impaired and leukocyte counts are more difficult to control with chemotherapy. Fatigue, weight loss, excessive sweating, bleeding from thrombocytopenia, abdominal pain.

- Blastic crisis: presents as **acute leukemia** and extramedullary tissue involvement (eg, lymph nodes, skin, and soft tissues).

DIAGNOSIS

- CBC with peripheral smear: **leukocytosis** (may be strikingly elevated) with **granulocytic cells** (eg, **neutrophilia, basophilia,** & eosinophilia). The cells look normal but are abnormal on immunochemistry.

- **Leukocyte alkaline phosphatase score**: **decreased** (LAP only found in functioning WBCs not leukemic cells).

- Bone marrow biopsy: granulocytic hyperplasia. Chronic: < 5% blasts. Accelerated: 5-30% blasts. Acute blast crisis: > 20% blasts.

- Cytogenetic analysis and fluorescence in situ hybridization (FISH) - genetic testing for the Philadelphia chromosome.

MANAGEMENT

- **Philadelphia +: Tyrosine kinase inhibitors first-line** (eg, **Imatinib,** Nilotinib, Dasatinib). They inhibit Philadelphia chromosome tyrosine kinase activity and myeloid leukemic cell proliferation.

- Hematopoietic stem cell transplant most effective cure.

	HODGKINS DISEASE (HD) LYMPHOMA	NON HODGKINS LYMPHOMA (NHL)
AGE	• ***Bimodal* peaks in 20s*** then in ***50s***	• ***>50y, Increased risk with immunosuppression: ex HIV, viral infection***
CELL TYPE	• ***REED STERNBERG CELLS pathognomonic**** ***B cell*** proliferation with bilobed or multilobar nucleus "owl eye."	• B CELL: ***Diffuse large B cell MC (more aggressive). Follicular (indolent but less curable); Mantle Cell,*** Burkitt's, Marginal zone ***MALT lymphoma*** is an extranodal type of marginal zone lymphoma), ***small cell lymphoma (SCL)*** & CLL thought to be same disease with different presentations (SCL primarily in the lymph nodes, CLL in the bone marrow/peripheral blood). • **T cell:** (T cell, T lymphoblastic), Natural Killer Cells.
LYMPH NODE INVOLVEMENT	• ***UPPER LYMPH NODE INVOLVEMENT*: neck, axilla,*** shoulder, chest (mediastinum). ± ***painful lymph nodes c ETOH ingestion**** Usually painless lymph nodes. • ***CONTIGUOUS spread*** to ***LOCAL LYMPH NODES. Usually Localized, single group of nodes (extranodal rare).***	• ***PERIPHERAL MULTIPLE NODE INVOLVEMENT*:*** axillary, abdominal, pelvic, inguinal, femoral. Waldeyer's ring (tonsils, base of tongue, nasopharynx) • ***NONCONTIGUOUS EXTRANODAL SPREAD*: GI MC, Skin 2nd MC*** (especially T cell), testes, bone marrow, GU, liver, spleen, thyroid, kidney, spine, CNS (headache, lethargy, spinal cord compression, focal neurologic symptoms).
ASSOCIATED SYMPTOMS	• ***B sx: fever, weight loss, anorexia, night sweats.*** Associated with a poorer prognosis. • ***PEL EBSTEIN FEVER: intermittent cyclical fevers x1-2 weeks****	• B symptoms not as common on presentation (but may be seen with advanced disease or aggressive disease). • Leukemic phase can be seen at times with NHL.
EBV ASSOCIATION (EPSTEIN-BARR VIRUS)	• ↑***associated with Epstein-Barr Virus**** (40%)	• Rare in most types of NHL. • ***EBV common in Burkitt's lymphoma – ❶ Endemic (Africa):*** associated with jaw involvement, ❷ Immunodeficient: ex. post transplant lymphoma & AIDS-associated lymphoma. ❸Sporadic (not associated with EBV).
MANAGEMENT	• ***Excellent 5y cure rate*** (60%)	• Variable.

	AML	CML	ALL	CLL
EPIDEMIOLOGY	• ***MC acute form of leukemia.*** **>50y**	• ***Older males***	• ***MC children* (peaks 3-7y)***	• ***MC Leukemia in adults***
DIAGNOSIS	***>20% blasts (immature WBCs).*** • **PROMYELOCYTIC** - ⊕***AUER RODS**** - Sudan Black & Myeloperoxidase ⊕ • **ACUTE MONOCYTIC:** - Gingival infiltration/hyperplasia • **MEGAKARYOCYTIC:** ↑Down syndrome	• ***PHILADELPHIA CHROMOSOME**** • ***Striking ↑WBC: >100,00*** • Chronic <5% blasts • Accelerated 5-30% blasts • Acute >30% blasts	• ***>30% blasts.*** PAS ⊕ • Precursor B-cell ALL (~85%) associated with CNS sx. • Precursor T cell MC associated with adolescents with mediastinal mass & CNS sx	• ***SMUDGE (SMEAR) CELLS**** • Well differentiated lymphocytes • ZAP-70 ⊕ ⇨ 8y survival. ZAP-70 negative ⇨ >25y.
MANAGEMENT	• ***Chemotherapy*** • ***Stem cell Transplant.*** • **Tumor Lysis syndrome** c chemotx: ↑K, ↓Ca, ↑Phos, Hyperuricemia & renal failure. Tx: Allopurinol, IV fluids.	• ***PO Chemotherapy*** (ex. Hydroxyurea, Imatinib). • ***Imatinib*** BCR-ABL tyrosine kinase inhibitor (Philadelphia ⊕).	• ***PO Chemotx*** in Philadelphia ⊕ • Induction: kills detectable disease for complete remission. • Consolidation: short term intensive therapy to sustain remission. • Maintenance: low dose to eradicate any remaining undetectable cells.	• Indolent: observation. • **Symptomatic or progressive:** ***Chemotherapy.*** • Allogeneic stem cell transplant is curative

	Bleeding Syndrome	Petechiae	Ecchymosis	Bleed after minor cuts	Bleeding after surgery
THROMBOCYTOPENIA (Quantitative/Qualitative)	***Mucocutaneous bleeding**** (oral, nasal, GI, GU), ***petechiae***	***Common****	Small superficial	***Yes***	Immediate
FACTOR DEFICIENCY: Hemophilias	***Deep bleeding**** (joint, muscles)	Uncommon	Large hematomas	Not usually	***Delayed****

HODGKIN LYMPHOMA

- Germinal or pregerminal **B-cell malignancy** originating in the lymphatic system.
- **Bimodal: peaks at 20 then again >50y.**
- Risk factors: **Epstein-Barr virus,** immunosuppression, smoking.

4 main types:

- **Nodular sclerosing: most common type overall** (64%). **Female predominance.**
- Mixed cellularity (25%). Associated with EBV.
- Lymphocyte rich/predominant: most common in males <35y. **Best prognosis.**
- Lymphocyte depleted: (4%). Most common in males >60y. Usually associated with other systemic diseases. Worst prognosis.

CLINICAL MANIFESTATIONS

- **Asymptomatic painless lymphadenopathy: most common presentation** (70%). Usually painless but **ETOH ingestion may induce lymph node pain** within minutes.

- **Upper body lymph nodes: neck most common site** (eg, **cervical and/or supraclavicular**), axilla, shoulder, mediastinum, & abdomen. Usually rubbery in consistency, not fixed (does not adhere to the skin), and may fluctuate in size.

- **Mediastinal lymphadenopathy or mass: second most common presentation** – incidental finding on chest radiograph. The mass may be large without producing local symptoms. If symptomatic - retrosternal chest pain, cough, or dyspnea may be experienced. Large mediastinal adenopathy is an adverse prognostic factor.

- Fatigue, pruritus, Intra-abdominal disease – **hepatomegaly, splenomegaly.** Cholestatic liver disease. Nephrotic syndrome, hypercalcemia.

- **Systemic "B" symptoms: fever** (> 100.4 F), **night sweats, weight loss** (> 10% of body weight over 6 months). **Pel-Ebstein fever** - **cyclical fever** that recurs at variable intervals of several days or weeks and lasts for 1-2 weeks before waning. Symptoms due to cytokine release by Reed-Sternberg cells. **B symptoms indicate advanced disease.**

DIAGNOSIS

- **Excisional whole lymph node biopsy: Reed-Sternberg cell pathognomonic** – large cells with bi- or multilobed nuclei ("**owl eye appearance**") & inclusions in the nucleoli. Reed-Sternberg cells are derived from an abnormal germinal B cell in the early stage of differentiation with CD15 & CD30 positivity.

- Imaging for staging: combined PET/CT scan of chest, thorax, & abdomen.

MANAGEMENT

- **Early stage disease (stage I or II): combination of chemotherapy + radiation** therapy. Chemotherapy alone is an acceptable alternative.

- **Advanced stage (III to IV): combination chemotherapy is the main treatment.** Radiation therapy may be used for select patients as consolidation. **"ABVD":** Adriamycin (Doxorubicin), Bleomycin, Vinblastine, Dacarbazine. "MOPP" Mustine, Oncovorin/Vincristine, Procarbazine, Prednisolone.

- Refractory (resistant): second-line high dose chemotherapy & autologous hematopoietic cell transplant are options.

NON HODGKIN LYMPHOMA

- Heterogenous group of lymphocyte neoplasms with proliferation in the lymph nodes & spleen.

MAJOR TYPES

- **Diffuse large B-cell: most common type of NHL. Fast growing, aggressive form (rapidly enlarging lymph nodes** of the neck, abdomen and groin). Most common in the middle aged & elderly (average age 70 years). Extranodal seen in 40%. Large size B cell proliferation. CD 20+.
- **Follicular:** second most common. Small cell proliferation in follicles (circular pattern) CD20+. Most common in adults. Presents with painless lymphadenopathy (especially in the neck, groin & axilla). **Follicular is usually indolent (slow growing) but hard to cure.** Sometimes not treated until symptomatic. Associated with t(14:18) mutation. Follicular may progress to large B cell lymphoma.
- **Mantle cell:** small cell proliferation surrounding the follicular zone (mantle). 5-15%. CD 20+, CD5+ (poorer prognosis). Most commonly seen in older adult population. Painless lymphadenopathy. GI, bone marrow & liver involvement common. T(11;14) mutation.
- **Marginal zone:** small B cell proliferation. 5-10% in the cells surrounding the mantle. CD 20+. Low grade (usually due to B-cell hyperplasia from chronic immune or inflammatory states: (eg, Hashimoto's thyroiditis, Sjogren syndrome). 3 subtypes: **Extranodal (Mucosal-Associated Lymphoid Tissue) MALT: Gastric MALT lymphomas often associated with *H-pylori* infections.** 8%. Nodal: originate in the lymph nodes. Splenic: originates in the spleen or bone marrow.
- **Burkitt Lymphoma:** intermediate-sized B cell proliferation. CD 20+. **Associated with Epstein-Barr virus infection** (except sporadic). Usually presents as extranodal mass. **Most commonly seen in pediatric/adolescent** & **HIV pts. Endemic (Africa):** usually **involves the jaw** & facial bones (especially with malaria). **Sporadic type:** GI & paraaortic involvement. **Immunodeficient type**: seen with HIV or immunosuppression (eg, post-transplant). Biopsy "starry sky" appearance. Burkitt's very aggressive (but highly curable). T(8:14) mutation.
- **Small lymphocytic:** spectrum of disease as Chronic lymphocytic leukemia. Small lymphocytic usually found in the lymph nodes & spleen (whereas CLL is found in the bone marrow and the blood). 7%.

RISK FACTORS

- **Increased age,** history of radiation therapy, family history. Chromosomal translocations.
- **Immunosuppression: HIV,** HCV, viral infection, organ transplantation
- **Infections: EBV, HHV-8, HIV. *H. pylori* associated with gastric lymphoma.**
- **Autoimmune disorders** (eg, Systemic lupus erythematosus, Dermatomyositis, Rheumatoid arthritis, Sjögren syndrome, Hashimoto thyroiditis).

CLINICAL MANIFESTATIONS

- The clinical presentation varies tremendously depending on the type of NHL & areas of involvement.
- Local: **painless lymphadenopathy.** Indolent lymphomas may present with slowly growing lymphadenopathy. Hepatosplenomegaly.
- Extranodal involvement: common. **GI tract most common site of extranodal involvement** (skin second most common). CNS also common.
- Systemic B symptoms: (fever, night sweats, weight loss) rarer in NHL but may be seen if advanced.

DIAGNOSIS

- Lymph node &/or tissue biopsy: required for the diagnosis and classification of NHL.
- Combined CT/PET scan of chest, abdomen and pelvis for staging

MANAGEMENT

- Low Grade: asymptomatic – no treatment. Localized disease (Stage I): radiation therapy. Chemotherapy: Chlorambucil, Fludarabine, 2-CdA (2-chloro-2'-deoxyadenosine). Rituximab (monoclonal antibody against CD20+). Stem cell transplant in refractory cases.
- Intermediate, High Grade (Aggressive): chemotherapy: eg, **R-CHOP: R**ituximab, **C**yclophosphamide, Doxorubicin, **H**ydrochloride, **O**ncovorin (Vincristine), **P**rednisolone.

CHEMOTHERAPEUTIC AGENTS FOR CANCER

ALKYLATING AGENTS	
Cyclophosphamide **Ifosfamide**	• Mechanism of action: inhibits DNA replication by **alkylating DNA** (requires bioactivation by the liver). • Indications: leukemia, lymphoma, multiple myeloma, ovarian and breast cancer, rheumatoid arthritis, rapidly-progressive glomerulonephritis. • Adverse effects: **hemorrhagic cystitis** (reduced by increased hydration, Mesna or N-acetylcysteine), GI mucosal damage (eg, nausea, vomiting, **stomatitis, diarrhea**), emesis, myelosuppression, SIADH, **bladder cancer.**
PLATINUM AGENTS	**(Alkylating Like Agents)**
Cisplatin **Carboplatin**	Mechanism of action: • Inhibits DNA synthesis similar to **alkylating-like agents.** • The platinum atom binds to DNA and crosslinks DNA. This interferes with DNA synthesis & cellular metabolism, triggering cell death. Indications: • Cisplatin: advanced metastatic testicular, ovarian and bladder cancers • Carboplatin: advanced ovarian cancer Adverse reactions: • **Neurotoxicity** – **ototoxicity** (acoustic nerve damage causes hearing loss usually bilateral and irreversible, tinnitus, vertigo), peripheral neuropathy. • **Nephrotoxicity** – Acute kidney injury may be reduced with hydration and Amifostine, a free radical scavenger. • **Highly emetogenic.** • Electrolyte disorders: eg, Hypomagnesemia, hypocalcemia.
ANTIMETABOLITES	
Methotrexate	• Mechanism of action: inhibits dihydrofolate reductase (**folic acid antagonist**) leading to decreased DNA and protein synthesis; inhibits lymphocyte proliferation. Indications: • Chemotherapy: non-Hodgkin lymphoma, trophoblastic tumors (eg, choriocarcinoma, hydatidiform mole), lung, breast, CNS, neck cancers, osteosarcoma. • Inflammatory arthritis: Rheumatoid arthritis, Psoriatic arthritis. • Reproductive: ectopic pregnancy and termination of pregnancy. Adverse effects: • GI side effects most common - **stomatitis,** nausea, vomiting, diarrhea. • 3 cardinal side effects of Methotrexate involve the **liver, lung, & marrow**: **hepatitis, interstitial pneumonitis, & marrow suppression**. • **Leukopenia (prevented by administration of Leucovorin/Folinic acid).** • Neurotoxicity, thrombocytopenia, nephrotoxicity. Drug interactions: • **Penicillins may increase toxicity of Methotrexate** (by decreasing elimination). • Aminoglycosides reduce GI absorption of Methotrexate. • Retinoids increase hepatotoxicity. • **Trimethoprim & sulfonamides increase hemotoxicity** (synergistic folate antagonism). • **Avoid NSAIDs with high-dose Methotrexate** (anti-neoplastic doses) due to increased toxicity from decreased renal excretion of Methotrexate. Contraindications: • **Pregnancy** (folic acid inhibition), severe liver or renal disease.

Fluorouracil (5-FU)	• Mechanism of action: antimetabolite - **pyrimidine analog** that inhibits RNA synthesis in cancer cells by uracil antagonism (uracil is essential for RNA synthesis). Inhibits thymidylate synthase, leading to decreased DNA and protein synthesis. Low emetogenic potential. Indications: • Topical: superficial basal cell cancer, actinic keratosis. • Metastatic colon and breast cancers, ovarian cancer, head or neck cancer. Adverse effects: • **GI** (eg, **nausea, vomiting, diarrhea**, anorexia, stomatitis) • Teratogenicity, **alopecia,** cardiotoxicity (eg, bradycardia, hypotension), ocular toxicity. • **Myelosuppression ("rescue" with Thymidine).** • Dermatitis & photosensitivity with topical.
Cytarabine	• Mechanism: inhibits DNA & RNA synthesis. • Indications: hematologic cancers (AML, ALL, blastic phase of CML), NHL. Poor activity vs. solid tumors. • Adverse effects: **CNS neurotoxicity** (cerebellar syndrome), myelosuppression, stomatitis, emetogenic, sloughing off of the skin on the palms & soles, **ocular toxicity, ototoxicity.**
Gemcitabine	• Mechanism: inhibits DNA synthesis. • Indications: advanced breast, ovarian, pancreatic & non-small cell lung cancers. • Adverse effects: emetogenic, hepatitis, myelosuppression.
MITOSIS INHIBITORS (TAXANES)	
• **Paclitaxel** • **Docetaxel**	• Mechanism of action: **stabilizes microtubules, preventing mitosis and cell division**. Indications: • **Paclitaxel: advanced ovarian cancer (with Cisplatin),** advanced breast and non-small cell lung cancers. Second-line for Kaposi sarcoma. • Docetaxel: advanced & metastatic breast, prostate, gastric, squamous cell, head, neck and non-small cell lung cancers. Adverse effects: • **Black box warning for hypersensitivity reactions and bone marrow suppression.** • **Hypersensitivity reaction** (may need to be treated with Dexamethasone, Diphenhydramine and H2 blocker, such as Ranitidine, prior to infusion to reduce the incidence). • Alopecia, nausea, vomiting, mucositis, anorexia, brittle nails, change in taste, leukopenia, neutropenia, myalgia, weakness, and peripheral neuropathy. • Hyaluronidase via the same IV line is the antidote for Paclitaxel toxicity due to extravasation.
MITOSIS INHIBITORS	
• **MOA:** destabilizes microtubules, **preventing mitosis and cell division**.	
Vincristine **Vinblastine**	Indications: • Vincristine used for leukemia, Hodgkin lymphoma, non-Hodgkin lymphoma, solid tumors. • Vinblastine used for lymphoma and testicular cancer. Adverse effects: • **Neurotoxicity most common side effect especially with Vincristine** (eg, **neuropathy such as foot drop**, cranial nerve palsies, demyelination, pain), myelosuppression, dermatologic (alopecia, rashes). • GI (**constipation,** nausea, vomiting, abdominal pain). • GU (eg, urinary retention, bladder dysfunction). • Oculotoxicity and hyperuricemia.

ANTHRACYCLINES	
• **Doxorubicin** • **Daunorubicin**	Mechanism of action: • **Intercalating agents** – inhibit nucleic acid & protein synthesis by intercalating and binding with DNA. Generate free radicals and inhibit topoisomerase (antibiotics derived from *Streptomyces* fungus). Indications: • Hematologic malignancies: AML, ALL, Hodgkin lymphoma (the A in ABVD) • Solid tumors: endometrial, lung, breast and ovarian cancer. Adverse effects: • **Cardiotoxicity: dilated cardiomyopathy,** myopericarditis. • GI side effects: nausea, vomiting, stomatitis. • Bone marrow suppression & alopecia. Monitoring: • **Echocardiogram or MUGA scan should be performed prior to initiation of therapy** to document the ejection fraction. Prevention of cardiotoxicity • Dexrazoxane is a cardioprotective agent against the toxic effects of anthracyclines used in select patients (prevents free radical formation).
OTHER AGENTS	
• **Bleomycin**	Mechanism of action: • Glycopeptide antibiotic that affects the G2 phase of cell division, generates free radicals, & inhibits DNA synthesis with lesser inhibition of protein and RNA synthesis. Indications: • **Hodgkin lymphoma** (the B in ABVD), non-Hodgkin lymphoma, squamous cell and testicular cancer. • Sclerosing agent for **pleurodesis in patients with malignant pleural effusions.** Adverse effects: • **Pulmonary toxicity: pulmonary fibrosis** & **pneumonitis** due to free radical production. • Dermatologic: alopecia, hyperpigmentation. • Raynaud phenomenon. • Myelosuppression not a significant side effect.
• **Hydroxyurea**	• Mechanism of action: **increases production of HbF** (which does not sickle and has a higher affinity for oxygen), increases RBC water, **reduces RBC sickling,** alters RBC adhesion to the endothelium. Inhibits ribonucleotide reductase. • **Indications**: **mainstay of treatment** in SCD - **reduces the frequency and severity of pain episodes, decreases hospitalization rates and prolongs survival.** Because it takes weeks to months to take full effect, it is not used for acute episodes. • Uses: Sickle cell disease, Polycythemia vera, Essential thrombocythemia. • The combination of Hydroxyurea and L-glutamine can have additive benefits. • Adverse effects: myelosuppression, GI (anorexia, nausea).

R-CHOP Rituximab (antibody vs. CD20), Cyclophosphamide, Hydroxydaunorubicin, Oncovin/Vincristine, Prednisone. Used in non-Hodgkin lymphoma.

ABVD Adriamycin (Doxorubicin), Bleomycin, Vinblastine, Dacarbazine. Used in Hodgkin lymphoma

MOPP Mustargen, Oncovin, Procarbazine, Prednisone. Older regimen for Hodgkin lymphoma

GENERAL CHEMOTOXICITIES

Gastrointestinal

- **Nausea/Vomiting:** Doxorubicin, Cytarabine, Cyclophosphamide, Methotrexate, Cisplatin.
- **Mucositis:** 5FU, Methotrexate.

Cardiovascular

- **Anthracyclines (eg, Doxorubicin) cause dilated cardiomyopathy.**

Pulmonary: Bleomycin (fibrosis), Methotrexate.

Neurologic: Vincristine, Methotrexate, Cytarabine, Cisplatin.

Renal: high-dose Methotrexate, Cisplatin (renal failure), Cyclophosphamide (bladder cancer & hemorrhagic cystitis)

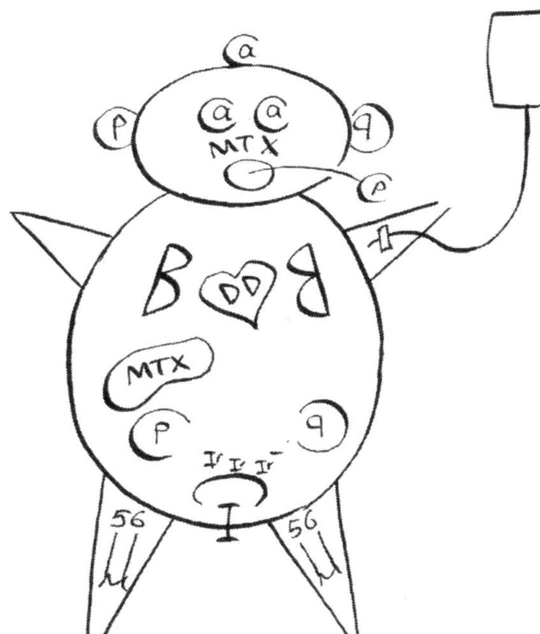

Ca = Cytarabine
- CNS toxicity, Ototoxicity

C^{p}= Cisplatin
- ototoxicity, highly emetogenic, renal failure

B = Bleomycin (pulmonary fibrosis)

MTX = Methotrexate
- Stomatitis, hepatotoxic,

D – Daunorubicin, Doxorubicin
- Dilated cardiomyopathy

C I = Cyclophosphamide, Ifosfamide
- Hemorrhagic cystitis

Irinotecan = acute & delayed diarrhea

Bone marrow toxicity:

5 = 5-FU; 6 = 6-Mercaptopurine, M = methotrexate

V of the arms & legs = Vincristine for peripheral neuropathy.

TUMOR MARKERS

TUMOR MARKER	MAIN ASSOCIATIONS
ALPHA FETOPROTEIN	• **Hepatocellular carcinoma** • **Nonseminomatous germ cell testicular cancer** • Decreased in Down syndrome "AFP is down in Down syndrome"
Beta-hCG	• **Nonseminomatous germ cell testicular cancer** • **Choriocarcinoma,** Teratomas • **Trophoblastic tumors** (eg, Hydatidiform molar pregnancy)
CA-125	• **Ovarian cancer**
CA 19-9	• **Pancreatic cancer** • GI – colorectal, esophageal, & hepatocellular cancers
CALCITONIN	• **Medullary thyroid cancer**
CEA	• **Colorectal cancer** • Medullary thyroid, pancreatic, gastric, lung, & breast cancers
PROSTATE SPECIFIC ANTIGEN	• **Prostate cancer** • Can also be elevated in BPH & Prostatitis

PHOTO CREDITS

Sickle Cell Anemia
By Ed Uthman from Houston, TX, USA (Sickle Cell Anemia Uploaded by CFCF) [CC-BY-2.0 (http://creativecommons.org/licenses/by/2.0)], via Wikimedia Commons
Rouleaux Formation
By Michail Charakidis, David Joseph Russell [CC-BY-2.0 (http://creativecommons.org/licenses/by/2.0)], via Wikimedia Commons
Peripheral Smear
By Ed Uthman from Houston, TX, USA [CC-BY-2.0 (http://creativecommons.org/licenses/by/2.0)], via Wikimedia Commons
Iron deficiency anemia
By Ed Uthman from Houston, TX, USA [CC-BY-2.0 (http://creativecommons.org/licenses/by/2.0)], via Wikimedia Commons
Howell Jolly Body
By Paulo Henrique Orlandi Mourao and Mikael Häggström [CC-BY-SA-3.0 (http://creativecommons.org/licenses/by-sa/3.0) or GFDL (http://www.gnu.org/copyleft/fdl.html)], via Wikimedia Commons
Acanthocyte
By Paulo Henrique Orlandi Mourao (Own work) [CC-BY-SA-3.0 (http://creativecommons.org/licenses/by-sa/3.0) or GFDL (http://www.gnu.org/copyleft/fdl.html)], via Wikimedia Commons
Shistocyte
By Paulo Henrique Orlandi Mourao (Own work) [CC-BY-SA-3.0 (http://creativecommons.org/licenses/by-sa/3.0) or GFDL (http://www.gnu.org/copyleft/fdl.html)], via Wikimedia Commons
Shistocyte
By Paulo Henrique Orlandi Mourao (Own work) [CC-BY-SA-3.0 (http://creativecommons.org/licenses/by-sa/3.0) or GFDL (http://www.gnu.org/copyleft/fdl.html)], via Wikimedia Commons
Bilobed Nucleus
By Paulo Henrique Orlandi Mourao (Own work) [CC-BY-SA-3.0 (http://creativecommons.org/licenses/by-sa/3.0) or GFDL (http://www.gnu.org/copyleft/fdl.html)], via Wikimedia Commons
Auer Rod
By Paulo Henrique Orlandi Mourao (Own work) [CC-BY-SA-3.0 (http://creativecommons.org/licenses/by-sa/3.0) or GFDL (http://www.gnu.org/copyleft/fdl.html)], via Wikimedia Commons
Atypical lymphocyte
By Ed Uthman, MD. [Public domain], via Wikimedia Commons
Target cells spherocytes
By Dr Graham Beards (Own work) [CC BY-SA 3.0 (http://creativecommons.org/licenses/by-sa/3.0)], via Wikimedia Commons. Basophilic stippling
By Herbert L. Fred, MD and Hendrik A. van Dijk (http://cnx.org/content/m15003/latest/) [CC BY 2.0 (http://creativecommons.org/licenses/by/2.0)], via Wikimedia Commons
Warm Immune Hemolytic Anemia
By E. Uthman, MD (http://www.flickr.com/photos/euthman/2989437967) [CC-BY-SA-2.0 (http://creativecommons.org/licenses/by-sa/2.0)], via Wikimedia Commons
NeutrophilBy Segmented_neutrophils.jpg: hematologist derivative work: patient-doc (Segmented_neutrophils.jpg) [CC-BY-SA-3.0 (http://creativecommons.org/licenses/by-sa/3.0/) or GFDL (http://www.gnu.org/copyleft/fdl.html)], via Wikimedia Commons
Acanthocytosis
By Rola Zamel, Razi Khan, Rebecca L Pollex and Robert A Hegele [CC-BY-2.0 (http://creativecommons.org/licenses/by/2.0)], via Wikimedia Commons
Sickle Cell disease
By Ed Uthman from Houston, TX, USA (Sickle Cell Anemia Uploaded by CFCF) [CC-BY-2.0 (http://creativecommons.org/licenses/by/2.0)], via Wikimedia Commons
Stem cell differentiation
By パタゴニア [CC-BY-SA-3.0 (http://creativecommons.org/licenses/by-sa/3.0)], via Wikimedia Commons
Hypersegmented Neutrophil
By Bobjgalindo (Own work) [GFDL (http://www.gnu.org/copyleft/fdl.html) or CC-BY-SA-3.0-2.5-2.0-1.0 (http://creativecommons.org/licenses/by-sa/3.0)], via Wikimedia Commons
Basophilic Stippling
By Herbert L. Fred, MD and Hendrik A. van Dijk (http://cnx.org/content/m15003/latest/) [CC-BY-2.0 (http://creativecommons.org/licenses/by/2.0)], via Wikimedia Commons

CHAPTER 15 - PEDIATRIC PEARLS

ERYTHEMA TOXICUM

- Thought to be due to immune system activation. Seen in up to 70% of neonates.

CLINICAL MANIFESTATIONS
- Small erythematous macules or papules ⇨ pustules on erythematous bases 3-5 days after birth. Does not involve the palms or soles. Individual lesions may spontaneously disappear.

MANAGEMENT
- Self-limited. Usually resolves spontaneously in 1-2 weeks.

MILIARIA

- **Blockage of eccrine sweat glands** (especially in hot & humid conditions). This leads to sweat into the epidermis & dermis.
- Increased counts of skin flora (*S. epidermis, S. aureus*).

TYPES
- Miliaria crystallina: tiny, friable clear vesicles (due to sweat in the superficial stratum corneum). **Most common in neonates** (especially in 1-week-old neonates).
- Miliaria rubra: severely pruritic papules (may develop pustules). Deeper in the epidermis.
- Miliaria profunda: flesh-colored papules (due to sweating in the papillary dermis).

MILIA

- 1-2mm pearly white-yellow papules (due to keratin retention within the dermis of immature skin) especially seen on the cheeks, forehead, chin & nose.

MANAGEMENT
- None. Usually disappears by the 1st month of life (may be seen up to 3 months).

CAFÉ AU LAIT MACULES

- Uniformly hyperpigmented macules or patches with sharp demarcation.
- They may be present at birth or develop early in childhood.

PATHOPHYSIOLOGY
- Due to increased number of melanocytes and melanin within the dermis.

ASSOCIATIONS
- **Neurofibromatosis I (6 or more macules, especially if associated with axillary or inguinal freckling)**
- Tuberous sclerosis
- McCune-Albright syndrome
- Bloom syndrome
- Fanconi anemia

PORT-WINE STAINS (CAPILLARY MALFORMATION, NEVUS FLAMMEUS)

- Vascular malformation of the skin due to superficial dilated dermal capillaries.

CLINICAL MANIFESTATIONS
- Pink-red, sharply demarcated, blanchable macules or papules in infancy. Over time, they **grow & darken to a purple (port wine) color and may develop a thickened surface.**

- Most commonly occurring on the face but can occur anywhere.

MANAGEMENT
- **Pulse dye laser treatment** (best used in infancy for best outcomes).

STURGE-WEBER SYNDROME:
- Congenital disorder associated with the triad of 1. **Facial port wine stains** (especially along the trigeminal nerve distribution area - forehead, cheeks) 2. **Leptomeningeal angiomatosis** & 3. **Ocular involvement** (eg, glaucoma).

- May develop hemiparesis contralateral to the facial lesion, seizures, intracranial calcification, or learning disabilities.

MONGOLIAN SPOTS

- Congenital dermal melanocytosis due to mid-dermal melanocytes that fail to migrate to the epidermis from the neural crest.

- May be seen in > 80% of Asians & East Indian infants. Increased in African-Americans.

CLINICAL MANIFESTATIONS
- **Blue or slate grey pigmented macular lesions with indefinite borders most commonly seen in the presacral, sacral-gluteal areas** but also can be seen on the shoulders, legs, back, and posterior thighs. May be solitary or multiple.

MANAGEMENT
- Usually fades over time in the first few years of life.

NEVUS SIMPLEX (STORK BITE)

- Areas of surface capillary dilation.

- Also known as a **stork bite** or Nevus flammeus nuchae.

CLINICAL MANIFESTATIONS
- **Pink-red, irregularly-shaped macular patches most commonly seen on the nape of the neck, eyelids & forehead.**

MANAGEMENT
- Observation: most will resolve spontaneously by age 2 and don't usually darken over time.

- Laser therapy can be used to reduce the appearance of persistent lesions.

STAPHYLOCOCCAL SCALDED SKIN SYNDROME (RITTER DISEASE)

- Superficial skin blistering condition due to dissemination of ***S. aureus*** **exfoliative toxins** (especially *S. aureus* strains 71 & 55).

PATHOPHYSIOLOGY

- Toxins cleave desmoglein-1, resulting in the formation of flaccid, fragile bullae.

- **Most common in infants** (3-7 days of age) or children < 5 years of age.

CLINICAL MANIFESTATIONS

- Erythema phase: fever, irritability, skin tenderness followed by **cutaneous blanching erythema** (often beginning at the mouth before becoming diffuse). The erythema is worse in the flexor areas and around orifices.

- **Bullae phase: sterile, flaccid blisters** occur about 1-2 days after the erythema, especially in areas of mechanical stress (eg, flexural areas, buttocks, hands, and feet). **Positive Nikolsky sign (gentle pressure applied to skin causes separation of the dermis and blister rupture).**

- Desquamative phase: skin that easily ruptures, leaving moist, denuded skin before healing.

- Conjunctivitis may be seen but mucous membranes are not involved.

DIAGNOSIS

- Clinical diagnosis. Cultures from blood or nasopharynx. Blisters are sterile.

- Skin biopsy: splitting of the lower stratum granulosum layer.

MANAGEMENT

- Antibiotics: **Penicillinase-resistant Penicillins** (eg, **Nafcillin, Oxacillin**). May add Clindamycin. Vancomycin if MRSA suspected or Penicillin allergy.

- Supportive care: maintain the skin clean and moist, emollients to improve barrier function, fluid & electrolyte replacement.

TURNER'S SYNDROME

- Group of X chromosome abnormalities characterized by **females with an absent or nonfunctional X sex chromosome.**

PATHOPHYSIOLOGY

- Mosaicism (67-90%) some cells have a combination of **X monosomy** (**45, XO** due to missing X chromosome), some cells are normal (46, XX), cells with partial monosomies (X/abnormal X) or cells that have a Y chromosome (46, XY).

CLINICAL MANIFESTATIONS

- **Hypogonadism:** 45, XO leads to **gonadal dysgenesis** (rudimentary fibrosed **streaked ovaries**) that can cause **early ovarian failure** (primary amenorrhea in 80% or early secondary amenorrhea), delayed secondary sex characteristics (eg, **absence of breasts**), and infertility.
- Physical examination: **short stature, webbed neck,** prominent ears, low posterior headline, **broad chest with widely spaced nipples,** short fourth metacarpals, high-arched palate, nail dysplasia, congenital lymphedema in neonates.
- Cardiovascular: **coarctation of the aorta** (30%), mitral valve prolapse, bicuspid aortic valves, aortic dissection, hypertension.
- Renal: congenital abnormalities (eg, horseshoe kidney), hydronephrosis.
- Endocrine: osteoporosis, hypothyroidism, Diabetes mellitus, dyslipidemias.
- GI: telangiectasias (may present with GI bleeding), inflammatory bowel disease, colon cancer.

DIAGNOSIS

- **Karyotyping – definitive diagnosis.** 45, XO mosaicism or X chromosomal abnormalities.
- **Low estrogen + high FSH and LH.**

MANAGEMENT

- Recombinant human growth hormone replacement (may increase final height).
- Estrogen/Progesterone replacement to cause pubertal development.

KLINEFELTER'S SYNDROME

- Genetic disorder seen in **males with an extra, inactive X chromosome (47 XXY)** karyotype (90%).

PATHOPHYSIOLOGY

- Extra sex chromosome due to failure of separation of sex chromosome or translocation.
- Most common chromosomal abnormality associated with hypogonadism.

CLINICAL MANIFESTATIONS

- Normal appearance before puberty onset, delayed puberty, followed by **tall stature** (thin & long-limbed with **Eunuchoid features**). Scoliosis, ataxia, mild developmental delays, & expressive language disorders.
- **Hypogonadism: small testicles, gynecomastia,** infertility (azoospermia), scarce pubic & axillary hair, decreased libido.
- **Obesity in adulthood.** Increased risk of Testicular cancer, Breast cancer, Extragonadal germ cell tumors and non-Hodgkin lymphoma.

DIAGNOSIS

- 47 XXY karyotype. Low serum testosterone, increased FSH, LH, and estradiol (due to loss of inhibin).

MANAGEMENT

- Testosterone may help with secondary sex characteristics

FRAGILE X SYNDROME

- X-linked genetic disorder associated with the loss of function of the fragile X mental retardation gene. (FMR1).
- **Most common gene-related cause of Autism spectrum disorder.**
- Pathophysiology: loss of function of the fragile X mental retardation gene leads to lack of production of the fragile X mental retardation protein.

CLINICAL MANIFESTATIONS
- Young males: mitral valve prolapse, hyperextensible joints, hypotonia, soft skin, flat feet, macrocephaly.
- Older males: long & narrow face, prominent forehead & chin, **large ears, macro-orchidism (enlarged testicles)**, flapping hands.
- Behavioral: expressive language deficits > receptive. **Severe intellectual disability.** Hyperactivity, seizures.

DIAGNOSIS
- Genetic studies: X chromosome in the q27 regions have an expanding repeating CGG segment

DOWN SYNDROME (TRISOMY 21)

- Genetic disorder due to 3 copies of chromosome 21 (**Trisomy 21**) or 3 copies of a region of the long arm of chromosome 21.
- **Most common chromosomal disorder and cause of mental developmental disability.**

CLINICAL MANIFESTATIONS
- Head and neck: low-set small ears, flat facial profile, flat nasal bridges, open mouth, protruding tongue, upslanting palpebral fissures, folded or dysplastic ears, brachycephalic, **prominent epicanthal folds**, excessive skin at the nape of the neck, short neck, almond-shaped eyes, **Brushfield spots** (white, grey or brown spots on the iris).
- Extremities: **transverse, singular palmar crease (Simian crease),** hyperflexibility of the joints, short broad hands, increased space between the first and second ties (sandal gap deformity).
- Neonates: poor Moro reflex, hypotonia, dysplasia of the pelvis, hypotonia, may develop transient neonatal leukemia.
- Congenital heart disease: **atrioventricular septal defects,** tetralogy of Fallot, patent ductus arteriosus.
- GI: duodenal or esophageal atresia, Hirschsprung disease.
- Complications: atlantoaxial instability (C1-C2), Acute lymphocytic leukemia, early onset of Alzheimer disease.

DIAGNOSIS
- Based on history, physical examination.
- Genetic testing used to confirm the diagnosis

PRENATAL SCREENING
- **Biochemical screening:** Free beta-hCG: abnormally high or low may be indicative of chromosomal abnormalities. PAPP-A: **low with fetal Down syndrome**.
- **Nuchal translucency ultrasound** at 10-13 weeks. Increased thickness can be seen with trisomies 13, 18 & 21 (Down syndrome).
- If increased thickness, chorionic villous sampling or amniocentesis is offered.

EHLERS DANLOS SYNDROME (EDS)

- Genetic disorder of collagen synthesis associated with **skin hyperextensibility, joint hypermobility, and fragile connective tissue.**
- 6 major types (eg, hypermobility most common, classical, vascular, kyphoscoliosis, arthrochalasia, & dermatosparaxis).

PATHOPHYSIOLOGY
- **Abnormal collagen production** (especially type IV EDS) affecting tendons, ligaments, skin, blood vessels, eyes and other organs.

CLINICAL MANIFESTATIONS
- **Skin hyperextensibility:** ability to stretch the skin > 4 cm in areas such as the neck and forearm.
- **Fragile connective tissue:** **mitral valve prolapse, Aneurysm rupture is a common cause of death.** Cervical insufficiency, rupture of internal organs.
- **Joint hypermobility:** joint dislocations and subluxations, pes planus, pectus excavatum. May develop myopia.

PHYSICAL EXAMINATION:
- **Smooth, velvety (doughy) fragile skin** that **bruises easily** or may split with trauma, widened atrophic scars, delayed wound healing, Metenier's sign (upper eyelid everts easily).

DIAGNOSIS: Clinical. Genetic or biochemical testing confirms the diagnosis.

MARFAN SYNDROME

- Autosomal dominant systemic connective tissue disorder that leads to cardiovascular, ocular, and musculoskeletal abnormalities.
- PATHOPHYSIOLOGY: **mutation of the fibrillin-1 gene**, leading to transforming growth factor beta mutation & misfolding of the protein fibrillin-1, resulting in **weakened connective tissue.**

CLINICAL MANIFESTATIONS
- Cardiovascular: **mitral valve prolapse** (85%), **progressive aortic root dilation (aortic regurgitation),** aortic dissection, & aortic aneurysms.
- Musculoskeletal: **tall stature, arachnodactyly** (long, lanky fingers, arms, & legs), scoliosis, anterior chest deformities (eg, **pectus carinatum,** pectus excavatum), spontaneous pneumothorax, **joint laxity.**
- Ocular: **ectopia lentis** (malposition or dislocation of the lens of the eyes), leading to reduced vision and extreme nearsightedness (**myopia**).

MANAGEMENT
- Treatment targeted at symptoms.
- Conservative: avoid high-contact sports. **Beta-blockers (first-line)** or angiotensin receptor blockers to halt the progression of aortic root dilation.
- Surgical: aortic aneurysm repair or cardiac valve repair if indicated.

- **EXAM TIP**
- Both: joint laxity, hypermobility, & aortic aneurysms.
- Marfan only: tall stature, arachnodactyly, dislocation of the lens, pectus carinatum and progressive aortic dilation.
- Ehlers-Danlos: skin hyperextensibility and the fragile connective tissue (eg, easy bruising, hypertrophic scar formation).

FETAL ALCOHOL SYNDROME

- Due to maternal alcohol use during pregnancy.

CLINICAL MANIFESTATIONS

- Children are often born small and remain relatively small throughout their lifetime. Associated with developmental delays & congenital abnormalities of internal organs.
- **Small physical findings:** microcephaly, thin upper lip, long & smooth philtrum, small palpebral fissures & small distal phalanges.

SMOKING DURING PREGNANCY

ADVERSE EFFECTS

- Preterm birth, miscarriage, stillbirth, reduction in birth weight, placental abnormalities, congenital malformations (eg, congenital heart defects, cleft lip, cleft palate, limb reduction defects, digital anomalies, bilateral renal hypoplasia or agenesis, anal atresia, etc.).

NEURAL TUBE DEFECTS

- Birth defects of the brain, spine, or spinal cord.
- **The two most common types are spina bifida and anencephaly.**
- **Increased incidence with maternal folate deficiency.**

PATHOPHYSIOLOGY

- Anencephaly: failure of closure of the portion of the neural tube that becomes the cerebrum.
- Spina bifida: incomplete closure of the embryonic neural tubule leads to non-fusion of some of the vertebrae overlying the spinal cords. This may lead to protrusion of the spinal cord through the opening. Most commonly seen at the lumbar and sacral areas of the spine.

TYPES OF SPINA BIFIDA

- **Spina bifida with myelomeningocele: most common type.** Meninges and spinal cord herniates thought the gap in the vertebrae. Often leads to disability.
- Spina bifida occulta: mildest form. No herniation of the spinal cord. The overlying skin may be normal or have some hair growing over it, dimpling of the skin or birthmark over the affected area.
- Spina bifida with meningocele: only the meninges herniate through the gap in the vertebrae

CLINICAL MANIFESTATIONS

- Sensory deficits, paralysis, hydrocephalus, hypotonia.

SCREENING

- Increased maternal serum alpha-fetoprotein followed by **amniocentesis showing increased alpha-fetoprotein & increased acetylcholinesterase.**

PRADER-WILLI SYNDROME

- Genetic disorder due to a small deletion or inexpression of genes in the paternal copy of chromosome 15 (15q 11-13).
- Characterized by **prenatal hypotonia, postnatal growth delay, developmental disabilities, hypogonadotropic hypogonadism, & obesity after infancy.**

CLINICAL MANIFESTATIONS

- **Neonates: severe hypotonia, floppy baby, weak cry, feeding difficulties,** trouble swallowing and suckling (nasogastric feeding may be needed). Genital hypoplasia, **cryptorchidism,** depigmentation of the skin, eyes, excessive sleeping, strabismus.
  Physical examination: almond-shaped eyes, high/narrow forehead, thin upper lip with small, down-turned mouth; prominent nasal bridges. Small feet & hands (with tapering of the fingers). Soft skin that easily bruises (may have extreme flexibility). Excess fat (especially *truncal obesity*).

- **Early childhood:** during the first year of life, muscle tone improves and child develops **voracious appetite (hyperphagia)** including **aggressive behavior related to eating, obesity**. Major milestone delays, behavioral and learning difficulties. Short stature, skin picking. Patients may have lighter hair and skin compared to other family members.

- Later childhood/adolescence: delay of secondary sex characteristics, increased incidence of epilepsy & scoliosis. Women are often sterile.

DIAGNOSIS

- DNA testing (DNA-based methylation studies).

MANAGEMENT

Growth hormone replacement, obesity control by monitoring food intake

BECKWITH-WIEDEMANN SYNDROME

- Abnormal gene expression affecting the chromosome 11p15.5 region.
- Large for gestational age, organomegaly, macroglossia, hypoglycemia in infancy, earlobe creases & pits, asymmetric limbs. **Increased risk of hepatoblastoma & Wilm's tumor.**

NEUROBLASTOMA

- Cancer of the peripheral sympathetic nervous system.
- 3rd most common pediatric cancer (90% diagnosed by age 5y).
- **Most common in the adrenal medulla & paraspinal region.**

CLINICAL MANIFESTATIONS

- Depends on tumor site. Most common in the abdomen (firm, irregular, nodular abdomen or flank mass). Unlike Nephroblastoma, **Neuroblastoma can cross the midline**.
- **Ataxia, opsoclonus myoclonus syndrome** (hypsarrhythmia/rapid "dancing eyes" & myoclonus/"dancing feet" – jerky movements), hypertension (especially diastolic), diarrhea.

DIAGNOSIS

- CT scan: tumor often seen with calcification & hemorrhaging. ↑vanillylmandelic acid.

MANAGEMENT

- Surgery, chemotherapy, or radiation depending on stage of disease & site of the tumor.

NEUROFIBROMATOSIS TYPE 1 (von Recklinghausen's disease)

- Autosomal dominant **neurocutaneous disorder** due to a mutated NF1 gene (chromosome 17q11.2 region) encoding for the protein neurofibromin (a tumor suppressor).
- **Most common type** (90%).

PATHOPHYSIOLOGY

- Loss of neurofibromin ⇨ increased risk of developing benign and malignant tumors. Mutations are highly variable between patients with NF1 and can appear at any age.

CLINICAL MANIFESTATIONS

Requires at least 2 of the following:

- **≥6 café-au-lait spots**: flat, uniformly hypopigmented macules that appear during the first year of birth and increase in number during early childhood.

- **Freckling:** especially **axillary or inguinal** freckling. May also be seen in intertriginous areas, & the neckline. Not usually present at birth but often appears by age 3 to 5 years.

- **Lisch nodules of the iris**: hamartomas of the iris seen on slit lamp examination. Often elevated and tan-colored.

- ≥2 neurofibromas or ≥1 plexiform neurofibroma. Neurofibromas are focal, benign peripheral nerve sheath tumors (often a combination of Schwann cells, fibroblasts, perineural cells and mast cells) described as small, rubbery lesions with a slight purplish discoloration of the overlying skin. Neurofibromas typically involve the skin but may be seen along peripheral nerves, blood vessels and viscera. Plexiform neurofibromas are located longitudinally along a nerve and involve multiple fascicles (may produce an overgrowth of an extremity).
  - **Optic pathway gliomas**: may involve the optic nerve, optic chiasm, and/or postchiasmal optic tracts. Most commonly occurs in younger children (ex. <6 years of age). May develop an afferent pupillary defect. If the tumor is large and involves the hypothalamus, it may be associated with delayed or premature onset of puberty.
  - Others: osseous lesions: scoliosis is common (especially thoracic spine), sphenoid dysplasia, long bone abnormalities. 1st degree relative with NF1 or short stature.

NEUROIMAGING

- **MRI**: unidentified bright objects = hyperintense T2-weighted signals (may be due to demyelination or focal areas of increased water content). Seen most commonly in the basal ganglia, brainstem, cerebellum, and subcortical white matter. There are no associated neurologic deficits. Increased brain volume often seen.

MANAGEMENT

- Optic pathway glioma: regular annual ophthalmologic screening. If any symptoms occur, an MRI of the brain & orbits should be performed.

- Neurofibromas: not removed unless there are associated complications.

NEUROFIBROMATOSIS TYPE 2

- Autosomal dominant associated with multiple CNS tumors **[bilateral CN VIII tumors** (also known as schwannomas, vestibular neuromas or acoustic neuromas), spinal tumors & intracranial tumors.

PATHOPHYSIOLOGY
- Mutation of the NF2 tumor suppressor gene (normally produces the protein schwannomin aka merlin).

CLINICAL MANIFESTATIONS
- **Neurologic lesions:**
  - BILATERAL VESTIBULAR SCHWANNOMAS (95%). Most develop by 30 years of age - hearing loss (usually gradual & progressive), tinnitus, and balance disturbances. Over a period of time, they can expand, causing hydrocephalus & brainstem compression.
  - Meningiomas: often multiple (especially in childhood), spinal & intramedullary tumors, neuropathy.

- **Optic lesions:** cataracts (may cause visual impairment early in childhood), retinal hamartomas.
- **Skin lesions:**
  - Cutaneous tumors, skin plaques (slightly raised and may be hyperpigmented), subcutaneous tumors that presents as nodules. Café-au-lait spots are seen with less frequency in NF2.

MANAGEMENT
Vestibular schwannomas:
- Surgery may be needed for complicated or symptomatic tumors.
- Bevacizumab: may cause shrinkage of the tumor and improvement in hearing.
  MOA: monoclonal antibody against vascular endothelial growth factor (VEGF).

TAY-SACHS DISEASE

- Rare, autosomal recessive genetic disorder most common in Ashkenazi Jewish families of Eastern European descent, Cajuns in Southern Louisiana & French Canadians.

PATHOPHYSIOLOGY
- Mutation of the HEXA gene on chromosome 15 ⇨ deficiency in β-hexosaminidase A ⇨ accumulation of gangliosides in the brain ⇨ premature neuron death & progressive degeneration of neurons.

CLINICAL MANIFESTATIONS
- **Infantile onset:** increased startle reaction, loss of motor skills. At 4-5 months of age ⇨ decreased eye contact, hyperacusis (exaggerated startle reaction to noise), paralysis, blindness, progressive developmental retardation & dementia. 2nd year: seizures and neurodegeneration. Death usually occurs between 3-4 years.
- Juvenile onset: symptoms occur between the ages of 2-10y ⇨ cognitive and motor skill deterioration, dysphagia, ataxia, spasticity. Death often occurs between the ages of 5-15y.
- Adult onset: usually develops symptoms during the 30s and 40s. Usually presents with unsteady, spastic gait and progressive neurological deterioration (leading to speech, swallowing difficulties), psychosis.

PHYSICAL EXAMINATION: Retinal examination: **cherry-red spots with macular pallor.** Macrocephaly.

DIAGNOSIS: enzymatic assay.

MANAGEMENT: No effective treatment.

TYPES OF VACCINES

1. LIVE, ATTENUATED VACCINES:

Contains a live, weakened version of the organism. Because it is the safest, closest thing to actually having the infection, it induces a good immune response of both *humoral (antibody) immunity* & *cell-mediated immunity.* No booster usually need. Cons: they are unstable & must be refrigerated. Because they may become virulent, **live attenuated vaccines are not given to immunocompromised or pregnant patients.**

- **MMR.** The only live, attenuated vaccine that can be given to HIV patients (if CD4 >200/μL).
- **Chicken pox (Varicella Zoster), Rotavirus.**
- Smallpox, yellow fever, oral typhoid, *Franciscella tularensis*, oral polio.

2. KILLED (INACTIVATED) VACCINES:

Killed organisms. These stimulate a weaker immune response compared to live attenuated vaccines so they only induce a humoral (antibody) immunity - may need booster shots.

- **Influenza, Rabies, Polio SalK (K= killed** - this is the primary form used in US), Vibrio cholerae, **Hepatitis A Vaccine.**

3. SUBUNIT CONJUGATE VACCINES:

Presents only the essential antigens needed to induce an immune system response (instead of giving the whole organism). Often contain multiple antigens that are linked or "conjugated" to toxoids or antigens that the immature immune system will recognize to identify bacterium that use their polysaccharide outer coating as a defense. **Made of capsular polysaccharides** so often used for many **encapsulated organisms "SHiN".**

- **S. pneumococcal** (infant version is conjugated so induces a helper T cell response).
- **H influenza** (capsular polysaccharide), **N. meningitidis,** PCV13 (pneumococcal vaccine).

4. SUBUNIT RECOMBINANT VACCINES:

A type of subunit vaccine in which recombinant DNA technology is used to manufacture the antigen molecules. Genes that encode for the important antigens are placed into Baker's yeast. The yeast reproduces the antigens that are processed & purified.

- **Hepatitis B vaccine** (HBsAg), **HPV vaccine** (6,11,16, & 18).

5. TOXOID VACCINES:

Chemically modified inactivated toxins from toxin-producing organisms to allow the body to recognize the harmless toxin. Later it has the ability to attack the natural toxin if exposed to it.

- **Tetanus, Diphtheria, Pertussis**

VACCINE CONTRAINDICATIONS

- **Baker's yeast: Hepatitis B** should be avoided (Think B for Baker's yeast & Hepatitis B).
- Gelatin: avoid varicella, influenza vaccines.
- Thimerosal: preservative used in vaccines so should be avoided in multi-dose vaccines.
- **Neomycin & Streptomycin allergy: MMR** (Measles Mumps Rubella) & **inactivated Polio vaccine** should be avoided (Neomycin & Streptomycin are preservatives in these vaccines).

PREGNANCY

Only vaccines safely given in pregnancy: diphtheria, tetanus, inactivated influenza, HBV, rabies, meningococcal.

Avoid live vaccines:

- Live vaccines: MMR, Varicella, Polio.
- Live attenuated vaccines: intranasal influenza vaccine.

Figure 1. Recommended immunization schedule for persons aged 0 through 18 years – United States, 2016.
(FOR THOSE WHO FALL BEHIND OR START LATE, SEE THE CATCH-UP SCHEDULE [FIGURE 2]).
These recommendations must be read with the footnotes that follow. For those who fall behind or start late, provide catch-up vaccination at the earliest opportunity as indicated by the green bars in Figure 1. To determine minimum intervals between doses, see the catch-up schedule (Figure 2). School entry and adolescent vaccine age groups are shaded.

Vaccine	Birth	1 mo	2 mos	4 mos	6 mos	9 mos	12 mos	15 mos	18 mos	19–23 mos	2-3 yrs	4-6 yrs	7-10 yrs	11-12 yrs	13-15 yrs	16-18 yrs
Hepatitis B[1] (HepB)	1st dose	← 2nd dose →			← 3rd dose →											
Rotavirus[2] (RV) RV1 (2-dose series); RV5 (3-dose series)			1st dose	2nd dose	See footnote 2											
Diphtheria, tetanus, & acellular pertussis[3] (DTaP: <7 yrs)			1st dose	2nd dose	3rd dose			← 4th dose →				5th dose				
Haemophilus influenzae type b[4] (Hib)			1st dose	2nd dose	See footnote 4		← 3rd or 4th dose, See footnote 4 →									
Pneumococcal conjugate[5] (PCV13)			1st dose	2nd dose	3rd dose		← 4th dose →									
Inactivated poliovirus[6] (IPV: <18 yrs)			1st dose	2nd dose	← 3rd dose →							4th dose				
Influenza[7] (IIV; LAIV)					Annual vaccination (IIV only) 1 or 2 doses						Annual vaccination (LAIV or IIV) 1 or 2 doses		Annual vaccination (LAIV or IIV) 1 dose only			
Measles, mumps, rubella[8] (MMR)					See footnote 8		← 1st dose →					2nd dose				
Varicella[9] (VAR)							← 1st dose →					2nd dose				
Hepatitis A[10] (HepA)							← 2-dose series, See footnote 10 →									
Meningococcal[11] (Hib-MenCY ≥ 6 weeks; MenACWY-D ≥9 mos; MenACWY-CRM ≥ 2 mos)			See footnote 11											1st dose		
Tetanus, diphtheria, & acellular pertussis[12] (Tdap: ≥7 yrs)														(Tdap)		
Human papillomavirus[13] (2vHPV: females only; 4vHPV, 9vHPV: males and females)														(3-dose series)		
Meningococcal B[11]														See footnote 11		
Pneumococcal polysaccharide[5] (PPSV23)											See footnote 5					

Range of recommended ages for all children; Range of recommended ages for catch-up immunization; Range of recommended ages for certain high-risk groups; Range of recommended ages for non-high-risk groups that may receive vaccine, subject to individual clinical decision making; No recommendation

This schedule includes recommendations in effect as of January 1, 2016. Any dose not administered at the recommended age should be administered at a subsequent visit, when indicated and feasible. The use of a combination vaccine generally is preferred over separate injections of its equivalent component vaccines. Vaccination providers should consult the relevant Advisory Committee on Immunization Practices (ACIP) statement for detailed recommendations, available online at http://www.cdc.gov/vaccines/hcp/acip-recs/index.html. Clinically significant adverse events that follow vaccination should be reported to the Vaccine Adverse Event Reporting System (VAERS) online (http://www.vaers.hhs.gov) or by telephone (800-822-7967). Suspected cases of vaccine-preventable diseases should be reported to the state or local health department. Additional information, including precautions and contraindications for vaccination, is available from CDC online

TANNER STAGE	2	3	4	5
Males	Age 11 - 12	Age 13	Age 14 – 15	Age 16-17
Pubic hair	Straight pubic hair at the base of penis	Coarse dark and curly pubic hair	Hair is almost completely full	Pubic hair achieves adult appearance
Females	Age 11	Age 12	Age 13	Age 14-15
Pubic Hair	Minimal straight pubic hair (long, downy)	Increased pubic hair (dark & coarse) lateral extension	Adult-like extends across pubis	Adult appearance (extends to medial thighs)
Breast	Breast buds palpable, areola enlarge	Elevation of areola contour, areola enlargement	Secondary mound of areola & papilla	Adult breast contour

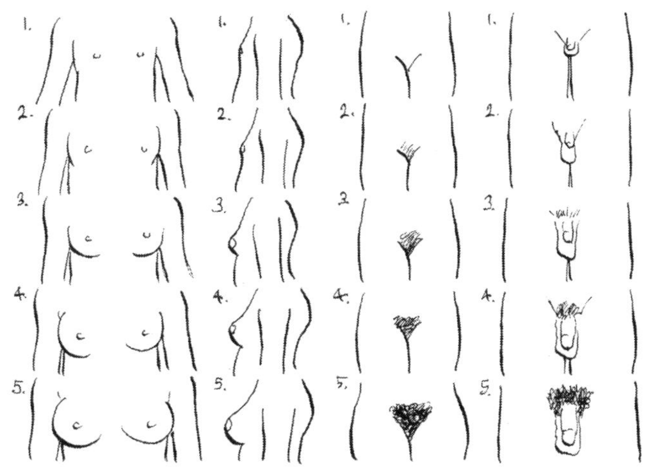

A

D

E

I

J

K

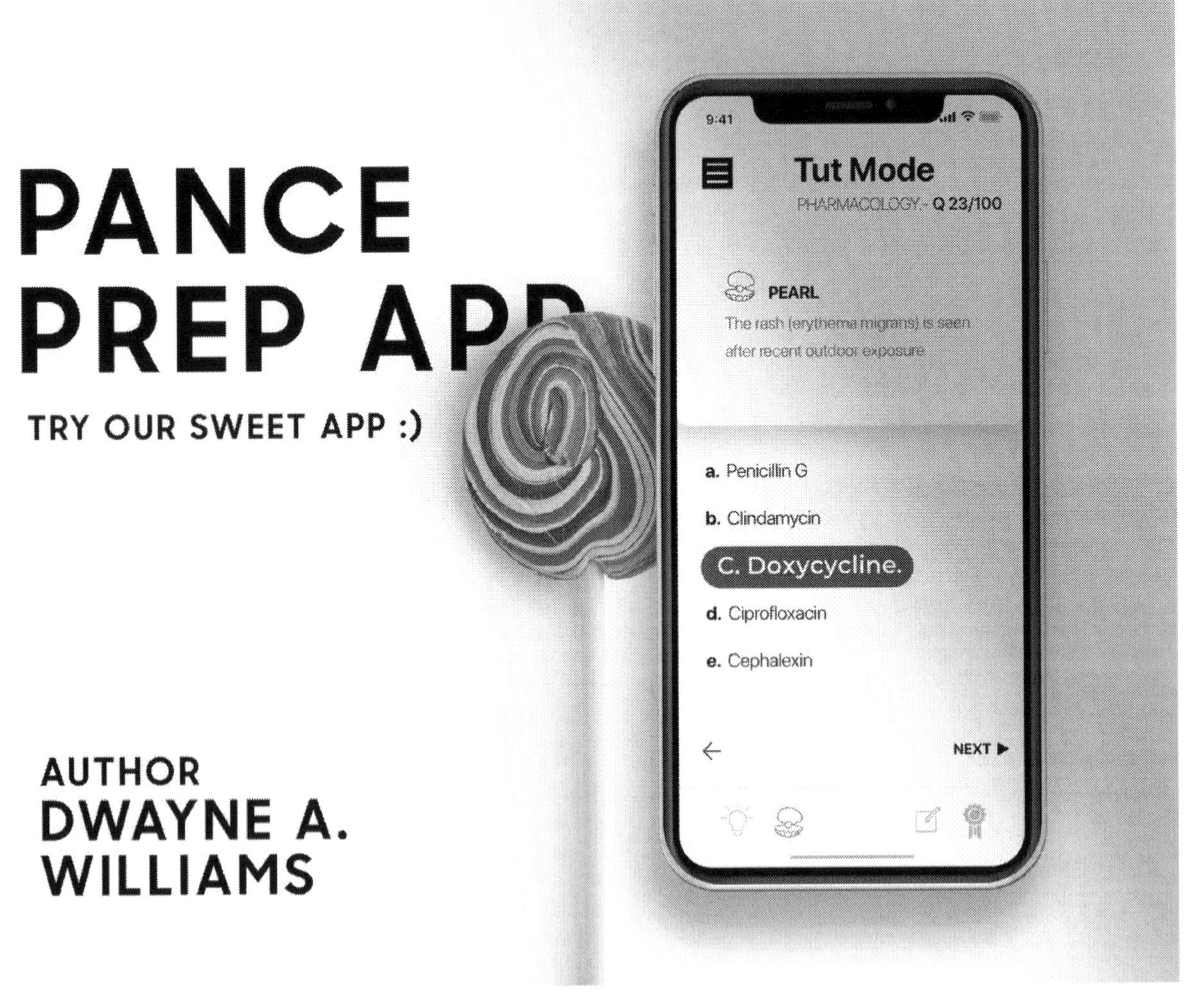

Over 8,600 clinically-based practice examination questions specifically formulated to enhance clinical skills and improve performance on examinations, such as the PANCE, PANRE, OSCES, USMLE, end of rotation examinations and comprehensive medical examinations.

This app will intuitively know your areas of weakness and give you a plan to improve your overall performance. Special clinical pearls, disease review, explanation of the answers, test taking strategies and much more.

3 modes,
Timed mode to simulate the exams
Tutor mode that allows you to review the disease states in addition to the questions and
improve mode to enhance your weak areas.

For every question in tutor mode, there is a feature for a hint to see if you are going in the right direction, answer explanation, a clinical pearl, and a bonus questions. Create your own examination based on organ systems or task areas. The ultimate study and exam preparation app!

ALSO AVAILABLE

CYTOCHROME P450 INDUCERS

John was **worth**y when referred & **inducted** into sainthood for giving up **chronic alcohol** use & placing him**self on a real** fast, **fend**ing off **greasy carbs**, leading to **less warfare** with **theo**logians.

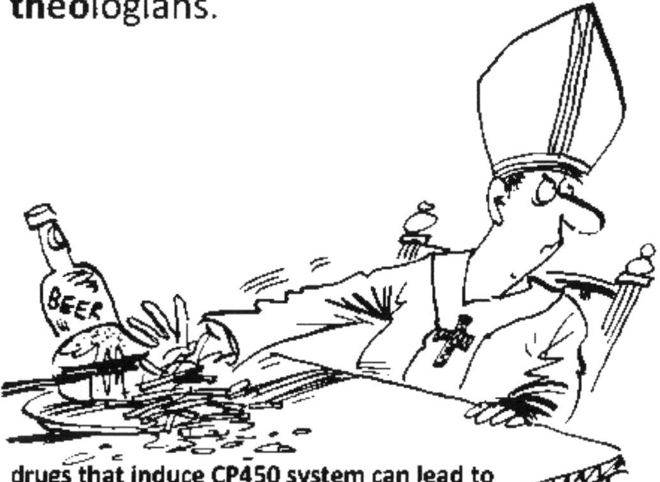

drugs that induce CP450 system can lead to decreased levels of certain drugs ex. warfarin (less warfare), theophylline (theologians) and phenytoin

INDUCERS OF THE P450

- **St. Johns Wort**
- **rifampin** (referred)
- **chronic alcohol use**
- **sulfonylureas** (self on a real)
- **Phenytoin**
- **Phenobarbital** (fend)
- **Griseofulvin** (greasy)
- **Carbamazepine** (carbs)

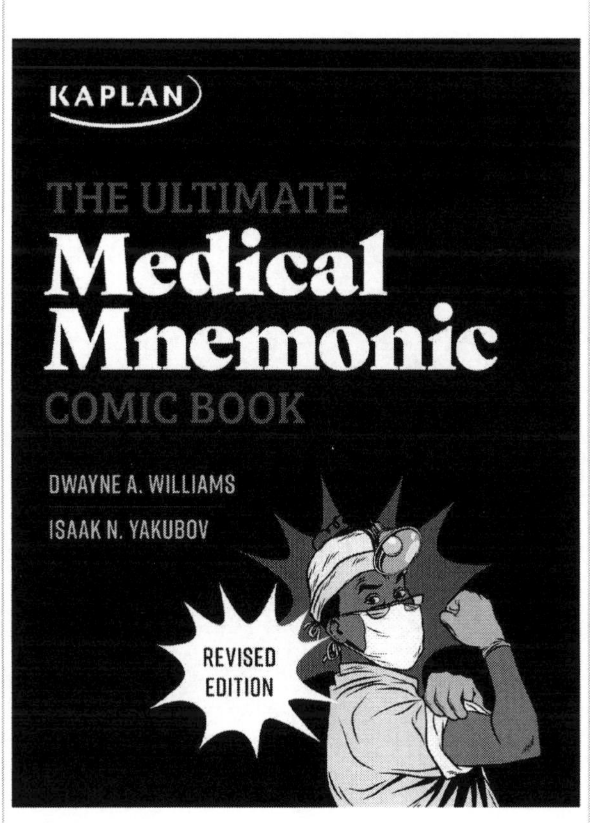